HEALTH PROMOTION IN NURSING PRACTICE

Fifth Edition

HEALTH PROMOTION IN NURSING PRACTICE

Fifth Edition

Nola J. Pender, PhD, RN, FAAN
Professor Emerita
University of Michigan
School of Nursing
Ann Arbor, Michigan

Carolyn L. Murdaugh, PhD, RN, FAAN
Professor and Associate Dean for Research
University of Arizona
College of Nursing
Tucson, Arizona

Mary Ann Parsons, PhD, RN, FAAN
Professor and Dean
University of South Carolina
College of Nursing
Columbia, South Carolina

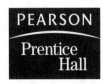

PEARSON
Prentice
Hall

Upper Saddle River, NJ 07458

Library of Congress Cataloging-in-Publication Data

Pender, Nola J. (date).
Health promotion in nursing practice / Nola J. Pender, Carolyn L. Murdaugh, Mary Ann Parsons.—4th ed.
   p.   ; cm.
 Includes bibliographical references and index.
 ISBN 0-13-031950-3 (paper)
1. Health promotion. 2. Preventive health services. 3. Nursing. I. Murdaugh, Carolyn L. II. Parsons, Mary Ann.
 III. Title.
   [DNLM: 1. Health Promotion—Nurses' Instruction. 2. Nursing Care—Nurses' Instruction. 3. Health
   Behavior—Nurses' Instruction. 4. Health Policy—Nurses' Instruction. WS 350.2 G798c 2001]
RT67 .P56 2001
613—dc21   2001016328

Publisher: Julie Levin Alexander
Publisher's Assistant: Regina Bruno
Editor-in-Chief: Maura Connor
Acquisitions Editor: Pamela Fuller
Editorial Assistant: Eileen Monaghan
Director of Manufacturing and Production:
Bruce Johnson
Managing Production Editor: Patrick Walsh
Production Liaison: Cathy O'Connell
Production Editor: Janet Kiefer, Carlisle Publishers
Services

Manufacturing Manager: Ilene Sanford
Manufacturing Buyer: Pat Brown
Design Director: Cheryl Asherman
Cover Designer: Anthony Gemmellaro
Senior Design Coordinator: Maria Gulielmo Walsh
Director of Marketing: Karen Allman
Executive Marketing Manager: Nicole Benson
Channel Marketing Manager: Rachele Strober
Composition: Carlisle Communications
Printer/Binder: Courier Stoughton
Cover Printer: Phoenix Color

Care has been taken to confirm the accuracy of information presented in this book. The authors, editors, and the publisher, however, cannot accept any responsibility for errors or omissions or for consequences from application of the information in this book and make no warranty, express or implied, with respect to its contents.

The authors and publisher have exerted every effort to ensure that drug selections and dosages set forth in this text are in accord with current recommendations and practice at time of publication. However, in view of ongoing research, changes in government regulations, and the constant flow of information relating to drug therapy and drug reactions, the reader is urged to check the package inserts of all drugs for any change in indications of dosage and for added warnings and precautions. This is particularly important when the recommended agent is a new and/or infrequently employed drug.

Pearson Education LTD.
Pearson Education Singapore, Pte. Ltd
Pearson Education, Canada, Ltd
Pearson Education–Japan

Pearson Education Australia PTY, Limited
Pearson Education North Asia Ltd
Pearson Educacion de Mexico, S.A. de C.V.
Pearson Education Malaysia, Pte. Ltd
Pearson Education Inc., Upper Saddle River, NJ

10 9 8 7 6 5 4 3 2 1
ISBN 0-13-119436-4

To my two sisters, Becky and Joanne, and their families for their love and support, for whom I wish a happy, healthy, and peaceful life.

C. Murdaugh

To George, my husband, Nicole and John Harwell, my daughter and son-in-law, Kent and Shannon, my son and daughter-in-law, and to our first grandchild, Blake Sterling Harwell, for a long, healthy, happy life.

M. A. Parsons

Contents

Foreword

It is a pleasure and an honor to write the Foreword for the fifth edition of *Health Promotion in Nursing Practice*. In past decades, lack of national attention to health promotion has resulted in sedentary lifestyles, escalating obesity, greater incidence of chronic diseases, and the limited capacity of many communities to support the well-being of their populations. Poor health practices and poor-quality environments limit the health potential of any nation. Fortunately, the health-promotion environment is changing drastically throughout the world. The governments of many countries now recognize the "added value" of health promotion to health care. Optimizing the health of a population is only possible through positive health policies and services that improve the quality of life and prevent premature morbidity and mortality. This book, intended for use by an international audience, presents important strategies for fostering healthy lifestyles and creating healthy home, work, school, and community environments for diverse populations.

Nurses as key health professionals provide guidance to individuals, families, and communities in making important health decisions. Therefore, nurses need skill in implementing effective health-promotion interventions. The authors of *Health Promotion in Nursing Practice* combine their expertise to create a high-quality text that is an important addition to the health-promotion interventions literature.

Dr. Carolyn Murdaugh and Dr. Mary Ann Parsons are ideal authors for this text. Dr. Carolyn Murdaugh, a well-known nurse scholar, is Associate Dean for Research at the University of Arizona and directed the Center for Health Promotion and Risk Reduction in Special Populations at the University of South Carolina. She has conducted research on promoting health and quality of life throughout her distinguished career. Dr. Parsons, nationally known for her publications in family practice and the health behavior of adolescents, is Dean of the College of Nursing at the University of South Carolina. She provides visionary leadership to other deans in schools of nursing regarding the integration of health-promotion and prevention concepts into nursing curricula.

Aspects of this new edition that are particularly noteworthy include: Adherence to an evidence-based approach to health promotion and prevention, focus on diverse populations, special attention to vulnerable populations, synthesis of an individual and a community focus, and provision of information on how to measure and evaluate the outcomes of health-promotion interventions. Carefully selected learning activities assist readers in developing expertise relative to the content of each chapter.

Baccalaureate and graduate education programs in nursing are responsible for preparing students of nursing with the expertise to excel in careers in health promotion. This book is an important resource to assist schools of nursing in achieving this goal.

Nola Pender, PhD, RN, FAAN
Professor Emerita
University of Michigan
School of Nursing

Preface

A major change has occurred in publishing the fifth edition of this book, as Dr. Nola Pender, founding author, has retired. Dr. Pender has been an international leader in research and scholarly writing to help develop and sustain the infrastructure for health-promotion efforts in this country and internationally. Her contributions to health promotion, academically, scientifically, and clinically, have resulted in a greater understanding of optimal health and how it can be obtained. The Health Promotion Model, developed by Dr. Pender, continues to be the guiding framework for studies that investigate the role of cognitive-perceptual and modifying factors in health behaviors. Although she has retired from academia and scholarly writing, Dr. Pender continues to be politically active, promoting consistent reimbursement for health-promotion and illness-prevention services as well as improving the delivery of culturally sensitive health-promotion services for diverse populations. We thank Dr. Pender for her contributions to health promotion through this book and hope that we, as authors, will continue to extend her scholarly work.

The purpose of the book has not changed and continues to be threefold: (a) to provide an overview of the major individual and community models and theories that guide health-promotion interventions; (b) to provide strategies and tools that can be used in practice settings to implement evidence-based health-promotion care for diverse populations; and (c) to foster critical thinking about future directions for health-promotion research and the most effective interventions for practice. We believe information in the book is the foundation on which to build the science and practice of health promotion.

The content of the book is organized into six parts. In Part 1, The Human Quest for Health, definitions of health are provided as well as an overview of both individual and community models to promote health. In Part 2, Planning for Health Promotion and Prevention, strategies are addressed that are needed to assess health, health beliefs, and health behaviors, as well as information to develop a health-promotion plan. Part 3, Interventions for Health Promotion and Prevention, addresses various topics, including physical activity, diet and nutrition, stress, and social support. In Part 4, Evaluating the Effectiveness of Health Promotion, strategies to evaluate health-promotion interventions are addressed, and Part 5, Health Promotion in Diverse Populations, describes health promotion across the life span, as well as strategies to promote health in vulnerable populations. In Part 6, Approaches for Promoting a Healthier Society, community partnerships for health promotion are described as well as policies and programs to promote social and environmental changes for a healthier society. New additions include objectives at the beginning of each chapter to guide the reader, and learning activities at the end of each chapter to promote application of the chapter content. The term *client* is used rather than *patient* throughout the book to refer to individuals, families, and communities who are active participants in health promotion. *Health* and *wellness* are used interchangeably. Finally, *health protection* and *prevention* are also used interchangeably throughout the book.

Sincere appreciation is extended to Malgorzata (Gosia) Jaros-White at Prentice Hall Health who has worked diligently with us in the preparation of the book. We are also indebted to Lisa Spruill, Administrative Assistant in the College of Nursing, University of South Carolina, who performed the manuscript formatting, prepared tables and figures, and proofed chapters, as well as coordinated communication between Prentice Hall Health and the authors. We also extend our appreciation to Shannon Lackey and Isabel Sanchez, who helped type and proof chapters.

Carolyn Murdaugh

Mary Ann Parsons

Reviewers

Margaret Christensen, PhD, RN
Associate Professor
Northeastern University
Bouve College of Health Sciences School
    of Nursing
Boston, Massachusetts

Barbara Cohen, EdD, RN
Professor Emeritus
College of Mount Saint Vincent
Riverdale, New York

Laurie Glover, MN, APRN, FNP
Adjunct Assistant Professor
Family Nurse Practitioner

Montana State University
College of Nursing
Great Falls, Montana

Patricia Leary, MA Ed
Instructor
Ferris State University
Mecosta—Osceola Career Center
Big Rapids, Michigan

Carol A. Smith, DSN, CRNP
Associate Professor
The Pennsylvania State University
School of Nursing
University Park, Pennsylvania

Introduction

Health Promotion and Disease Prevention: Challenges of the 21st Century

Institutionalizing health promotion and disease prevention as integral aspects of health care continues to present challenges for all nations. Accumulating evidence indicates that health promotion holds promise for maintaining vigor, vitality, and productivity into the eighth and ninth decades of life for an increasing proportion of the world population. Governments of many countries are developing national health-promotion plans to shape the future directions of health care as they recognize the link between a healthy and productive population and national welfare and economic prosperity. The overall goals of these plans are to help people of all ages stay healthy, to optimize health in the presence of chronic disease or disability, and to create healthy environments in which to live. According to the World Health Organization (WHO) health promotion includes encouraging healthy lifestyles, creating supportive environments for health, strengthening community action, reorienting health services to place primary focus on promoting health and preventing disease, and building healthy public policy (Turner, 1986). Health promotion must be geared not only to individuals but also to families and the communities in which they live. Healthy public policy facilitates positive changes in health behavior norms, and also provides health-enhancing environments on a national and international scale (Jamner & Stokols, 2000; Kumanyika, 2001; Turner, 1986).

Unfortunately the gap between the generation of knowledge about health promotion and prevention and its application in practice continues to exist (Minkler, 2000). A number of theories and models to guide health-promotion interventions for individuals, families, and communities have been proposed and tested. However, education for health professionals has been slow to promulgate curricula to ensure development of knowledge and expertise in delivering theory-based health promotion and prevention care to clients. Greater expediency is needed in moving scientific breakthroughs into evidence-based practice in order for the public to benefit in a timely manner from new knowledge. One challenge of the 21st century is to provide access to knowledge and services that promote health for all segments of an increasingly diverse population. This must be accomplished in an environment of economic constraints requiring that resources spent on health care be balanced with other resource demands.

Another challenge is to address social problems that compromise health and well-being. Early development of positive health behaviors such as caring interpersonal relationships, community service participation, and responsible sexuality can decrease social problems such as violence, suicide, and sexually transmitted diseases that are of increasing prevalence worldwide. Youths are a valuable global asset, yet this is the population in which many social problems are most prevalent. Healthy behaviors need to be supported by families and communities to optimize health for all (Hofmann, 2000; Wallack, 2000; Wilson, Rodrigue, & Taylor, 1997). Gender-specific health promotion frameworks need further development to address issues of gender socialization that impact health behaviors as well as the physical and mental health of adolescents (Guthrie, Caldwell, & Hunter, 1997).

In an age of rapid advances in information technology, electronic media offer unprecedented opportunities to provide health-related information to the public. Innovative use of interactive computer technology and interactive television through worldwide networks is enabling health professionals and consumers to collaborate as never before in tailoring health communications to the special needs of individuals and families from diverse populations (Kreuter, Farrell, Olevitch, & Brennan, 2000; Kreuter, Strecher, & Glassman, 1999; Skinner, Campbell, Rimer, Curry, & Prochaska, 1999). Innovative use of communication networks such as the World Wide Web provides open access to the latest health knowledge, creating a national and international resource for informed health care decision making by both providers and consumers. Care must be taken to provide access to computerized information systems for vulnerable populations. It is encouraging to note that research examining the acceptability of computerized assessments of smoking behavior in low-income populations indicated that 92% of the study participants found the programs either "very easy" or "easy" to use (Bock, Niaura, Fontes, & Bock, 1999).

Nurses need to be at the forefront in developing interactive health education counseling programs and behavioral interventions that capitalize on emerging information technology breakthroughs. A "one size fits all" approach to health-promotion programming has become outdated. Technology offers nurses new tools for further developing the individualized health care to which they have long been committed. Breakthroughs in understanding the human genome have the potential to markedly enhance health and prevent disease. Molecular prevention is fast becoming a reality. Nurses are pivotal in helping clients combine knowledge about personal genetic makeup, genetic prevention techniques, and behavior change strategies to prevent illnesses for which they are at high risk. Nursing research agendas as well as nursing education programs must embrace evolving scientific discoveries in the health sciences, and pioneer and test innovative biopsychosocial nursing care strategies.

Toward a Global Health Agenda

All people of the world must be recognized as a global community, a health megasystem. What affects one country does not happen in isolation but affects other countries as well. Strategies suggested to achieve health for all on a global scale include: (a) empowering people by providing the latest health information and decision-making opportunities;

(b) strengthening local systems of primary health care; (c) improving education and training programs in health promotion and prevention for health professionals; (d) applying science and technology to critical health problems; (e) using new approaches to problems such as violence that have resisted solution; (f) providing culturally appropriate assistance to the least developed countries; and (g) establishing a process for examination of the world challenges that must be addressed to make good health a reality for the masses (WHO, 1988). The health-promoting and health-damaging features of social policies, organizations, and environments are receiving increased attention. As early as the mid-1980s, WHO emphasized the necessity of going beyond the education of individuals to include organizational changes, community development, and legislation (WHO, 1984). This broader approach to health promotion is well illustrated by the Healthy Cities Project that WHO initiated in Europe in 1984. The project stresses a municipal approach to health promotion through extensive community participation, intersectoral cooperation, and the implementation of comprehensive city plans for health promotion. The target endpoints evaluated were not only the traditional morbidity and mortality outcomes, but also included prevalence of health-promoting behaviors, quality of the physical and social environment, and extent of community empowerment and action (Ashton, Grey, & Barnard, 1986). The Healthy Cities Project focused on health as a central concern. Building healthy cities is an ecological approach that has yet to reach its full potential for improving the health of the masses. Many lessons have been learned from the WHO project that enable cities and nations to make health a priority and improve well-being throughout the life span, especially for vulnerable populations. Web sites for up-to-date information about Healthy Cities are noted at the end of each chapter.

A challenge for scientists is to develop credible, widely recognized, high-quality standards to evaluate the effectiveness of multisectoral health-promotion interventions. This task presents a formidable challenge given the complexity of health-promotion interventions ranging from changing behaviors of individuals and collectives to changing policies that set norms for behavior (McQueen, 2000). Use of behavioral surveillance systems will be critical to assessing progress toward health-promotion objectives, as will time-sensitive strategies for analyzing data and using data to make strategic decisions about "what works." These strategies are essential to further the public health agenda for prevention and health promotion (McQueen, 1999).

A progressive step toward international collaboration among nurses for health promotion and prevention was the establishment of World Health Organization Collaborating Centers. Nurses from centers throughout the world share information about innovative models for delivery of health promotion and prevention services, curricula content at the undergraduate and graduate levels to prepare nursing students to deliver quality health education counseling and behavioral interventions, approaches to developing strategic national plans for health promotion, and directions for research to build scientific knowledge upon which successful health-promotion and prevention nursing interventions are based. Nurses play a pivotal role throughout the world in mobilizing forces for change in individual, family, and organizational health behaviors. Thus, the development of nurses for leadership in health promotion is an international priority.

National Progress Toward Health

Unhealthy lifestyles and the environment are responsible for a major percentage of the morbidity and mortality in the United States (U.S. Department of Health and Human Services, 2000). Unless the health care system is significantly changed to influence lifestyles and environments, the nation's health profile will continue to deteriorate. Demographic changes toward an older population and a more ethnically diverse population create new demands for health promotion and prevention services in primary care and public health (U.S. Department of Health and Human Services, 1997).

In 1979, the report *Healthy People: The Surgeon General's Report on Health Promotion and Disease Prevention* (1979) introduced a set of broad national goals for improving the health of Americans by 1990. In 1980, a companion document, *Promoting Health—Preventing Disease: Objectives for the Nation* (1980), was published and identified 226 specific health goals in three major areas: health promotion, health protection, and preventive health services. The greatest gains were made in the areas of control of high blood pressure, injury prevention, smoking reduction, immunization, and dental health. Death rates for both heart attacks and strokes also decreased. Because the 1990 objectives were effective in drawing the nation's attention to the potential of disease prevention and health promotion to increase longevity and improve the quality of lives, national objectives were also set for the year 2000. In 1990, *Healthy People 2000: National Health Promotion and Disease Prevention Objectives* (1990) was published. It identified three broad goals: Increase the span of healthy life for Americans, reduce health disparities among Americans, and achieve access to preventive services for all Americans. The plan organized 300 national objectives into 22 priorities for action. These were placed in the categories of health promotion, health protection, preventive services, and surveillance and data systems (*Healthy People 2000*, 1990). Surveillance and data systems were put in place to better track achievement of national goals and greater attention was given to tracking the health status of groups by race and ethnicity. Successes included increasing immunization levels among children and older adults, reducing infant mortality, decreasing unintended pregnancies among adolescents, increasing use of seat belts, decreasing driving while impaired by alcohol or drugs, and leveling off of tobacco, alcohol, and illicit drug use (U.S. Department of Health and Human Services, 2000). An excellent overview of the status of the nation on six different health behaviors was provided by a series of articles in the *American Journal of Health Promotion* (Babor, Aguirre-Molina, Marlatt, & Clayton, 1999; Carey, 1999; Glanz, 1999; Gutman & Clayton, 1999; Marcus & Forsyth, 1999; Orleans & Cummings, 1999; Orleans, Gruman, Ulmer, Emont, & Hollendonner, 1999).

Healthy people in healthy communities is the vision of *Healthy People 2010* (U.S. Department of Health and Human Services, 2000), the blueprint for health services in the United States in the new millennium. The two major goals include increasing quality and years of healthy life and eliminating health disparities. The goal change from *decreasing health disparities* to *eliminating health disparities* is an important change for our country in that it indicates that health disparities that characterize our diverse populations will no longer be tolerated. The document includes 467 objectives in 28 focus areas offering an exciting array of goals to be pursued in primary care as well as by schools, work sites, and other public health settings. Critical health indicators have been identified to track progress toward the overall goals. These include physical activity, overweight and obesity, tobacco use, substance abuse, responsible sexual behavior, mental health, injury and violence, environmental quality, immunization, and access to health care (U.S. Department of Health and Human Services, 2000). Of particular concern are vulnerable populations who often have inadequate health care, low-paying jobs without health insurance coverage, and chronic exposure to hazardous environments. Successful collaboration with communities to improve the health and environment of vulnerable populations will be a major challenge for health care providers in the next decade. Health-promotion and illness prevention programs for these populations should be culturally appropriate and integrated into the contexts in which they spend their daily lives.

Public support continues to grow for coverage of health-promotion and illness prevention services by third-party payers. Managed care organizations are demonstrating more interest in offering health-promotion and preventive services that have been shown to be effective in promoting positive behavior change and decreasing health care costs. The federal government and private insurers must continue to evaluate the impact of providing an array of prevention and health-promotion services to individuals and families including the millions of U.S. citizens who are currently uninsured or underinsured.

Health Promotion and Disease Prevention: Is There a Difference?

The most important difference between health promotion and disease or illness prevention is in the underlying motivation for the behavior on the part of individuals and aggregates. *Health promotion* is behavior motivated by the desire to increase well-being and actualize human health potential. *Disease prevention*, also called *health protection*, is behavior motivated by a desire to actively avoid illness, detect it early, or maintain functioning within the constraints of illness. The *actualizing tendency* underlying health promotion increases states of positive tension in order to promote change and growth. This increase in tension is often experienced as a challenge and facilitates behaviors expressive of human potential. The *stabilizing tendency* underlying disease prevention is evident in the functioning of homeokinetic mechanisms and is directed toward maintaining balance and equilibrium. The stabilizing tendency is responsible for protective maneuvers, primarily maintaining the internal and external environments within a range compatible with continuing existence.

Probably the purest form of motivation for health promotion exists in childhood through young adulthood when energy, vitality, and vigor are important to attain but the threat of chronic illness seems remote. Youth may engage in health behaviors for the pure pleasure of doing so or for the improvement of physical appearance and attractiveness to others. In the adult years, when human vulnerabilities become more apparent, the two motivations for health behavior usually coexist. For example, an older adult may be motivated to jog in order to improve stamina and energy (health promotion) but also to avoid cardiovascular disease (disease prevention). Regulatory measures for clean air may be passed to prevent exposure to asbestos as a cancer risk factor (disease prevention) but also to improve the overall quality of the environment (health promotion).

Three important theoretical differences between health promotion and disease prevention are presented. First, health promotion is not illness- or injury-specific; prevention is. Second, health promotion is "approach" motivated, whereas prevention is "avoidance" motivated. Third, health promotion seeks to expand positive potential for health, whereas prevention seeks to thwart the occurrence of insults to health and well-being. When interventions are tailored to particular clients, a distinction between the *motivational dynamics* of health promotion and prevention is likely to be helpful. In reality, health promotion and prevention are complementary processes. Both are critical to the quality of life at all developmental stages. More attention will be given to these two concepts throughout the rest of the book.

The Multidimensional Nature of Health Promotion

The health of individuals and families is affected markedly by the community, environment, and society in which they live. The context for living either sustains and expands health potential or inhibits the emergence of health and well-being. It is important that nurses appreciate and consider the complexity of health-promotion endeavors. Dunn (1973) in his early classic writings on high-level wellness provided the following schema for health-promotion efforts:

- Individual wellness
- Family wellness
- Community wellness
- Environmental wellness
- Societal wellness

Individual Wellness

Individuals play a critical role in the determination of their own health status because self-care represents the dominant mode of health care in our society. Many personal decisions are made daily that shape lifestyle and the social and physical environments. Health promotion at the individual level improves personal decision making and health practices. Throughout this book, the frame of reference for individual prevention and health-promotion activities is the total life span from childhood to the older adult years. Every developmental stage must be considered in formulating national health policy and programs if the quality of life for people of all ages is to be significantly enhanced through health-promotion efforts.

Family Wellness

Although the family plays a critical role in the development of health beliefs and health behaviors, there is limited research on the health-promoting role of the family. Almost all individuals identify with a family group in which members influence one another's ideas and actions. Each family has a characteristic value, role, and power structure as well as unique communication patterns. In addition, families fulfill affective, socialization, health care, and coping functions in varying ways. Parenting styles and family environments encourage healthy or unhealthy behaviors that may persist throughout the life span. Much more attention should be given to the development of strategies to promote family wellness.

Community Wellness

Community wellness is achieved by multiple actions that improve the conditions of family and community life (Dunn, 1973). A number of benefits of community-based health-promotion programs are identified:

1. Enhanced opportunities for information exchange and social support among members of the target population.
2. Reduced unit cost of programming because large groups, rather than individuals, receive health-promotion services.
3. Availability of networks that facilitate and coordinate health-promotion efforts.
4. Potential for widespread change in social norms regarding health and health behavior.
5. Coordinated rather than piecemeal approach to the promotion of health in large populations.
6. Access to a broad array of media for dissemination of health information.
7. Availability of aggregate indices to be used for tracking the health status of the population.
8. Use of the talents and resources of community residents resulting in a sense of commitment to health-promotion programming.

Community programming for prevention and health promotion will result in rapid dissemination of health information and in marked changes in cultural norms relevant to health and health behavior.

Environmental Wellness

The level of environmental wellness affects the extent to which individuals, families, and communities achieve their optimum potential. *Environment* is a comprehensive term meaning the physical, interpersonal, and economic circumstances in which we live. The quality of the environment is dependent on the absence of toxic substances, the availability of aesthetic or restorative experiences, and the accessibility of human and economic resources needed for healthful and productive living. Socioeconomic conditions such as unemployment, poverty, crime, prejudice, and isolation have adverse effects on health. Environmental wellness is manifest in harmony and balance between human beings and their surroundings.

Societal Wellness

The wellness of a society depends largely on the passage of laws and the establishment of policies that protect the health and welfare of all age groups. A well society is one in which all members have a standard of living and way of life that enables them to meet basic human needs and engage in activities that express their human potential. Essential to a well society is the collective citizenry's willingness to accept responsibility for health and to foster a level of education commensurate with informed decision making. A well society recognizes the dignity of all human beings, adopts policies to maintain that dignity, and avoids policies and programs that are demeaning or belittling to its members. A well society empowers its members to use their talents throughout the life span without premature retirement or relegation to a status of less value with age. Societal wellness requires involvement of a number of sectors, including those of education, food production, housing, and employment, as well as the health sector, in joint efforts to improve a population's health profile. Prerequisites for a well society include:

1. A belief that disease and illness are not inevitable consequences of human existence.
2. A vision for the population beyond that of immediate survival.
3. Awareness of the close relationship between individual, family, and community health assets and the well-being and productivity of a society.
4. Acceptance of high-level wellness as the goal of the society.

Societal wellness provides the framework in which individual, family, community, and environmental wellness exist. Decisions made at all levels of bureaucracy in the public and private sectors affect the range of health-promoting options available.

Coordinated interventions at all five levels are likely to be the most cost-efficient and effective approach to health promotion. Such interventions are complex and synergistic, optimizing ultimate chances of success.

The Contribution of Nurses to the Prevention and Health-Promotion Team

Nurses, because of their biopsychosocial expertise and frequent, continuing contact with clients, have the unique opportunity of providing global leadership to health professionals in the promotion of better health for the world community. Nurses should serve as role models of health-promoting lifestyles and as leaders to activate communities for health promotion. Nurses, as the largest single group of health care providers, continue to play a vital role in making health-promotion and illness prevention services available to all population groups, including those who are underserved and vulnerable. Payers are increasingly willing to reimburse for health-promotion and prevention services that add value to health care (Atkins, Best, & Shapiro, 2001). Many managed-care organizations already provide selected prevention and health-promotion services to their members. This trend will escalate in the future. Primary care and community care delivery systems must be reorganized to continue to eliminate any system barriers to delivery of quality health-promotion and illness prevention services. These barriers include lack of trained personnel, lack of tracking systems, absence of reminder systems for systematic follow-up, and inadequate intervention materials (Solberg, Kottke, & Brekke, 1998; Solberg, Kottke, Conn, et al., 1997). Nurses as major health care providers must continue to work toward the redistribution of health care resources so that quality health-promotion and illness prevention services are available to all.

REFERENCES

Ashton, J., Grey, P., & Barnard, K. (1986). Healthy cities: WHO's new public health initiative. *Health Prom, 1*, 319–324.

Atkins, D., Best, D., & Shapiro, E. N. (2001, April). The Third U.S. Preventive Services Task Force: Background, methods, and first recommendations. *Am J Prev Med, 20*(35), 1–107.

Babor, T. F., Aguirre-Molina, M., Marlatt, G. A., & Clayton, R. (1999). Managing alcohol problems and risky drinking. *Am J Health Prom, 14*(2), 98–103.

Bock, B., Niaura, R., Fontes, A., & Bock, F. (1999). Acceptability of computer assessments among ethnically diverse, low-income smokers. *Am J Health Prom, 13*(5), 299–304.

Carey, M. P. (1999). Prevention of HIV infection through changes in sexual behavior. *Am J Health Prom, 14*(2), 104–111.

Dunn, H. L. (1973). *High-level wellness.* Arlington, VA: R. W. Beatty Co.

Glanz, K. (1999). Progress in dietary behavior change. *Am J Health Prom, 14*(2), 112–117.

Guthrie, B. J., Caldwell, C. H., & Hunter, A. G. (1997). Minority adolescent female health: Strategies for the next millennium. In D. K. Wilson, J. R. Rodrigue, & W. C. Taylor (Eds.), *Health-promoting and health-compromising behaviors among minority adolescents* (pp. 153–171). Washington, DC: American Psychological Association.

Gutman, M., & Clayton, R. (1999). Treatment and prevention of use and abuse of illegal drugs: Progress on intervention and future directions. *Am J Health Prom, 14*(2), 92–97.

Healthy People: The Surgeon General's Report on Health Promotion and Disease Prevention. (1979). Washington, DC: U.S. Public Health Service; U.S. Department of Health, Education, and Welfare publication PHS 79-55071.

Healthy People 2000: National Health Promotion and Disease Prevention Objectives. (1990). Washington, DC: U.S. Public Health Service.

Hofmann, A. D. (2000). Adolescent sexuality and health care reform. In M. S. Jamner & D. Stokols (Eds.), *Promoting human wellness: New frontiers for research, practice and policy* (pp. 541–585). Berkeley: University of California Press.

Jamner, M. S., & Stokols, D. (Eds.). (2001). *Promoting human wellness: New frontiers for research, practice, and policy.* Berkeley: University of California Press.

Kreuter, M., Farrell, D., Olevitch, L., & Brennan, L. (2000). *Tailoring health messages: Customizing communication with computer technology.* Mahwah, NJ: Lawrence Erlbaum Associates, Inc.

Kreuter, M. W., Strecher, V. J., & Glassman, B. (1999). One size does not fit all: The case for tailoring print materials. *Annals of Behavioral Medicine, 21*(4), 276–283.

Kumanyika, S. K. (2001). Minisymposium on obesity: Overview and some strategic considerations. *Annu Rev Public Health, 22*, 293–308.

Marcus, B. H., & Forsyth, L. H. (1999). How are we doing with physical activity? *Am J Health Prom, 14*(2), 118–124.

McQueen, D. (1999). A world behaving badly: The global challenge for behavioral surveillance. *American Journal of Public Health, 89*(9), 1312–1314.

McQueen, D. (2000). *Strengthening the evidence base for health promotion.* Technical Report #1. Fifth Global Conference on Health Promotion. Sponsored by World Health Organization, Pan American Health Organization, and Ministry of Health of Mexico. Mexico City, Mexico, June 5–9, 2000.

Minkler, M. (2000). Health promotion at the dawn of the 21st century: Challenges and dilemmas. In M. S. Jamner & D. Stokols (Eds.), *Promoting human wellness: New frontiers for research, practice and policy* (pp. 349–377). Berkeley: University of California Press.

Orleans, C. T., & Cummings, K. M. (1999). Population-based tobacco control: Progress and prospects. *Am J Health Prom, 14*(2), 83–91.

Orleans, C. T., Gruman, J., Ulmer, C., Emont, S. L., & Hollendonner, J. K. (1999). Rating our progress in population health promotion: Report card on six behaviors. *Am J Health Prom, 14*(2), 75–82.

23. *Promoting Health–Preventing Disease: Objectives for the Nation.* (1980). Washington, DC: U.S. Public Health Service.

Skinner, C. S., Campbell, M. K., Rimer, B. K., Curry, S., & Prochaska, J. O. (1999). How effective is tailored print communication? *Annals of Behavioral Medicine, 21*(4), 290–298.

Solberg, L. I., Kottke, T. E., & Brekke, M. L. (1998). Will primary care clinics organize themselves to improve the delivery of preventive services? A randomized controlled trial. *Prev Med, 27,* 623–631.

Solberg, L. I., Kottke, T. E., Conn, S. A., et al. (1997). Delivering clinical preventive services is a systems problem. *Annals of Behavioral Medicine, 19*(3), 271–278.

Turner, J. (1986). World Health Organization—Charter for health promotion. *Lancet, 2,* 1407.

U.S. Department of Health and Human Services. (1997). *Developing objectives for Healthy People 2010.* Washington, DC: Office of Disease Prevention and Health Promotion.

U.S. Department of Health and Human Services. (2000, January). *Healthy People 2010* (Conference Edition, in two volumes). Washington, DC: U.S. Government Printing Office.

Wallack, L. (2000). Strategies for reducing youth violence: Media, community, and policy. In M. S. Jamner & D. Stokols (Eds.), *Promoting human wellness: New frontiers for research, practice and policy* (pp. 507–540). Berkeley: University of California Press.

Wilson, D. K., Rodrigue, J. R., & Taylor, W. C. (Eds.). (1997). *Health-promoting and health-compromising behaviors among minority adolescents.* Washington, DC: American Psychological Association.

World Health Organization. (1984). *Report of the working group on concepts and principles of health promotion.* Copenhagen, Denmark: WHO.

World Health Organization. (1988). *From alma-ata to the year 2000: Reflections at midpoint.* Geneva, Switzerland: WHO.

Part 1

The Human Quest for Health

1

Toward a Definition of Health

OBJECTIVES

1. Compare traditional and holistic definitions of health.
2. Contrast conceptions of individual health as stability and health as actualization.
3. Describe conceptions of health by nurse theorists.
4. Discuss family and community definitions of health.
5. Describe common approaches to measuring the meaning of health.

OUTLINE

- Health as an Evolving Concept
- Health and Illness: Distinct Entities or Opposite Ends of a Continuum?
- Definitions of Health That Focus on Individuals
  A. Health as Stability
  B. Health as Actualization
  C. Health as Actualization and Stability
  D. The Need for an Integrated View of Health
- Definitions of Health That Focus on the Family
- Definitions of Health That Focus on the Community
- Measurement of the Meaning of Health
- Directions for Research on the Meaning of Health
- Directions for Practice in the Context of Holistic Health

- Summary
- Learning Activities
- Selected Web Site
- References

Health, person, environment, and nursing constitute the commonly accepted meta-paradigm of the discipline of nursing (American Nurses Association, 2003; Faucet, 2000). Although health is the frequently articulated goal of nursing, different conceptions about the meaning of health are common. These differences may result from the increasingly diverse social values and norms that shape conceptualizations of health in societies with many distinct ethnic, religious, or cultural groups. What many health professionals once assumed was a universally accepted definition of health, the absence of diagnosable disease, is actually only one of many views of health held today. All people who are free of disease are not equally healthy. Furthermore, health can exist without illness, but illness never exists without health as its context (Pender, 1990).

The emergence of health promotion as the central strategy for improving health has shifted the paradigm from defining health in traditional medical terms (the curative model within a biologic perspective) to a multidimensional definition of health with biopsychosocial, spiritual, environmental, and cultural dimensions. In a multidimensional model of health, benefits can potentially be achieved from positive changes in any one of the health dimensions (Benson, 1996). This expanded perspective of health is empowering, as it opens up multiple options for improving health.

During the course of human development, the definition of health changes over the life span. As children mature and move into adolescence, their definition of health becomes more inclusive and more abstract (Millstein, 1994). Health definitions of adolescents show a trend toward greater thematic diversity (physical, mental, social, and emotional health) and less emphasis on the absence of illness with increasing age (Millstein, 1987). Older adults hold a definition of health that integrates the physical, mental, spiritual, and social aspects of health, reflecting how health is embedded in everyday experiences (Arcury, Quandt, & Bell, 2001). In addition, gender differences in health have been described. Perceived determinants of health differ between men and women (Denton, Prus, & Walters, 2004). However, reasons for these differences are not clear. Conceptions of health as well as gender differences in health over the life span need further exploration to understand developmental variations across genders, races, and cultures.

In a positive model of health, emphasis is placed on strengths, resiliencies, resources, potentials, and capabilities rather than on existing pathology. Despite a philosophic and conceptual shift in thinking about health, the nature of health as a positive life process is less understood empirically. Morbidity (prevalence of illness) and mortality (death) are still commonly used to define the health of a population. These indicators are problematic, as they more accurately reflect the disease burden and the need for health care, not health (Congdon, 2001). Health is determined by complex interwoven forces embedded in the social context of people's lives. For example, life conditions, such as neighborhood, food, work, and leisure, which lie outside the realm of health practice, positively or negatively influence health long before morbid states are evident.

Health as an Evolving Concept

A brief review of the historical development of the concept of health provides the background for examining definitions of health found in the professional literature. The word *health* as it is commonly used did not appear in writing until approximately AD 1000. It is derived from the Old English word *health*, meaning being safe or sound and whole of body (Sorochan, 1970). Historically, physical wholeness was of major importance for acceptance in social groups. Persons suffering from disfiguring diseases, like leprosy, or from congenital malformations were ostracized from society. Not only was there fear of contagion of physically obvious disease, but there was also repulsion at the grotesque appearance. Being healthy was construed as natural or in harmony with nature, while being unhealthy was thought of as unnatural or contrary to nature (Dolfman, 1973).

With the advent of the scientific era and the resultant increase in medical discoveries, illness came to be regarded with less disgust, and society became concerned about assisting individuals in their escape from its catastrophic effects. *Health* in this context was defined as "freedom from disease." Because disease could be traced to a specific cause, often microbial, it could be diagnosed. The notion of health as a disease-free state was extremely popular into the first half of the 20th century and was recognized by many as *the* definition of health (Wylie, 1970). Health and illness were viewed as extremes on a continuum; the absence of one indicated the presence of the other. This gave rise to "ruling out disease" to assess health, an approach still prevalent in the medical community today. The underlying erroneous assumption is that a disease-free population is a healthy population.

The concept of mental health as we now know it did not exist until the latter part of the 19th century. Individuals who exhibited unpredictable or hostile behavior were labeled "lunatics" and ostracized in much the same way as those with disfiguring physical ailments. Being put away with little if any human care was considered their "just due," because mental illness was often ascribed to evil spirits or satanic powers. The visibility of the ill only served as a reminder of personal vulnerability and mortality, aspects of human existence that society wished to ignore.

For several decades, the importance of mental health became obscured in the rapid barrage of medical discoveries for treatment of physical disorders. However, the psychologic trauma resulting from the high-stress situations of combat during World War II expanded the scope of health as a concept to include consideration of the mental status of the individual. Mental health was manifest in the ability of an individual to withstand stresses imposed by the environment. When individuals succumbed to the rigors of life around them and could no longer carry out the functions of daily living, they were declared to be mentally ill. Despite efforts to develop a more holistic definition of health, the dichotomy between individuals suffering from physical illness and those suffering from mental illness persisted (Congdon, 2001; Sorochan, 1970).

In 1974, the World Health Organization (WHO) proposed a definition of health that emphasized "wholeness" and the positive qualities of health: "Health is a state of complete physical, mental, and social well-being and not merely the absence of disease and infirmity" (WHO, 1986a, 1996). This definition increased the number of components to take into consideration in assessing health. The definition was revolutionary in that it did

(a) reflect concern for the individual as a total person; (b) place health in the context of the social environment; and (c) equate health with productive and creative living.

The WHO definition called attention to the multiple dimensions of health. However, the definition has been criticized by many who state that the definition is utopian, too broad, too abstract, and not subject to scientific application (Larson, 1999). Despite these criticisms, the WHO definition of health is the most popular and most comprehensive definition of health worldwide. In the Healthy People 2010 initiative, health indicators that comprise 10 areas of health were unveiled (U.S. Department of Health and Human Services, 2000). These health indicators reflect individual behaviors (physical activity, overweight and obesity, tobacco use, substance abuse, sexual behavior, mental health), the physical and social environment (injury and violence, environmental quality), and important health system issues (immunizations, access to health care) that affect health.

Nine "images" of health have been proposed by Arnold and Breen (1998), which include health as the antithesis of disease, a balanced state, a growth phenomenon, functional capacity, goodness of fit, wholeness, well-being, transcendence, and empowerment. Each of these images reflect a different view or frame of reference for health, based on the life history of the beholder, which in turn are reflected in different personal preferences, programs, and policies.

Health is now recognized as a concept that is not only multidimensional but also applicable to both individuals and aggregates. In the following sections, definitions of health will be discussed that focus on the individual, the family, and the community. In the past, defining health for individuals received more attention in nursing and other health disciplines than defining health for families and communities. However, it has become clear that individual health is linked closely to both family and community health. The underlying premise of Healthy People 2010 is that the health of individuals is almost inseparable from the health of the larger community, and the health of every community determines the overall health status of the nation (U.S. Department of Health and Human Services, 2000).

Health and Illness: Distinct Entities or Opposite Ends of a Continuum?

The issue of whether health and illness are separate entities or opposite ends of a continuum continues to be debated by scientists. Are health and illness quantitatively or qualitatively different concepts? Are they bipolar?

Theorists who present health and illness as a continuum usually identify possible reference points such as (a) optimum health, (b) suboptimal health or incipient illness, (c) overt illness and disability, and (d) very serious illness or approaching death (Dunn, 1959). Such scales have only one point representing health, whereas three points on the scale represent varying states of illness. Dunn's model of wellness maintained that health and illness are separate concepts and proposed construction of continua that allow the differentiation of varying levels of health as well as varying levels of illness (Dunn, 1975).

When health and illness are assumed to represent a single continuum, it is difficult to discuss healthy aspects of the ill individual. The presence of illness ascribes the "sick role," and the individual is expected to direct all energies toward finding the cause of the illness and engaging in behaviors that will result in a return to health as soon as possible.

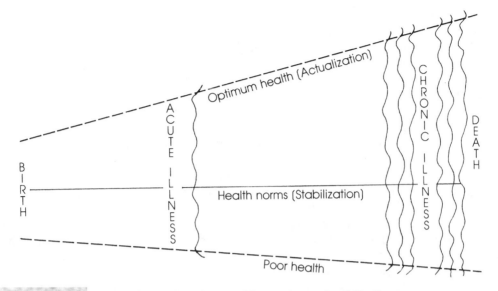

FIGURE 1–1 **The Health Continuum Throughout the Life Span**

Health can be manifested in the presence of illness, so a case can be made for separate but parallel continua for health and illness. Poor health can exist even if disease is not present and good health can be present in spite of disease (Tamm, 1993). Oelbaum (1974) stressed the interrelationship of health and illness, even though she considers the concepts to be separate entities rather than opposite ends of a continuum. She stated that apathy toward the work of wellness is the precursor of disease. The particular health behaviors or functions that are poorly performed will influence the type of disease, disorder, or damage that will follow (Oelbaum, 1974).

The authors of this book believe health and illness are qualitatively different, interrelated concepts that may coexist (Sullivan, 2003). In Figure 1–1, multiple levels of health are depicted in interaction with the experience of illness. Illness, which may be of short (acute) or long (chronic) duration, is represented as discrete events within the life span. Health can still be an aspiration to those with a chronic illness, and health can be achieved despite being diagnosed with a disease (Hwu, Coates, & Boore, 2001). These illness experiences can either hinder or facilitate one's continuing quest for health. Thus, good health or poor health can exist with or without overt illness (Neuman, 1995).

Definitions of Health That Focus on Individuals

Health as Stability

For individuals, stability-based definitions of health derive primarily from the physiologic concepts of homeostasis and adaptation. Dubos (1965), an early advocate of the stability position, defined health as a state or condition that enables the individual to adapt to the environment. The degree of health experienced is dependent on one's ability to adjust to the various internal and external tensions that one faces. Dubos (1965) considered optimum health to be a mirage because in the real world individuals must face the physical and social forces that are forever changing, frequently unpredictable, and often dangerous. According to Dubos, the closest approach to optimum or high-level health is a physical and mental state free of discomfort and pain that permits one to function effectively within the environment.

Definitions of health based on normality can be described as stability oriented. Statistical norms for a variety of human functions are already well defined. A major problem with normative definitions of health is that they predict "what could be" based on "what is," leaving little room for incorporating growth, maturation, and evolutionary emergence into a definition of health. In addition, norms represent average or middle-range effectiveness rather than excellence or exceptional effectiveness in human functioning.

Environmental-focused models of health can also be described as stability oriented, as the essence of these models is adaptation of individuals to their environment. Health is related to the ability of individuals to maintain a balance with the environment, with relative freedom from pain, disability, or limitations, including social limitations. Health exists when one is able to adapt to the environment successfully and is able to grow, function, and thrive. In contrast, lack of adaptation is seen as a gap between one's ability and the demands of the environment (Verbrugge & Jette, 1994).

Parson's (1958) conceptualization of health is compatible with an environmental model, as health is defined in terms of social norms rather than physiologic norms. More than 40 years ago he described health as "the effective performance of valued roles and tasks for which an individual has been socialized."

Similar to Parsons' sociologic model of health, Patrick, Bush, and Chen (1973) and Feeney et al. (2002) have defined health in terms of functional norms. Their conception of health is the ability to perform socially valued activities usual for a person's age and social roles with a minimum probability of change to less valued function levels. The desirability of the immediate function level, as well as the probability that the current condition or state will change to a higher or lower preference function level, must be considered in assessing one's present health status.

A number of nurse-theorists have proposed definitions of health emphasizing stability. Levine defined health as a state in which there is balance between input and output of energy and in which structural, personal, and social integrity exist (Feeney et al., 2002). Johnson, in her behavioral system model, does not explicitly define health. A conception of health that focuses on stability can, however, be inferred from her conceptualization of internal homeostasis. Health or wellness is balance and stability among the following behavioral systems: attachment or affiliative, dependency, ingestive, eliminative, sexual, aggressive, and achievement. Behavioral system stability is demonstrated by efficient and effective behavior that is purposeful, goal-directed, orderly, and predictable (Schaefer & Pond, 1991). Neuman (1995) has defined health or wellness as a condition in which all subsystems—physiologic, psychologic, and sociocultural—are in balance and in harmony with the whole of man. Health is a state of saturation, of inertness, free of disruptive needs. Disrupting forces or noxious stressors with which individuals cannot cope create disharmony, reducing the level of wellness. In a wellness state, total needs are met and more energy is generated and stored than expended. A strong, flexible line of defense is maintained, providing the individual with considerable resistance to disequilibrium (Loveland-Cherry & Wilkerson, 1989).

Roy (Roy & Andrews, 1999) also subscribed to a stability definition of health. The central concept in Roy's model is adaptation. Health is a state and process of successful adaptation that promotes being and becoming an integrated whole person. The four adaptive modes through which coping energies are expressed are: physiologic, self-concept, role performance, and interdependence modes. Adaptation promotes integrity. Integrity implies soundness or an unimpaired condition that can lead to completeness and unity. The person in an adapted state is freed from ineffective coping attempts that deplete energy. Available energy can be used to enhance health (Roy & Andrews, 1999).

Tripp-Reimer (1984) also proposed a model for health that is stability oriented. The conceptualization of health is based on a two-dimensional perspective: an *etic* dimension (disease-nondisease), which reflects a quantitative, objective interpretation of health by a health care professional; and an *emic* dimension (wellness-illness), which represents the subjective perception and experiences of health by an individual. The etic-emic approach has been further described by Arcury et al. (2001), who state that the etic dimension focuses on a medical model of normality or homeostasis, while the emic approach, which focuses on the lay perspective, is well suited to social scientists who understand the interactions concerning health. The model is especially useful cross-culturally as it sheds light on reasons disagreements about the concept of health are often found between medical personnel and clients of differing ethnic backgrounds (Tripp-Reimer, 1984).

Health as Actualization

When individual health is defined more broadly as actualization of human potential, some scholars have proposed a different term, *wellness*. Wellness is considered an expanded term not as restricted as the concept of health. Despite this difference, *health* and *wellness* tend to be used interchangeably in the health-promotion literature and will be used interchangeably in this text.

Halbert Dunn was one of the early advocates for emphasizing actualization in definitions of health. Dunn coined the term *high-level wellness*, which he described as integrated human functioning that is oriented toward maximizing the potential of which the individual is capable. This requires that individuals maintain balance and purpose within the environment where they are functioning (Dunn, 1980). Though the definition identifies balance as a dimension of health, major emphasis is on the realization of human potential through purposeful activity. There is a single optimum level of wellness, as individuals move toward their personal optimum level based on their capabilities and potential.

Dunn (1959; 1975) stated that high-level wellness, or an ideal state of optimum health, involves three components: (a) progress in a forward and upward direction toward a higher potential of functioning, (b) an open-ended and ever-expanding challenge to live at a fuller potential, and (c) progressive maturation of the individual at increasingly higher levels throughout the life cycle. Dunn proposes that high-level wellness can only emerge in a favorable environment. Health, according to Dunn (1980), is not simply a passive state of freedom from illness; it is an emergent process characteristic of the entire life span.

Orem (1995) used health and well-being to refer to two different but related human states in her self-care theory. She defined health as a state characterized by soundness or wholeness of human structures and bodily and mental functions. Well-being was defined as an ideal state characterized by experiences of contentment, pleasure, and happiness; by spiritual experiences; by movement toward fulfillment of one's self-ideal; and by continuing personalization. Personalization is movement toward maturation and achievement of human potential. Engaging in responsible self-care and continuing development of self-care competency are facets of the process of personalization. Individuals can experience well-being even under conditions of adversity, including disorders of human structure and function.

Parse (1981), in describing her man-living-health theory of nursing, presents five assumptions about health that essentially define the term from her perspective:

1. Health is an open process of becoming, experienced by individuals.
2. Health is a rhythmically coconstituting process of the individual-environment relationship.
3. Health is an individual's patterns of relating value priorities.
4. Health is an intersubjective process of transcending with the possibles.
5. Health is an individual's negentropic (toward increasing order, complexity, and heterogeneity) unfolding.

Newman (1991), building on the work of Martha Rogers, defined health as the totality of the life process, which is evolving toward expanded consciousness. This definition emphasizes the actualizing properties of individuals throughout the life span. Four dimensions of health as a concept are identified:

1. Health is a fusion of disease and nondisease.
2. Health is the manifestation of an individual's unique pattern.
3. Health is the expansion of consciousness. Time is a measure of consciousness, and movement is a reflection of consciousness.
4. Health encompasses the entire life process, which evolves toward higher and greater frequency of energy exchange.

Key life-process phenomena include: consciousness, movement, space, and time. Newman's model of health addresses holistic characteristics of human beings. However, because there is no intent to create empirical referents for many of the terms within the model that focus on health as experience and not as a state, potential testing or applying the model empirically is not appropriate.

Both Newman and Parse build on Martha Rogers' theory of unitary man. Both represent early attempts to define health in terms of holism as opposed to defining health in terms of component parts. The emergent nature or actualization potential of the healthy individual and the capacity for open energy exchange with the environment are characteristics of both Newman's definitions of health.

Actualization or wellness models have been criticized because of the difficulties in measuring subjective perceptions. In addition, perceptions of health and wellness vary according to age and cultural context (U.S. Department of Health and Human Services, 2000). Another criticism is that the expanded definitions of health in these models do not distinguish health from happiness, quality of life, and other global concepts (Saracci, 1997). In spite of these criticisms the wellness models provide a focus on the whole person and promote the positive aspects of health. Also, persons who accept the wellness model of health are more likely to seek alternative sources of therapy, not because of dissatisfaction with conventional medicine, but because of their different beliefs and values about life and health (Astin, 1998). They are also more likely to view themselves as healthy in the presence of illness.

Health as Actualization and Stability

Models of individual health also incorporate both stability and actualization. For example, Wu (1973) has described health as a feeling of well-being, a capacity to perform to the best of one's ability, and the flexibility to adapt and adjust to varying situations created by the systems in which they exist. Wu proposed that wellness and illness represent distinct entities, with a repertory of behaviors for each. Within this frame of reference, both wellness and illness can exist simultaneously, so an evaluation of both wellness and illness are critical to a comprehensive health assessment.

King (1983) proposed a definition of health that emphasized both stabilizing and actualizing tendencies. She defined health as a dynamic state in a person's life cycle that implies adjustment to stressors in the environment through optimum use of resources to achieve maximum potential for daily living. In King's model (1983) a holistic health perspective relates to the way individuals handle stressors while functioning within the culture to which they were born and attempt to conform. King (1990) viewed health as a functional state in the life cycle, with illness defined as interference in the life cycle.

Smith (1983) proposed a model of health encompassing four dimensions; three focus on stability and one on actualization. Each health dimension is defined by the extremes on the health-illness continuum identified by the dimension.

- *Clinical Dimension*: Health extreme: absence of signs or symptoms of disease or disability as identified by medical science; illness extreme: presence of signs or symptoms or obvious disability.
- *Role-Performance Dimension*: Health extreme: performance of social roles with maximum expected output; illness extreme: failure to perform one's social roles.
- *Adaptive Dimension*: Health extreme: flexible adaptation to the environment, interaction with environment with maximum advantage; illness extreme: alienation of the person from environment, failure of self-corrective responses.
- *Eudaimonistic Dimension*: Health extreme: exuberant well-being; illness extreme: devitalized, languishing debility.

Each dimension requires a distinct approach and a different mode of intervention, depending on which dimension is used as the guiding framework for care.

A definition of health needs to be applicable to everyone: to the well, to those with a treatable disease or illness, and to those with chronic disease or disability (Institute of the Future, 2000). The authors of this text believe a definition of health should incorporate both actualizing and stabilizing tendencies and define health as the actualization of inherent and acquired human potential through goal-directed behavior, competent self-care, and satisfying relationships with others, while making adjustments as needed to maintain structural integrity and harmony with relevant environments. This broad, conceptual definition has led to a classification system that describes affective and behavioral expressions of health by

TABLE 1–1 Classification System for Affective and Behavioral Expressions of Health

Affect

Serenity	Harmony	Vitality	Sensitivity
Calm	Spiritual	Energetic	Aware
Relaxed	Contemplative	Vigorous	Connected
Peaceful	At one with the universe	Zestful	Intimate
Content		Alert	Loving
Comfortable			Warm

Attitudes

Optimism	Relevancy	Competency
Hopeful	Useful	Purposive
Enthusiastic	Contributing	Initiating
Open	Valued	Self-motivating
Reverent	Committed	Self-affirming
Resilient	Involved	Innovative

Activity

Positive Life Patterns	Meaningful Work	Invigorating Play
Healthy eating	Realistic goals	Meaningful hobbies
Regular exercise	Varied activities	Satisfying leisure activities
Stress management	Challenging tasks	Energizing diversions
Adequate rest	Collaboration	
Positive relationships		
Health monitoring		
Constructive coping		

Aspirations

Self-Actualization	Social Contribution
Growth	Global harmony and interdependence enhancement
Personal mastery	Environmental preservation

Accomplishments

Enjoyment	Creativity	Transcendence
Pleasure from daily living	Maximum use of capacities	Freedom, harmony
Sense of achievement	Innovative contribution	Purpose in life

individuals (Table 1–1). The major culture-free dimensions of health expression include: affect, attitudes, activity, aspirations, and accomplishments. The physical, mental, social, and spiritual components of health that are now cited in expanded definitions of health, including the WHO definition, are encompassed in this classification. The dimensions are further divided into 15 subcategories that may be culture-specific. The system is based on the assumptions that health is a manifestation of person and environment interactional patterns that become increasingly complex throughout the life span. The classification system provides a framework for a comprehensive assessment of health that is consistent with a positive, unitary, humanistic view.

The Need for an Integrated View of Health

Health is a holistic experience and only becomes fragmented in the minds of health professionals. The biological model has provided for technological excellence and sophisticated medical care, but it has led to a narrow focus on disease. An expansive view of health and its mental, social, and spiritual, as well as physical, dimensions are positive, holistic, and humanistic and can be integrated with traditional biomedical models (disease) and public health models (mortality, morbidity, risks) of health to provide a holistic biopsychosocial view (Engel, 1997; Institute of the Future, 2000). The biopsychosocial view eliminates the need to reject one view of health at the cost of another and enables clinicians and researchers to work with health and disease together rather than separating the concepts (Engel, 1997). Last, the social context is now recognized as a powerful determinant of health (Institute of the Future, 2000; U.S. Department of Health and Human Services, 2000). Therefore, understanding the relevance of a broad definition of health to individuals in their everyday experiences in different social contexts is critical to improving their health.

Definitions of Health That Focus on the Family

The complexity of the family and the diversity of family life in different ethnic and geographic settings pose a challenge for defining and promoting family health. The traditional definition of family as two or more persons living together who are related by marriage, blood, or adoption is no longer adequate in American society. A broad definition of family now accepted is two or more persons who depend on one another for emotional, physical, or financial support (Hanson & Boyd, 1996). In this definition family members are self-defined and may include any individuals who make a significant commitment to each other outside of marriage. It is critical that variation in family structure be taken into consideration in defining and measuring family health.

Conceptual frameworks of family health are evolving with the changing definition. Family nursing conceptual frameworks and theories are emerging from the family social science disciplines, family therapy theory, and nursing theories (Klein & White, 1996). The nursing theories originated with the individual as a focus. However, a few, such as Rogers, Roy, King, and Neuman, have expanded to include the family. Four major social science theories that have provided direction for the development of nursing knowledge in family health include developmental theory, systems theory, structural functional theory, and interactional theory.

Loveland-Cherry (2000) has observed that family health is a concept often referred to as a goal of nursing but seldom defined. She defines family health as possessing the abilities and resources to accomplish the development tasks of the family. Adapting Smith's (1983) models of health to families, she has proposed the following dimensions of family health (Loveland-Cherry, 2000):

- *Clinical Model*: Lack of evidence of physical, mental, or social disease, deterioration, or dysfunction of family system.
- *Role-Performance Model*: Ability of family system to carry on family functions effectively and to achieve family developmental tasks.
- *Adaptive Model*: Family patterns of interaction with the physical and social environment, characterized by flexible, effective adaptation or ability to change and grow.
- *Eudaimonistic Model*: Ongoing provision of resources, guidance, and support to realize the family's maximum well-being and potential throughout the life span.

This framework specifies the critical dimensions of family health conceptually and enables the nurse to be able to assess each of the dimensions.

Other approaches to family nursing have been proposed to promote health (McCubbin, 1999). These include the family as context, family as client, family as system, and family as a component of society. A model of family reciprocal determinism has been proposed to take into account the complexity of the family environment in promoting health (Baranowski, Perry, & Parcel, 2002). Within the model, behavior is a function of the shared environment with other family members and their behavior and personal characteristics. The family plays an important role in the promotion of health because health information is shared and behaviors are learned, practiced, and reinforced in the daily routine, which are facilitated or hindered by family values and beliefs (Wingood & Keltner, 1999). All of the perspectives move the basic unit of analysis from the individual to the family system, as the interaction of the individual with other members of the family or other units in society is emphasized.

A biopsychosocial definition of family health has been proposed which states that family health is a dynamic changing state of well-being, including biologic, psychological, sociological, spiritual, and cultural factors of the family system (Engel, 1997). In this definition an individual's health affects the functioning of the family, and in turn, family functioning affects the health of the individual. Both the family system and the individual members must be part of the health assessment.

Characteristics of healthy families have been described. These characteristics include affirmation and support for one another, shared sense of responsibility, shared leisure time, shared religious core, respect, trust, and family rituals and traditions. These qualities address the stability of family functioning and balance in interaction among family members. Family typologies have also been developed to identify a common profile that may be linked to health in families. For example, four family types (balanced, traditional, disconnected, emotionally strained) have differentiated among health measures in two community-based samples (Fisher et al., 1998). These typologies also suggest that health-promotion interventions need to be implemented in ways that are compatible with family values, beliefs, and orientations. Additional research is needed to evaluate the effects of health-related interventions based on family type.

Many factors influence how family health is defined. Social, cultural, environmental, and religious factors play a central role in determining how families view their health. Families' strengths, resources, and competencies are also an integral part of a positive conceptualization of health. Family health processes are being given increased attention by nurse researchers as well as scientists in other disciplines. Development and testing of theoretical models to describe family health will assist health professionals to identify determinants of family well-being to promote the health of families.

Definitions of Health That Focus on the Community

Communities are usually defined within one of two frameworks: geographical area or relational. Geographical definitions are based on legal or geopolitical areas such as cities, towns, or census tracts. Relational definitions are based on how people interact to achieve common goals. The WHO (1974) defines *community* as a social group determined by both geographical area and common values, with members who know each other and interact within a social structure. Members of the community create norms, values, and social institution for its members. The WHO definition focuses on the spatial, personal, and functional dimensions of a community.

Social-ecological theories of community health emphasize the interaction and interdependence of the individual with the family, community, social structure, and physical environment (Green, 1999). A social ecology model described in the Ottawa Charter for Health Promotion, a landmark policy statement, outlines the essential dimensions of community health (WHO, 1986b). Fundamental to community health are peace, shelter, education, food, income, a stable ecosystem, sustainable resources, social justice, and equity. Flynn, whose Healthy Cities project is based on a social ecological view, notes that the responsibility for health is widely shared in the community with collaborative decision making about health issues (Flynn, 1997). Informed political action and healthy public policies are essential to a healthy community.

Three major dimensions have been identified in an effort to develop a broad understanding of community health. These dimensions, which can be assessed by multiple measures, provide information that is complementary for developing a clear picture of the health of the community (Shuster & Goeppinger, 2000).

1. *Status Dimension*: Biological, emotional, and social components, measured by morbidity, mortality, life expectancy, risk factors, consumer satisfaction, mental health, crime rates, functional levels, worker absenteeism, and infant mortality.

2. *Structural Dimension*: Community health services and resources measured by utilization patterns, treatment data, and provider/population ratios; social indicators measured by socioeconomic and racial distributions, and median education level.

3. *Process Dimension*: Effective community functioning or problem solving that results in community competence as evidenced by commitment, self–other awareness, effective communication, conflict containment and accommodation, participation, management of relations with larger society, and mechanisms to facilitate interaction and decision making.

Based on these dimensions, community health can be defined as meeting the collective needs of its members through identifying problems and managing interactions within the community and between the community and the larger society (Hemstrom, 1995).

Community health is more than the sum of the health states of its individual members; it encompasses the characteristics of the community as a whole. Individual, family, and community health are intimately related. The health of the community depends on individual health as well as whether the social, physical, and political aspects enable individuals to live healthy lives. Research indicates that the characteristics of communities have an important influence on health and individual risk behaviors (DiClemente, Cresby, Sionean, & Holtgrave, 2004). Studies have also documented the relationship between social and economic conditions and the health of individuals in a community. *Social capital* has also been described as a major determinant of health in communities. This term, which includes trust, reciprocity, and cooperation among families, neighborhoods, and entire communities, will be discussed in more detail in Chapter 3 (Putnam, 2000). Healthy communities support healthy lifestyles. Likewise the collective attitudes, beliefs, and behaviors of individuals who live in the community influence community health (U.S. Department of Health and Human Services, 2000). Healthy People 2010 objectives focus on determinants of health that include the effects of the individual, physical, and social community environments, and policies and interventions to promote health and access to care. All of these components must be assessed prior to developing strategies to create healthier communities.

The traditional focus on an individual, curative model, while successful in the care of chronic diseases, unintentionally relegated individual and community health to a position of secondary importance. However, the focus is shifting to an ecological model that goes beyond the individual to include community level factors (Reppucci, Woolard, & Fried, 1999). Evidence supports an expanded view of individual health that is inseparable from the community. Effective health-promotion interventions are beginning to be based on the assessment of a community's competence and actualizing potential, as recommended by Healthy People 2010.

Measurement of the Meaning of Health

In general, few health measures incorporate the holistic and expansive views of health to which nurses claim to subscribe. Instead, nurses, just as other professionals, choose health status measures that are derived from an illness or curative model (Hinshaw, 1999). Many commonly used measures of health status continue to focus primarily on mortality or on morbidity-related indices such as dysfunction, disability, or impairment. Such "measures of health" are really "measures of illness." Measures of health need to encompass the complexity of health. They should (a) characterize health by conditions that define its presence rather than its absence, (b) identify a spectrum of health states, and (c) reflect a life-span developmental perspective.

Based on the WHO definition, Ware (1987) proposed five distinct dimensions as a minimum standard for a comprehensive health measure: physical health (functional and structural integrity), mental health (emotional and intellectual functioning), social functioning, role functioning, and general perceptions of well-being, which are now widely accepted measures of health status. Another classification has more recently been proposed that includes subjective health status, or individuals' global assessment of their health; chronic health problems, or illnesses diagnosed by a physician that are expected to last 6 months or more; and functional health, or characteristics of the individuals' health in eight domains (vision, hearing, speech, mobility, cognition, emotion, pain/discomfort and distress or an unpleasant subjective state; Denton et al., 2004). As can be seen in both of these classifications measuring health status, there is a greater focus on limitations in performance or functioning and/or disease, reflecting the illness model of health.

Two views of self-rated health assessments have been proposed: spontaneous assessment and enduring self-concept. In the spontaneous assessment view, self-rated assessments of health are considered responsive to observable indicators of illness and bear a relationship to future reports of illness and functional limitations. Global self-evaluations of health have been shown to take a wide range of factors into consideration, including functional ability, lifestyle and health practices, sociocultural constructions of health, and physical symptoms (Ballis, Segall, & Chipperfield, 2004). Individual ratings of health may be transitory, with respect to multiple dimensions of one's health status as well as available social support. The enduring self-concept view characterizes self-rated health as a reflection of one's established beliefs about one's health. In this view, self-rated health is stable over time, and is based on one's self-concept. Therefore, self-rated health may not reflect more objective indicators of health, as it is independent of one's physical status. This view is more congruent with an expansive definition of health, as an individual's self-evaluation of global health is more related to an overall sense of well-being.

Measurement of health is complex, and becomes even more so when the individual's perspective is taken into account. This issue results in measurement challenges, as there is no gold standard on which to validate self-report measures of health. However, this does not negate an individual-centered perspective assessment of the meaning of health, as individual values must be the base on which to develop interventions to promote health.

Directions for Research on the Meaning of Health

The fundamental mechanisms underlying human health processes are now receiving attention from nurse scientists. However, many questions remain to be addressed. How is human health expressed biologically and behaviorally? What are the gender, culture, and racial differences in the expressions of health? How does health qualitatively differ at varying points of life-span development? What is the maximum human health potential? What interactive conditions between the person and the environment enhance or deplete health? Which health dimensions are critical to assess the health of families? Which health dimensions are key to evaluating the health of communities? Generating knowledge relevant to these questions will advance nursing science and provide an empirical base to guide effective health-promoting interventions.

Models of health that incorporate ethnic, cultural, social, environmental, and political factors are needed to examine the diversity of health conceptions. Attention should be given to developing more rigorous, consistent definitions of family health and community health. Furthermore, longitudinal studies are needed to determine the developmental variations in health definitions across the life span. Multidisciplinary research teams are suggested to test theories that incorporate a clear, expanded definition of health. Measures that assess the expanded conceptualizations of health can then be constructed that will provide information needed to guide the design of interventions to improve individual, family, and community health. In addition, culturally sensitive, age-appropriate, objective measures need to be developed to assess the expanded definition that has been proposed in order to advance knowledge about an integrated holistic view of health.

Directions for Practice in the Context of Holistic Health

The definition of health has evolved from traditional usage in a medical, curative model to a multidimensional phenomenon with biopsychosocial, spiritual, environmental, and cultural dimensions. The increasing acceptance of a holistic view of health has major implications for nursing (Hwu et al., 2001). Nurses and other health care professionals need to understand and assess all of these multiple dimensions in their health assessments. The assessment information can then be used to develop intervention strategies. For example, the traditional biomedical assessment may be useful in guiding genetic counseling or screening interventions. Information gleaned from a spiritual and cultural assessment can provide valuable knowledge in developing health-promotion interventions for diverse populations. An assessment of the social and physical environment will provide useful information about aspects of the environment that may be positively or negatively affecting the health of the individual or community. In a holistic view of health, an assessment is not complete unless it involves the individual as well as the family and community in which the individual resides. Nurses work in partnership with clients to teach the knowledge and skills needed to empower them to achieve their health goals. Last, health needs to be viewed from a positive perspective when conducting an assessment or designing health promotion strategies. This means that the nurse should focus on available resources, potentials, and capabilities as well as dysfunction and potential risks. When health is viewed in a positive model, strategies can be developed that concentrate on strengthening resources as well as decreasing negative risks.

SUMMARY

Varying definitions of health have been presented that provide the foundation on which health-promotion programs for individuals, families, and communities can be based. To address the promotion of health, one must know how health, the desired outcome, is defined and how achievement of health can be measured at individual, family, and community levels. The shift from rigid adherence to a biomedical model to a view of health that encompasses mental, social, and spiritual well-being as well as a focus on family and community has begun to occur. Supporters of this shift advocate a proactive approach to health that includes building strengths, enhancing resources, and fostering resilience to enhance prospects for effective living (WHO, 1974). A shift to this broader perspective of health will also facilitate development of proactive policy to improve the nation's health.

LEARNING ACTIVITIES

1. Write your own definition of health and describe factors you considered in developing the definition.
2. Interview three persons at varying points in the life span to obtain their perspective of their health and things they do to stay healthy.
3. Categorize the three conceptions of health based on the information obtained in interviews as stability, actualization, or traditional.
4. Using Table 1–1, generate additional adjectives to describe the affective and behavioral expressions of health that might be helpful for your clients.

SELECTED WEB SITE

Healthy People 2010

http://www.health.gov/healthypeople

REFERENCES

American Nurses Association. (2003). *Nursing's social policy statement: Second edition.* Pub # 03NSPS.

Arcury, T. A., Quandt, S. A., & Bell, R. A. (2001). Staying healthy: The salience and meaning of health maintenance behaviors among rural older adults in North Carolina. *Social Science and Medicine, 53,* 1541–1556.

Arnold, J., & Breen, L. J. (1998). Images of health. In S. S. Gorin & J. Arnold (Eds.), *Health promotion handbook.* St. Louis: Mosby.

Astin, J. (1998). Why patients use alternative medicine: Results of a national study. *JAMA, 279,* 1548–1553.

Bailis, D. S., Segall, A., & Chipperfield, J. G. (2004). Two views of self-rated general health status. *Social Science and Medicine, 56*(2), 203–217.

Baranowski, T., Perry, C. L., & Parcel, G. S. (2002). How individuals, environments and health behavior interact: Social cognitive theory. In K. Glanz, F. M. Lewis, & B. K. Rimer (Eds.), *Health behavior and health education* (2nd ed., pp. 153–178). San Francisco: Jossey-Bass.

Benson, H. (1996). *Timeless healing: The power and biology of belief.* New York: Scribner.

Congdon, P. (2001). Health status and healthy life measures for population health need assessment: Modeling variability and uncertainty. *Health & Place, 7,* 13–25.

Denton, M., Prus, S., & Walters, V. (2004). Gender differences in health: A Canadian study of the psychosocial, structural and behavioral determinants of health. *Social Science and Medicine, 58*(12), 2585–2600.

DiClemente, R. J., Crosby, R. A., Sionean, C., & Holtgrave, D. (2004). Community intervention trials: Theoretical and methodological considerations. In D. S. Blumenthal & R. J. DiClemente (Eds.), *Community-based health research* (pp. 171–198). New York: Springer.

Dolfman, M. L. (1973). The concept of health: An historic and analytic examination. *J Sch Health, 43,* 493.

Dubos, R. (1965). *Man adapting.* New Haven, CT: Yale University Press.

Dunn, H. L. (1959, November). What high-level wellness means. *Can J Public Health, 50*(11), 447–457.

Dunn, H. L. (1975). Points of attack for raising the level of wellness. *J Nat Med Assoc., 49,* 223–235.

Dunn, H. L. (1980). *High-level wellness.* Theofare, NJ: Charles B. Slack, Inc.

Engel, G. (1997). From biomedical to biopsychosocial. Being scientific in the human domain. *Psychosomatics, 38*(6), 521–526.

Faucet, J. (2000). *Analysis and evaluation of contemporary nursing knowledge: Nursing models and theories.* Philadelphia, PA: FA Davis Co.

Feeney, D., Furlong, W., Torrance, G. W., Goldsmith, C. H., et al. (2002). Multiattribution and single attribute utility functions for the health utilities index mark 3 system. *Medical Care, 40,* 113–128.

Fisher, L., Paradis, G., Soubhi, H., Mansai, O., Gauvin, L., & Potvin, L. (1998). Family process in health research: Extending a family topology to a new cultural context. *Health Psychology, 17*(4), 358–366.

Flynn, B. C. (1997). Partnerships in healthy cities and communities: A social commitment for advanced practice nurses. *Advanced Practice Nursing Quarterly, 2*(4), 1–6.

Green, L. (1999). Health education's contribution to public health in the twentieth century: A glimpse through health promotion's rear-view mirror. *Annual Review of Public Health, 20,* 67–88.

Hanson, S. M., & Boyd, S. T. (1996). *Family healthcare nursing: Theory, practice and research.* Philadelphia, PA: FA Davis.

Hemstrom, M. M. (1995). Application as scholarship: A community client experience. *Public Health Nursing, 12*(30), 279–283.

Hinshaw, A. S. (1999). Evolving nursing research traditions: Influencing factors. In A. S. Hinshaw, S. L. Feetham, & J. Shaver, *Handbook of clinical nursing research* (pp. 19–38). Thousand Oaks: Sage.

Hwu, Y., Coates, V., & Boore, J. (2001). The evolving concept of health in nursing research: 1988-1998. *Patient Education and Counseling, 42,* 105–114.

Institute of the Future. (2000). *Health and healthcare 2010.* San Francisco: Jossey-Bass.

King, I. M. (1983). *A theory for nursing: Systems, concepts, processes.* New York: Teachers College Press.

King, I. M. (1990). Health as the goal for nursing. *Nurs Sci Q, 3*(3), 123–128.

Klein, D. M., & White, J. M. (1996). *Family theories: An introduction.* Thousand Oaks: Sage.

Larson, J. S. (1999). The conceptualization of health. *Medical Care Research and Review, 56*(2), 123–136.

Loveland-Cherry, C. J. (2000). Family health risks. In M. Stanhope & J. Lancaster (Eds.), *Community & public health nursing* (5th ed., pp. 506–525). St. Louis: Mosby.

Loveland-Cherry, C., & Wilkerson, S. A. (1989). Dorothy Johnson's behavioral system model. In J. Fitzpatrick & A. Whall (Eds.), *Conceptual models of nursing: Analysis and application* (2nd ed.). Norwalk, CT: Appleton & Lange.

McCubbin, M. M. (1999). Normative family transitions and health outcomes. In A. Hinshaw, S. Feetham, & J. Shaver (Eds.), *Handbook of clinical nursing research* (pp. 201–230). Thousand Oaks: Sage.

Millstein, S. G. (1994). A view of health from the adolescent's perspective. In S. G. Millstein, A. C. Petersen, & E. O. Nightingale (Eds.), *Promoting the health of adolescents: New directions for the twenty-first century* (pp. 97–118). New York: Oxford University Press, Inc.

Millstein, S. G., & Irwin, C. E. (1987). Concepts of health and illness: Different constructs or variation in a theme. *Health Psychol, 6*, 515–524.

Neuman, B. (1995). *The Neuman Systems Model: Applications to nursing education and practice* (2nd ed.). Norwalk, CT: Appleton & Lange.

Newman, M. A. (1991). Health conceptualization. In J. Fitzpatrick, R. L. Taunton, & A. K. Jacox (Eds.), *Annual review of research* (pp. 221–243). New York: Springer Publishing Co.

Oelbaum, C. H. (1974). Hallmarks of adult wellness. *Am J Nurs, 74*, 1623.

Orem, D. E. (1995). *Nursing: Concepts of practice* (5th ed.). New York: McGraw-Hill, Inc.

Parse, R. R. (1981). *Man-living health: A theory of nursing.* New York: John Wiley & Sons.

Parsons, T. (1958). Definitions of health and illness in the light of American values and social structure. In E. G. Jaco (Ed.), *Patients, physicians and illness* (p. 176). New York: Free Press.

Patrick, D. L., Bush, J. W., & Chen, M. M. (1973). Toward an operational definition of health. *J Health Soc Behav, 14*, 6.

Pender, N. J. (1990). Expressing health through lifestyle patterns. *Nurs Sci Q, 3*(3), 115–122.

Putnam, R. D. (2000). *Bowling alone: The collapse and retrieval of American communities.* New York: Simon & Schuster.

Reppucci, N. D., Woolard, J. L., & Fried, C. S. (1999). Social, community and preventive interventions. *Annual Review of Psychology, 50*, 387–418.

Roy, C., & Andrews, H. A. (1999). *The Roy adaptation model.* Norwalk, CT: Appleton & Lange.

Saracci, R. (1997). The World Health Organization needs to reconsider its definition of health. *British Medical Journal, 314*, 1409–1410.

Schaefer, K. M., & Pond, J. B. (1991). *Levine's conservation model: A framework for nursing practice.* Philadelphia, PA: FA Davis Co.

Shuster, G. F., & Goeppinger, J. (2000). Community as client: Using the nursing process to promote health. In M. Stanhope & J. Lancaster (Eds.), *Community & public health nursing* (5th ed., pp. 306–329). St. Louis: Mosby.

Smith, J. (1983). *The idea of health: Implications for the nursing profession.* New York: Teachers College Press.

Sorochan, W. (1970). Health concepts as a basis for orthobiosis. In E. Hart & W. Sechrist (Eds.), *The dynamics of wellness.* Belmont, CA: Wadsworth, Inc.

Sullivan, M. (2003). The new subjective medicine: Taking the patient's point of view on health care and health. *Social Science and Medicine, 56*, 1595–1604.

Tamm, M. E. (1993). Models of health and disease. *British Journal of Medical Psychology, 66*, 213–228.

Tripp-Reimer, T. (1984). Reconceptualizing the concept of health: Integrating emic and etic perspectives. *Res Nurs Health, 7*, 101–109.

U.S. Department of Health and Human Services. (2000). *Healthy People 2010: Understanding and improving health.* Washington, DC: U.S. Government Printing Office.

Verbrugge, L., & Jette, A. (1994). The disablement process. *Social Science & Medicine, 38*, 1–14.

Ware, J. E. (1987). Standards for validating health measures: Definition and content. *J Chronic Dis, 40*, 473–480.

Wingood, G. M., & Keltner, B. (1999). Sociocultural factors and prevention programs affecting the health of ethnic minorities. In J. M. Raczynski & R. J. DiClemente (Eds.), *Handbook of health promotion and diseases prevention* (pp. 561–578). New York: Kluwer Academic/Plenum Publishers.

World Health Organization. (1974). Community health nursing: Report of a WHO expert committee. *Technical Report Series No. 558.* Geneva, Switzerland: WHO.

World Health Organization. (1986a). *Alma Alta 1978: Primary health care.* Geneva, Switzerland: WHO.

World Health Organization. (1986b). Ottawa charter for health promotion. *Health Prom, 1*(4), ii–v.

World Health Organization. (1996). *Basic document* (36th ed.). Geneva, Switzerland: WHO.

Wu, R. (1973). *Behavior and illness.* Englewood Cliffs, NJ: Prentice-Hall, Inc.

Wylie, C. M. (1970, February). The definition and measurement of health and disease. *Public Health Rep, 85*, 100–104.

2

Individual Models
to Promote Health Behavior

Services provided by health professionals in the United States are increasingly directed toward the goal of assisting individuals, families, and populations to achieve their full health potential through the adoption of healthy behaviors. Although early detection of disease, referred to as secondary prevention, is extremely important, it has produced limited health, quality-of-life, and economic benefits. Secondary prevention is based on a disease model of health care. Health promotion and primary prevention (action to avoid illness/disease) have been shown to have substantial benefits in improving quality of life and longevity. In contrast to secondary prevention, primary prevention and health promotion are based on behavioral or sociopolitical models of health care that recognize the effects of multiple systems on health outcomes. The goal of improving the health of the population is best served by emphasizing health promotion and primary prevention throughout the life span (Brown & Garber, 1998; Kaplan, 2000; McKinlay, 1993). In this book, prevention is used to represent the concept of health protection as well. Progress toward this goal requires an understanding of the motivational dynamics of actions that enhance health. This chapter focuses on models and theories useful in explaining and predicting individual health behaviors—those actions motivated by the desire to prevent disease or promote health. Specific theory-based strategies that nurses use to assist individuals in making health-behavior changes are presented also.

Health behavior may be motivated by an individual's desire to protect health by avoiding illness or a desire to increase one's level of health in either the presence or absence of illness. *Health promotion* is directed toward increasing the level of well-being and self-actualization of a given individual or group. Health promotion focuses on efforts to approach or move toward a positive valance state of high-level health and well-being. In reality, for many health behaviors, both "approaching a positive state" and "avoiding a negative state" serve as sources of motivation for behavior. A *mixed* motivation model (approach and avoidance) explains most health behaviors of adults who are middle age or older. In contrast, healthy children are motivated toward positive healthy behaviors because negative illness events possible in the future lack the relevancy needed to motivate behavior.

Human Potential for Change

Individuals have tremendous plasticity and potential for change. Because of human beings' capacity for self-knowledge, self-regulation, decision making, and creative problem solving, self-directed change is possible. Self-change is defined as new behaviors that clients willingly undertake to achieve self-selected goals or desired outcomes. Clients have the power and skill to change health behaviors or modify health-related lifestyles. The nurse's role is to promote a positive climate for change, serve as a catalyst for change, assist the client with various steps of the change process, and increase the client's capacity to maintain change.

Use of Multiple Theories in Behavior Change

The models and theories presented in this chapter focus primarily on individual, intrapersonal, and interpersonal influences to promote health. These models have their origins in theories such as stimulus response, expectancy-value, social cognitive, and decision making. Key concepts in these theories include cognition, motivation, behavior, and environment. Cognitive processing of information is important in all of the models because individuals' perceptions and interpretations of what they experience directly affect their behaviors. Further, the models recognize the potential of individuals to alter their environment as well as respond to it. Knowledge of the elements of behavior-change theories that are documented to influence health behavior enables nurses and other health care providers to optimize their effectiveness in counseling and structuring behavioral interventions for clients (Elder, Ayala, & Harris, 1999).

A Prevention Model

A prevention model is presented because illness frequently thwarts the attainment of high-level wellness. Maintaining an illness-free state through prevention is highly desirable because freedom from illness and the resultant stresses and strains allows individuals and families to direct more energy toward the promotion of health. Understanding the determinants of prevention is critical for the development of effective interventions that health professionals use to assist clients in altering behaviors that increase risk for illness. The Health Belief Model is an example of a prevention model that has been empirically tested.

The Health Belief Model

The Health Belief Model (HBM) was proposed in the 1960s as a framework for exploring why some people who are illness-free take actions to avoid illness, whereas others fail to take preventive actions (Rosenstock, 1960; Strecher & Rosenstock, 2002). At the time, a major public health concern was the widespread reluctance of individuals to accept screening for tuberculosis, Pap smear for detection of cervical cancer, immunizations, and other preventive measures that were often free or provided at nominal charge. The model was viewed as potentially useful to predict individuals who would or would not use preventive measures and to suggest interventions that might increase the predisposition of resistant individuals to engage in preventive behaviors.

The HBM is derived from cognitive theory, primarily the work of Lewin (Lewin et al., 1994). He conceptualized the life space in which an individual exists as composed of regions, some having negative valence, some having positive valence, and others being relatively neutral. Illnesses are conceived to be regions of negative valence exerting a force moving the person away from the region. Preventive behaviors are strategies for avoiding the negative valence regions of illness. The model, as modified by Becker et al., (1977), is presented in Figure 2–1. Variables proposed to directly affect predisposition to take action are: (a) a perceived threat to personal health, and (b) the conviction that the benefits of taking action to protect health outweigh the barriers that will be encountered. Beliefs about personal susceptibility and the seriousness of a specific illness combine to produce the degree of threat or negative valence of that illness. Perceived susceptibility reflects an individual's feelings of personal vulnerability to a specific health problem. Perceived seriousness or severity of a given health problem may be judged either by the degree of emotional arousal created by the thought of having the disease, or by the medical, clinical, or social difficulties (e.g., family and work life) that individuals believe a given health condition would create for them. Perceived benefits are beliefs about the effectiveness of recommended actions in preventing the health threat. Perceived barriers are perceptions concerning the potential negative aspects of taking action such as expense, danger, unpleasantness, inconvenience, and time required. Modifying factors such as demographic, social, psychological, and structural variables as well as cues to action, affect action tendencies only indirectly through their relationship with the perception of threat. The HBM is appropriate as a model for disease-preventing behavior but is clearly inappropriate as a model for health-promoting behavior.

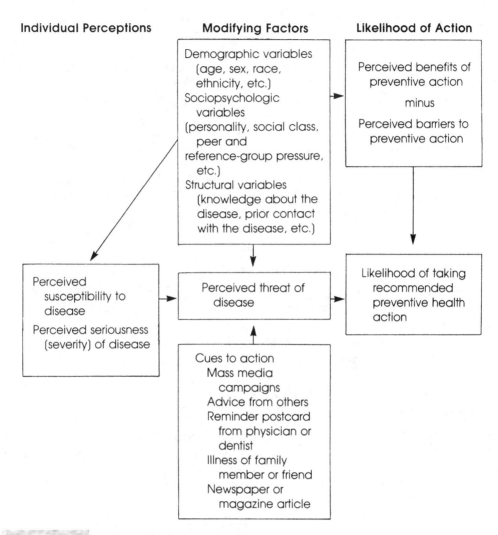

FIGURE 2–1 **The Health Belief Model**

(From M. H. Becker, D. P. Haefner, and S. V. Kasl, et al., 1997, "Selected Psychosocial Models and Correlates of Individual Health-Related Behaviors," *Med Care*, *15*, 27–46. Used with permission.)

Numerous studies, both retrospective and prospective, show perceived barriers to be the most powerful HBM dimension in explaining or predicting various preventive behaviors. Perceived susceptibility has also been an important predictor of preventive behaviors. Both perceived benefits of taking action and perceived severity of illness lacked power to explain or predict preventive behavior (Strecher & Rosenstock, 2002). Only two component variables in the model, *perceived barriers* and *perceived susceptibility to disease*, rather than the whole model, are supported by research as relevant to designing preventive interventions. Rosenstock and associates proposed adding self-efficacy (judgment of person's capabilities) from social cognitive theory to the HBM as an explanatory variable and suggested that it be incorporated in interventions based on the model (Rosenstock, Strecher, & Becker, 1988). They indicated that when the HBM was first developed, it was intended for application to one-time behaviors such as immunization. However, application of the model to more complex behavioral risks such as smoking and unsafe sexual practices necessitates attending to individual perceptions of competence or self-efficacy to repeatedly engage in preventive behaviors over a long period of time. Further research is needed to test whether the addition of self-efficacy to the model increases its value in structuring preventive interventions. Other applications of the model have been targeted to prediction of perceived and actual dietary quality (Sapp & Jensen, 1998), tuberculosis screening behaviors of Mexican migrant farm workers (Poss, 1999), perceived susceptibility to breast cancer, and benefits and barriers for mammography screening (Champion, 1999).

Mixed Models and Theories of Health Promotion and Prevention

The models and theories discussed in this section are used to understand both health-promoting and preventive behaviors. Thus, they are applicable in research and clinical settings across a wide range of health behaviors.

Theory of Reasoned Action and Theory of Planned Behavior

Ajzen and Fishbein (1975) proposed the Theory of Reasoned Action (TRA) in which attitudes and subjective norms, both intrapersonal factors, constitute the fundamental building blocks of the theory. Attitudes and subjective norms influence behavioral intention, which is the immediate determinant of behavior. These relationships are depicted as follows:

Behavior ≈ Intention to Perform the Behavior
Intention = Attitude Toward Behavior + Subjective Norm for Behavior
(≈ means a function of)

The first determinant of intention, attitude toward a behavior, is a function of beliefs concerning the consequences of performing the behavior and evaluation of each of these consequences as either positive or negative. When the evaluation of outcomes of a behavior is primarily desirable the result is a positive attitude, whereas a negative attitude results when the evaluation of outcomes is primarily undesirable. The second determinant of intention, subjective norms, is a function of what significant others expect a person to do—that is, what they would approve or disapprove of—and the motivation of the individual to comply with their expectations. The relative importance of attitudes and subjective norms in predicting any given behavior varies depending on the target behavior, the context, and the population being studied (Montano, Kasprzyk, & Taplin, 2002).

The TRA is based on the assumption that both attitudes and subjective norms are amenable to change. Interventions by health care professionals may target attitudes by addressing beliefs about outcomes and values related to the outcomes, or subjective norms by focusing on perceptions concerning normative expectations of others and motivation to comply with what others expect. Research has tested the applicability of the TRA to various health behaviors. An overview of related research findings indicates that intentions are, for the most part, moderately to highly correlated with behavior, attitudes are moderately correlated with behavior, and subjective norms are only modestly correlated with behavior. Thus, attitudes and intentions have been the only components of the model clearly supported by research. Recent research has shown that components of the TRA influence a range of health behaviors such as increasing milk consumption among women (Brewer, Blake, & Rankin, 1999), increasing physical activity (Hausenblas, Carron, & Mack, 1997), and promoting the practice of HIV-preventive behaviors (Jemmot & Jemmott, 2000).

The TRA assumes that behavior is under volitional control; that is, there are no barriers to performance of the intended behavior. Ajzen (1991), in a critique of the TRA, commented that behavior is not completely under the control of the individual. Thus, he added a third variable, perceived behavioral control, to the original Fishbein and Ajzen concepts of attitude and subjective norms. He labeled the extended theory the Theory of Planned Behavior (TPB). Perceived behavioral control is measured by beliefs concerning the opportunities to engage in the behavior as well as the power of various factors to inhibit or facilitate the behavior. An example of a control belief is "How likely is it that I can get a ride to the gym tomorrow with my friend?" An inhibiting factor is illustrated by "If I cannot get a ride to the gym tomorrow, how likely am I to walk in my neighborhood?" In a study of fifth- and eighth-graders' intentions to participate in physical activity, perceived behavioral control predicted behavioral intentions (Craig, Goldberg, & Dietz, 1996). Likewise, in a study of health care workers, perceived behavioral control predicted the intention to use gloves to prevent the risk of exposure to bloodborne pathogens (Levin, 1999).

Social Cognitive Theory

Social cognitive theory is a broad theoretical approach to explaining human behavior that has been the most frequently used framework to design individual behavior change interventions. In social cognitive theory, environmental events, personal factors, and behavior act as reciprocal determinants of each other. The theory places major emphasis on self-direction, self-regulation, and perceptions of self-efficacy. Social cognitive theory proposes that human beings possess the following basic capabilities (Bandura, 1985):

1. *Symbolization:* Processing and transforming transient experiences into internal models that guide future action.
2. *Forethought:* Anticipating likely consequences of prospective actions and planning future courses of action to achieve valued goals.
3. *Vicarious Learning:* Acquiring rules to generate and regulate behavior through observing others without the need to engage in extensive trial and error.

4. *Self-Regulation:* Using internal standards and self-evaluative reactions to motivate and regulate behavior; arranging the external environment to create incentives for action.

5. *Self-Reflection:* Thinking about one's own thought processes and actively modifying them.

Given these basic capabilities, behavior is neither solely driven by inner forces nor automatically shaped by external stimuli. Instead, cognitions and other personal factors, behavior, and environmental events are interactive. Behavior may modify cognitions and other personal factors as well as change the environment. The environment may also augment or constrain behavior. This dynamic interactional causality provides a rich array of human possibilities (Bandura, 1977).

According to social cognitive theory, self-beliefs formed through self-observation and self-reflective thought greatly influence human functioning. These self-beliefs include self-attribution, self-evaluation, and self-efficacy. Beliefs concerning self-efficacy are particularly important. Perceived self-efficacy is a judgment of one's ability to carry out a particular course of action. Perceptions of self-efficacy develop through mastery experiences, vicarious learning, verbal persuasion, and somatic responses to particular situations. Marked overestimation of one's competencies may result in failure and marked underestimation may result in lack of challenge and resultant growth. Efficacy judgments that appear to be most effective are those that slightly exceed present capabilities. Such judgments facilitate undertaking realistically demanding tasks that build competencies and confidence. The greater the perceived efficacy, the more vigorous and persistent individuals will engage in a behavior, even in the face of obstacles and aversive experiences (Bandura, 1997). Individuals derive their sense of self-efficacy for a given behavior by weighing and integrating efficacy information from these diverse sources. According to social cognitive theory, the cumulative perception of efficacy determines the predisposition to undertake a given behavior (Siela & Wieseke, 2000). Nurse scientists have developed instruments to measure self-efficacy for a wide range of health behaviors including the prevention of osteoporosis (Horan, Kim, Gendler, Froman, & Patel, 1998) and successful breast-feeding (Dennis & Faux, 1999). The interaction of self-efficacy with other predictors of health behaviors needs to be explored further to understand the intricate nature of the motivational dynamics underlying health behavior. For a comprehensive description of social cognitive theory, the reader is referred to Bandura's book (1985) *Social Foundations of Thought and Action.*

Transtheoretical Model

Prochaska and DiClemente (1984) developed the transtheoretical model based on their extensive research on smoking cessation among adults. They propose that health-related behavior change progresses through five stages, regardless of whether the client is trying to quit a health-threatening behavior or adopt a healthy behavior. These stages are:

- *Precontemplation:* A client is not thinking about quitting or adopting a particular behavior, at least not *within the next 6 months* (not intending to make changes).
- *Contemplation:* A client is seriously thinking about quitting or adopting a particular behavior *in the next 6 months* (considering a change).

- *Planning or Preparation*: A client who has tried to quit a negative behavior or adopt a positive behavior in the past year is seriously thinking about engaging in the contemplated change *within the next month* (making small or sporadic changes).
- *Action*: The client has made the behavior change and it has persisted *for a period of 6 months* (actively engaged in behavior change).
- *Maintenance*: This is the period beginning 6 months after action has started and continuing indefinitely. The client has continued and stabilized the change beginning 6 months after the action started and continuing indefinitely (sustaining the change over time; Prochaska & Diclemente, 1984).

An attempt has been made to integrate various core concepts from other models of behavior change into the transtheoretical model. In particular, the concept of *decisional balance* from Janis and Mann's decision-making model (1985) is integral to the theory. The Janis and Mann conflict model assumes sound decision making involves comparison of all potential gains and losses, which are entered into a balance sheet. Behavior should occur when the potential gains of engaging in the behavior outweigh the losses. Decisional balance has been shown to have particular patterns across behavior change stages. Cross-sectional studies of 12 health behaviors indicated that during precontemplation, the cons of changing the behavior were higher than the pros. During either contemplation or preparation, depending on the behavior, the pros increase was followed by a decrease in the cons so that there was a crossover in decision balance. For the majority of behaviors studied, the balance between the pros and cons had reversed before action occurred. During the maintenance stage, the pros of engaging in the desirable behavior or not engaging in the undesirable behavior continued to outweigh the cons (Prochaska, 1994; Prochaska, Velicer, Rossi, et al., 1994). It has been suggested that self-efficacy needs to be integrated into the transtheoretical model, based on shifts in self-efficacy in a predictable way across the stages of behavior change, with clients progressively becoming more efficacious (Marcus, Selby, Niaura, et al., 1992).

Prochaska proposed that different processes of change are appropriate at different stages of behavior change. The 10 processes of change, presented in Table 2–1, are categorized as either experiential or behavioral processes or strategies. Experiential processes are more important than behavioral processes in the early stages of change for understanding and predicting progress. Behavioral processes are more important for understanding and predicting transition from preparation to action and from action to maintenance. Experiential processes are to a large extent internally focused on behavior-linked emotions, values, and cognitions. Behavioral processes focus directly on behavioral change (Prochaska, Velicer, et al., 1994). Once an individual's stage has been assessed, the nurse may select appropriate processes to help the client progress from stage to stage. Peterson and Aldana (1999) tested the model in an intervention designed to increase physical activity among working adults. Participants were randomly assigned to one of three groups: stage-based information, generic information, and a no-information control group. Six weeks after the intervention, a 13% increase in physical activity in the stage-based information group, a 1% increase in the generic information group, and an 8% decrease in the control group were reported. Abrams described a unique intervention model for cessation of smoking combining stepped-care and stage matching to derive personalized intervention strategies (Abrams, Orleans, Niaura, et al., 1996). For more information on processes of

TABLE 2–1 Processes of Change

Process	Definition
Experiential Processes	
Consciousness raising	Efforts by the individual to seek new information and to gain understanding and feedback about the problem
Dramatic relief	Affective aspects of change, often involving intense emotional experiences related to the problem behavior
Environmental reevaluation	Consideration and assessment by the individual of how the problem affects the physical and social environments
Self-reevaluation	Emotional and cognitive reappraisal of values by the individual with respect to the problem behavior.
Social liberation	Awareness, availability, and acceptance by the individual of alternative lifestyles in society
Behavioral Processes	
Counterconditioning	Substitution of alternative behaviors for the problem behavior
Helping relationships	Trusting, accepting, and utilizing the support of caring others during attempts to change the problem behavior
Reinforcement management	Changing the contingencies that control or maintain the problem behavior
Self-liberation	The individual's choice and commitment to change the problem behavior, including the belief that one *can* change
Stimulus control	Control of situations and other causes that trigger the problem behavior

(From B. H. Marcus, J. S. Rossi, & V. C. Selby, et al., 1992, "The Stages and Processes of Exercise Adoption and Maintenance in a Worksite Sample," *Health Psychol*, *11*, 387. Used with permission.)

change proposed in the transtheoretical model, the reader is referred to other sources (Prochaska, Diclemente, & Norcross, 1992; Prochaska, Norcross, & Diclemente, 1994).

Interaction Model of Client Health Behavior

The Interaction Model of Client Health Behavior (IMCHB) focuses on both characteristics of the client and factors external to the client to provide a comprehensive explanation of actions directed toward risk reduction and health promotion. Client background variables included in the model are demographic characteristics, social influence, previous health care experience, and environmental resources. These background variables and the intrinsic motivation, cognitive appraisal, and affective response of the client in regard to a particular behavior interface with elements of client–professional interaction (affective support, health information, decisional control, and professional–technical competencies) to affect health outcomes (Cox, 1982). Based on the Cognitive Evaluation Theory proposed by Deci and Ryan (1985), Cox (1985) indicated that intrinsic motivation, or doing an activity for its own sake because of interest or positive cognitive or emotional responses, is an important source of motivation for health behavior. Critical health outcomes are the use of health care services, clinical health status indicators, severity of health care problems, adherence to the recommended care regimen, and satisfaction with care. The model is depicted in Figure 2–2.

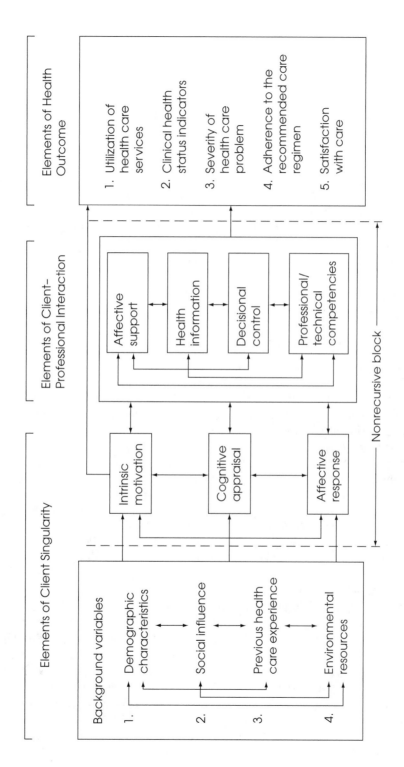

FIGURE 2–2 Interaction Model of Client Health Behavior

(From Cox with permission from Aspen Publishers.)

45

The Health Self-Determinism Index (HSDI) is derived from the Cognitive Evaluation Theory as an approach to measuring intrinsic motivation. The instrument measures self-determined health judgments, self-determined health behavior, perceived competency in health matters, and internal and external cue responsivesness (Cox, 1985). The Health Self-Determinism Index for Children (HSDI-C) measures intrinsic motivation in health behavior. The psychometric characteristics of both instruments are reported elsewhere (Cox, Cowell, Marion, et al., 1990).

A number of tests of the model have been published. Troumbley and Lenz (1992) applied the IMCHB to explain relationships between client singularity variables (demographic characteristics, intrinsic motivation, cognitive appraisal of designating self as overweight or normal weight, and affective response of psychological distress to weight concerns) and health outcomes (health risk and health status) among enlisted U.S. Army soldiers. Client singularity variables explained both health status and health risk (Troumbley & Lenz, 1992). The IMCHB was tested with 260 fourth-grade children and their mothers to determine its explanatory potential for 36 health behaviors. Health perception exerted the only direct effect on health behaviors among both girls and boys (Farrand & Cox, 1993). The IMCHB merits further exploration in prospective studies to determine its explanatory potential for health behaviors.

Relapse Prevention Model

Marlatt and Gordon (1985) proposed a model of relapse prevention for addictive behaviors such as alcoholism, smoking, obesity, and drug dependency. Because of the addictive nature of these behaviors and the high rates of recidivism, researchers have focused on understanding various factors affecting relapse to health-damaging behaviors and on designing interventions to prevent relapse.

In understanding the natural history of relapse, it is important to differentiate between lapses and relapse. A lapse is a "slip" that results in a single repeat of the addictive behavior. In relapse, the client returns to the addictive behavior, often engaging in it with increased frequency. By allowing room for mistakes to occur but providing clients with preparatory training (coping responses) to manage lapses, relapses are prevented (Marlatt & Gordon, 1985). For example, a client in a smoking cessation program who has been abstinent and suddenly smokes a cigarette, if taught appropriate coping responses, may smoke no additional cigarettes and feel efficacious or competent in being able to stop after one smoke. According to the theory, this should result in a decreased probability of experiencing relapse. In contrast, the client who lapses and has no coping responses to draw upon is likely to experience decreased self-efficacy for quitting, positive effects from return to substance use, and the abstinence violation effect (AVE) of feeling guilty and "out of control." Shiffman and colleagues (1997) provided evidence about the occurrence of AVE following smoking lapses. The cognitive–behavioral model of the relapse process appears in Figure 2–3.

Individuals experience enhanced self-efficacy and personal control when abstinence is maintained. Perceived control continues to strengthen but is threatened by high-risk situations. A high-risk situation is defined as one that threatens self-control and may potentially trigger relapse. Three categories of events associated with high rates of relapse are negative emotional states (anger, frustration, depression, boredom), social situations (negative situations such as interpersonal conflict or positive situations such as partying

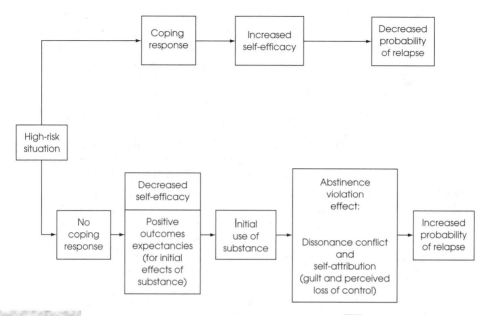

FIGURE 2–3 **A Cognitive Behavioral Model of the Relapse Process**

(From G. A. Marlatt and J. R. Gordon, 1985, *Relapse Prevention: Maintenance Strategies in the Treatment of Addictive Behaviors* (pp. 38), New York: Guilford Press. Used with permission.)

or relaxing with friends), and physical craving (withdrawal symptoms and physical response to cues). In these situations, use of coping responses that have been learned and rehearsed in relapse-prevention training may prevent a lapse from becoming a relapse. Specific relapse-prevention strategies include self-monitoring, relaxation training, and relapse rehearsal (Brownell, Marlatt, Lichtenstein, et al., 1986; Marlatt & Gordon, 1985; Shiffman et al., 1997). Combining relapse prevention strategies with strategies to enhance self-efficacy is promising for maintaining cessation of addictive behaviors (Velicer, Diclemente, Rossi, et al., 1990).

Health Promotion Model

In the early 1980s, the initial version of Pender's Health Promotion Model (HPM) appeared in nursing literature (Pender, 1982). The HPM proposed a framework for integrating nursing and behavioral science perspectives on factors influencing health behaviors. The framework offered a guide for exploration of the complex biopsychosocial processes that motivate individuals to engage in behaviors directed toward the enhancement of health. The term *health behavior* was being used with increasing frequency in health literature, and there was renewed interest in earlier work by Dunn (1959a, 1959b) on high-level wellness and behavior that was motivated by a desire to promote personal health and well-being.

The initial HPM stimulated a number of studies to describe the potential of seven cognitive–perceptual factors and five modifying factors to explain and predict health behaviors. The cognitive–perceptual factors were importance of health, perceived control of health, definition of health, perceived health status, perceived self-efficacy, perceived benefits, and perceived barriers. The modifying factors were demographic and biologic characteristics, interpersonal influences, situational influences, and behavioral factors. Assumptions and theoretical propositions, a summary of empirical support for constructs in the HPM, and intervention studies using the HPM may be reviewed in the fourth edition of this book (Pender, Murdaugh, & Parsons, 2002).

The HPM is a competence- or approach-oriented model. Unlike the Health Belief Model, the HPM does not include "fear" or "threat" as a source of motivation for health behavior. Although immediate threats to health have been shown to motivate action, threats in the distant future lack the same motivational strength. Thus, avoidance-oriented models of health behavior are of limited usefulness in motivating overall healthy lifestyles, particularly in children, youths, and young adults, who often perceive themselves to be invulnerable to illness. Because the HPM does not rely on personal threat as a primary source of health motivation, it is a model with applicability across the life span. The HPM is applicable to any health behavior in which threat is not proposed as a major source of motivation for the behavior. Findings from studies using the HPM are available in Table 2–2. The initial model (Pender, 1987, 1996) has since been replaced by the Health Promotion Model (revised) depicted in Figure 2–4.

TABLE 2–2 **Selected Findings from Studies Using the Health Promotion Model**

Author	Population	Dependent Variable	Variables Studied	Variance Explained
Health-Specific Outcome Measures				
Pender et al., 1990	White-collar workers	Health-promoting lifestyle	1,5,6,7,8,9,10	31%
Moore, 1992	Older adults	Health-promoting lifestyle	1, 8, 10	————
Warren, 1993	Adult males in cardiac rehabilitation	Health-promoting lifestyle	8, 10	38%
Gillis, 1993	Adolescent females	Health-promoting lifestyle	1, 3, 8, 9, 10	41%
Harrison, 1993	HIV seropositive males	Health-promoting lifestyle	10	12%
Hutchinson, 1996	Black university students	Health-promoting lifestyle	1, 6, 7, 8, 9, 10	34%
Nikulich-Barrett, 1997	Rural, older black and white females	Health-promoting lifestyle	8, 10	22%—Blacks 33%—Whites
Millard, 1998	Older adults (Seventh-day Adventists)	Health-promoting lifestyle	1, 7, 10	19%
Bolio, 1999	Incarcerated males	Health-promoting lifestyle	1, 3, 8	9–20%

Author	Population	Dependent Variable	Variables Studied	Variance Explained
Suwonnaroop, 1999	Black and white older adults	Health-promoting lifestyle	1, 3, 10	31%
Lucus et al., 2000	Elderly women	Health-promoting lifestyle	1, 10, 11, 12	———
Agazio et al., 2002	Military women with children	Health-promoting lifestyle	1, 4, 8, 9, 10	44%
Hulme et al., 2003	Spanish-speaking Hispanic adults	Health-promoting lifestyle	1, 3, 10	12%

Behavior-Specific Outcome Measures

Author	Population	Dependent Variable	Variables Studied	Variance Explained
Pender et al., 1990	White-collar workers	Exercise (total group with stages combined)	1, 2, 3, 4, 5, 6, 7, 8, 9, 10, 11, 12	59%
Jeffries, 1996	Expatriates in Indonesia	Nutrition	1, 6, 7, 8, 9, 10, 11, 12	———
Chen, 1995	Taiwanese elderly	Physical activity	1, 6, 8, 10, 11, 12	46%
Stutts, 1999	Adult males and females	Exercise	1, 8, 11, 12	10%
Piazzi et al., 2001	Female nurses	Exercise	1, 7, 8, 10	———
McCullagh, 2002	Farmers	Use of hearing protection	1, 3, 4, 11, 12	———
Wu & Pender, 2002	Taiwanese adolescents	Exercise	3, 5, 8, 11, 12	30%
Lusk et al., 1995	Blue-collar workers (manufacturing plant)	Use of hearing protection	6, 7, 8, 9, 10, 11, 12	42%
Lusk et al., 1999	Construction workers	Use of hearing protection	1, 3, 4, 7, 8, 9, 10, 11, 12	46%
Kerr et al., 2002	Mexican American industrial workers	Use of hearing protection	1, 2, 3, 4, 7, 8, 9, 10, 11, 12	25–50%
Martinelli, 1996	Young adults	Environmental tobacco smoke exposure	1, 2, 4, 7, 8	34%
Tober, 1997	Obese adults	Weight loss	7, 8	———
Sample et al., 2002	Black & white adults	Colorectal cancer prevention	1, 11, 12	———
Lohse, 2003	Parents of young children	Bicycle helmet use	11, 12	———

KEY
1 = Demographic characteristics
2 = Biologic characteristics
3 = Interpersonal influences
4 = Situational influences
5 = Behavioral factors (prior behavior)
6 = Importance of health

7 = Perceived control of health
8 = Perceived self-efficacy
9 = Definition of health
10 = Perceived health status
11 = Perceived benefits
12 = Perceived barriers

Individual
Characteristics
and Experiences

Behavior-Specific
Cognitions
and Affect

Behavioral
Outcome

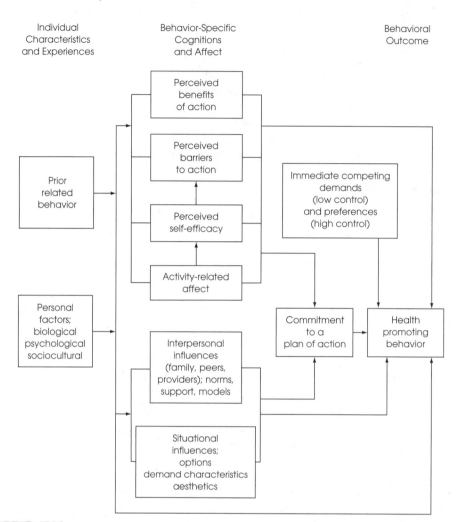

FIGURE 2–4 Health Promotion Model (revised)

The Theoretical Basis for the Health Promotion Model

The HPM is an attempt to depict the multidimensional nature of persons interacting with their interpersonal and physical environments as they pursue health. The HPM integrates a number of constructs from expectancy-value theory and social cognitive theory, within a nursing perspective of holistic human functioning. Social cognitive theory was discussed earlier in this chapter. Expectancy-value theory is briefly described next.

Expectancy-Value Theory

Many conceptions of goal-directed behavior, including social cognitive theory, are based on the expectancy-value model of human motivation described by Feather (1982). According to the expectancy-value model, behavior is rational and economical. Specifically, a person engages in a given action and persists in it (a) to the extent that the outcome of taking action is of positive personal value, and (b) to the degree that based on available information, taking the course of action is likely to bring about the desired outcome. Thus, individuals will not invest their effort and personal resources in working toward goals that are of little or no value to them. Furthermore, most individuals will not invest their efforts in goals that, despite their attractiveness, are perceived as impossible to achieve. Personal change is best understood within this theoretical framework by considering the subjective value of the change and the subjective expectancy of achieving it. The motivational significance of the *subjective value of change* is based on the supposition that the more a person is dissatisfied with his or her present situation in a particular domain, the greater the rewards or benefits associated with favorable change. This subjective value of change is viewed as comparable to the perceived benefits of engaging in a given health behavior. The motivational significance of the *subjective expectancy of successfully obtaining the change* is based on prior knowledge of personal successes or the successes of others in attaining the change and the personal confidence that one's success will be the same or even superior to others (Klar, Nader, & Mallor, 1992).

The Health Promotion Model (Revised)

The revised HPM (Figure 2–4) first appeared in the third edition of *Health Promotion in Nursing Practice* (Pender, 1996). The variables in the revised HPM and their interrelationships are described below. Three new variables appear in the revised model: activity-related affect, commitment to a plan of action, and immediate competing demands and preferences. It is beyond the scope of this chapter to describe approaches to measuring each variable in the model, but information regarding measurement of variables that is not already reported in the literature may be obtained from the first author.

Individual Characteristics and Experiences

Each person has unique personal characteristics and experiences that affect subsequent actions. The importance of their effect depends on the target behavior being considered. Individual characteristics or aspects of past experience selected provide flexibility in the HPM to capture variables that may be highly relevant to a particular health behavior but not to all health behaviors or in a particular target population but not in all populations.

Prior Related Behavior

Behavioral factors have been retained in the HPM as "prior related behavior." Of the HPM studies that were reviewed (Table 2–2), 75% supported its importance in determining subsequent behavior. Research indicates that often the best predictor of behavior is the frequency of the same or a similar behavior in the past. Prior behavior is proposed as having both direct and indirect effects on the likelihood of engaging in health-promoting behaviors. The direct effect of past behavior on current health-promoting behavior may be due to habit formation, predisposing one to engage in the behavior automatically, with little attention to the specific details of its execution. Habit strength accrues each time the behavior occurs and is particularly augmented by concentrated, repetitive practice of the behavior.

Consistent with social cognitive theory, prior behavior is proposed to indirectly influence health-promoting behavior through perceptions of self-efficacy, benefits, barriers, and activity-related affect. According to Bandura (1985), actual enactments of a behavior and its associated feedback are a major source of efficacy or "skill" information. Anticipated or experienced benefits from engaging in the behavior are referred to by Bandura as outcome expectations. If desired short-term benefits are experienced early in the course of the behavior, the behavior is more likely to be repeated. Barriers to a given behavior are experienced and stored in memory as "hurdles" that need to be overcome to successfully engage in the behavior. Every incident of a behavior is also accompanied by emotions or affect. Positive or negative affect either before, during, or following the behavior is encoded into memory as information that is retrieved when engaging in the behavior is contemplated at a later point in time. Prior behavior is proposed as shaping all of these behavior-specific cognitions and affect. The nurse helps the client shape a positive behavioral history for the future by focusing on the benefits of a behavior, teaching clients how to overcome hurdles to carrying out the behavior, and engendering high levels of efficacy and positive affect through successful performance experience and positive feedback.

Personal Factors

The relevant personal factors predictive of a given behavior are shaped by the nature of the target behavior being considered. In the revised HPM, personal factors are categorized as biologic, psychological, and sociocultural. Biologic factors include age, body mass index, pubertal status, menopausal status, aerobic capacity, strength, agility, or balance. Psychological factors include self-esteem, self-motivation, and perceived health status. Sociocultural factors include race, ethnicity, acculturation, education, and socioeconomic status. Personal factors should be limited to those that are theoretically relevant to explain or predict a given target behavior. Although personal factors may influence cognitions, affect, and health behaviors, some personal factors cannot be changed; thus, nursing interventions cannot modify them.

Behavior-Specific Cognitions and Affect

Behavior-specific variables within the HPM are considered to have major motivational significance. Thus, these variables constitute a critical "core" for intervention, because they are subject to modification through nursing actions. Measuring change in these variables is essential to determine if such changes actually result from the intervention and, in turn, influence changes in commitment or in the occurrence of health-promoting behaviors.

Perceived Benefits of Action

Of the studies reviewed that tested the HPM (Table 2–2), 61% supported the importance of perceived benefits in influencing health behaviors, providing moderate support for the construct. An individual's expectations to engage in a particular behavior hinge on the anticipated benefits that it will occur. In the HPM, perceived benefits are proposed to directly motivate behavior as well as indirectly motivate behavior through determining the extent of commitment to a plan of action to engage in the behaviors from which the anticipated benefits will result. Anticipated benefits of action are mental representations of the positive or reinforcing consequences of a behavior. According to the expectancy-value theory, the motivational importance of anticipated benefits is based on personal outcomes from prior direct experience with the behavior or vicarious experience through observing others engaging in the behavior. Individuals tend to invest time and resources in activities that have a high likelihood of increasing their experience of positive outcomes. Benefits from performance of the behavior may be intrinsic or extrinsic. Examples of intrinsic benefits include increased alertness and decreased feelings of fatigue. Extrinsic benefits include monetary rewards or social interactions possible as a result of engaging in the behavior. Initially, extrinsic benefits of health behaviors may be highly significant, whereas intrinsic benefits may be more powerful in motivating continuation of health behaviors. The expected magnitude of benefits and the temporal relation of benefits to action impact the potency of anticipated benefits as a determinant of health behavior. Beliefs in benefits or positive outcome expectations have generally been shown to be a necessary although not sufficient condition to engage in a specific health behavior.

Perceived Barriers to Action

Anticipated barriers have been repeatedly found to affect intentions to engage in a particular behavior and to execute the behavior. Of the studies testing the HPM (Table 2–2), 79% provided support for barriers as a determinant of health-promoting behavior. Barriers may be imagined or real. They consist of perceptions concerning the unavailability, inconvenience, expense, difficulty, or time-consuming nature of a particular action. Barriers are often viewed as mental blocks, hurdles, and personal costs of undertaking a given behavior. Loss of satisfaction from giving up health-damaging behaviors such as smoking or eating high-fat foods to adopt a healthier lifestyle may also constitute a barrier. Barriers usually arouse motives of avoidance in relation to a given behavior.

When readiness to act is low and barriers are high, action is unlikely to occur. When readiness to act is high and barriers are low, the probability of action is much greater. Perceived barriers to action in the revised HPM affect health-promoting behavior directly by serving as blocks to action as well as indirectly through decreasing commitment to a plan of action.

Perceived Self-Efficacy

Self-efficacy is the judgment of personal capability to organize and carry out a particular course of action. Self-efficacy is not concerned with the skill one has but with judgments of what one can do with whatever skills one possesses. Judgments of personal efficacy are distinguished from outcome expectations. Perceived self-efficacy is a judgment of one's abilities to accomplish a certain level of performance, whereas an outcome expectation is a judgment of the likely consequences (e.g., benefits, costs) such behavior will produce (Siela & Wieseke, 2000). Perceptions of skill and competence in a particular domain motivate individuals to engage in those behaviors in which they excel. Feeling efficacious and skilled in one's performance is likely to encourage one to engage in the target behavior more frequently than is feeling inept and unskilled. Of the HPM studies reviewed (Table 2–2), 86% provided support for the importance of self-efficacy as a determinant of health-promoting behavior.

Personal knowledge about one's self-efficacy is based on four types of information: (a) performance attainments from actually engaging in the behavior and evaluating performance in relation to some self-standard or external feedback given by others, (b) vicarious experiences of observing the performance of others and their related self-evaluation and feedback, (c) verbal persuasion on the part of others that one does possess the ability to carry out a particular course of action, and (d) physiologic states (e.g., anxiety, fear, calm, tranquility) from which people judge their competencies (Bandura, 1997). In the HPM, perceived self-efficacy is proposed to be influenced by activity-related affect. The more positive the affect, the greater the perceptions of efficacy is present. However, in reality this relationship is reciprocal with greater perceptions of efficacy, in turn increasing positive affect. Self-efficacy influences perceived barriers to action, with higher efficacy resulting in lowered perception of barriers. Self-efficacy motivates health-promoting behavior directly by efficacy expectations and indirectly by affecting perceived barriers and level of commitment or persistence in pursuing a plan of action.

Activity-Related Affect

Subjective feeling states occur prior to, during, and following an activity, based on the stimulus properties associated with the behavioral event. These affective responses may be mild, moderate, or strong and are cognitively labeled, stored in memory, and associated with subsequent thoughts of the behavior. Activity-related affect consists of three components: emotional arousal to the act itself (act related), the self-acting (self-related), or the environment in which the action takes place (context related). The resultant feeling state is likely to affect whether an individual will repeat the behavior again or maintain the behavior long term (Gauvin & Rejeski, 1993). Behavior-contingent feeling states have been explored as determinants of health behaviors in recent studies (Gauvin & Rejeski, 1993; Godin, 1987; Hardy & Rejeski, 1989; McAuley & Courneya, 1992; Rejeski, Gauvin, Hobson, et al., 1995). The affect associated with the behavior reflects a direct emotional reaction or gut-level response to the thought of the behavior, which can be positive or negative—is it fun, delightful, enjoyable, disgusting, or unpleasant? Behaviors associated with positive affect are likely to be repeated, whereas those associated with negative affect are likely to be avoided. For some behaviors, both positive and negative feeling states are induced. Thus, the relative balance between positive and negative affect prior to, during, and following the behavior is important to ascertain. Activity-related affect is different from the evaluative dimension of attitude proposed by Fishbein and Ajzen (1975). The evaluative dimension of attitude reflects affective evaluation of the specific outcomes of a behavior rather than the response to the stimulus properties of the behavioral event itself.

For any given behavior, the full range of negative and positive feeling states in relation to the act, self as actor, and context for action should be measured. In many instruments proposed to measure affect, negative feelings are elaborated more extensively than positive feelings. This is not surprising because anxiety, fear, and depression have been studied much more than have joy, elation, and calm. Based on social cognitive theory, there is a relationship between self-efficacy and activity-related affect. McAuley and Courneya (1992) found that positive affective response during exercise was a significant predictor of post-exercise efficacy. This is consistent with Bandura's proposal (1985) that emotional responses and their induced physiologic states during a behavior serve as sources of efficacy information. Thus, activity-related affect is proposed to influence health behavior directly as well as indirectly through self-efficacy and commitment to a plan of action.

Because of the recent addition of activity-related affect to the HPM, few studies have explored its contribution to the explanatory and predictive power of the model. Further studies are needed to determine the importance of activity-related affect in regard to various health behaviors.

Interpersonal Influences

According to the HPM, interpersonal influences are cognitions concerning the behaviors, beliefs, or attitudes of others. These cognitions may or may not correspond with reality. Primary sources of interpersonal influence on health-promoting behaviors are family (parents or siblings), peers, and health care providers. Interpersonal influences include norms (expectations of significant others), social support (instrumental and emotional encouragement), and modeling (vicarious learning through observing others engaged in a particular behavior). These three interpersonal processes affect individuals' predisposition to engage in health-promoting behaviors.

Social norms set standards for performance that individuals may adopt or reject. Social support for a behavior taps the sustaining resources offered by others. Modeling portrays the sequential components of a health behavior and is an important strategy for behavior change in social cognitive theory. In the HPM, interpersonal interaction influences health-promoting behavior directly as well as indirectly through social pressures or encouragement to commit to a plan of action. Individuals vary in the extent to which they are sensitive to the wishes, examples, and praise of others. However, given sufficient motivation to behave in a way consistent with interpersonal influences, individuals are likely to undertake behaviors for which they will be admired and socially reinforced. In order for interpersonal influences to have an effect, individuals must attend to the behaviors, wishes, and inputs of others; comprehend them; and assimilate them into cognitive representations related to given behaviors. Susceptibility to the influence of others may vary developmentally and be particularly evident in adolescence. Some cultures may place more emphasis on interpersonal influences than others. For example, *familismo* among Hispanic populations may encourage individuals to engage in a particular behavior for the good of the family rather than for personal gain.

In studies based on the HPM (Table 2–2), 57% provided support for interpersonal influences as determinants of health-promoting behavior, indicating moderate support for the construct. More rigorous measures of interpersonal influences need to be developed and tested so that its usefulness may be determined across diverse populations.

Situational Influences

Personal perceptions and cognitions of any situation or context facilitate or impede behavior. Situational influences on health-promoting behavior include perceptions of options available, demand characteristics, and aesthetic features of the environment in which a given behavior is proposed to take place. Kaplan and Kaplan (1989), in their work on restorative natural environments, have heightened awareness of how environments or situational contexts influence health and health-related behaviors. Individuals are drawn to and perform more competently in situations or environmental contexts in which they feel compatible rather than incompatible, related rather than alienated, safe and reassured rather than unsafe and threatened. Environments that are fascinating and interesting are also desirable contexts for the performance of health behaviors.

In the revised HPM, situational influences have been reconceptualized to directly and indirectly influence health behavior. Situations may directly affect behaviors by presenting an environment "loaded" with cues that trigger action. For example, a "no smoking" environment creates demand characteristics for nonsmoking behavior. Company regulations for hearing protection to be worn create demand characteristics that employees comply with regulations. Both situations enforce commitment to health actions.

Situational influences have received moderate support as determinants of health behavior. Of the HPM studies reviewed (Table 2–2), 56% reported situational influences as significant predictors of health-promoting behavior. Situational influences may be an important key to developing new and more effective strategies for facilitating the acquisition and maintenance of health-promoting behaviors in diverse populations.

Commitment to a Plan of Action

Commitment to a plan of action initiates a behavioral event. This commitment propels the individual into and through the behavior unless a competing demand that cannot be avoided or a competing preference that is not resisted occurs. Human beings generally engage in organized rather than disorganized behavior. According to Fishbein and Ajzen (1975), intentionality is a major determinant of volitional behavior. *Commitment to a plan of action* in the revised HPM implies the following underlying cognitive processes: (a) commitment to carry out a specific action at a given time and place and with specified persons or alone, irrespective of competing preferences; and (b) identification of definitive strategies for eliciting, carrying out, and reinforcing the behavior. Identification of specific strategies to be used at different points in the behavioral sequence goes beyond intentionality to further the likelihood that the plan of action will be successfully implemented. For example, the strategy of contracting consists of a mutually agreed-upon set of actions to which one party commits with the understanding that the other party will provide some tangible reward or reinforcement if the commitment is sustained. Strategies are selected by clients to energize and reinforce health behaviors according to their own preferences and stage of change. Commitment alone without associated strategies often results in "good intentions" but failure to perform a valued health behavior.

Immediate Competing Demands and Preferences

Immediate competing demands or preferences refer to alternative behaviors that intrude into consciousness as possible courses of action immediately prior to the intended occurrence of a planned health-promoting behavior. Competing demands are viewed as alternative behaviors over which individuals have a relatively low level of control because of environmental contingencies such as work or family care responsibilities. Failure to respond to a competing demand may have untoward effects for the self or for significant others. Competing preferences are viewed as alternative behaviors with powerful reinforcing properties over which individuals exert a relatively high level of control. They may derail a health-promoting behavior in favor of the competing behavior (Vara & Epstein, 1995). The extent to which an individual resists competing preferences depends on the ability to be self-regulating. Examples of "giving in" to competing preferences are selecting a food high in fat rather than low in fat because of taste or flavor preferences, or driving past the recreation center where one usually exercises to stop at the mall (a preference for browsing or shopping rather than physical activity). Both competing demands and preferences can derail a plan of action. Competing demands are differentiated from barriers in that the individual must carry out an alternative behavior based on unanticipated external demand. Competing preferences are differentiated from barriers such as lack of time, because competing preferences are last-minute urges based on one's preference hierarchy that derail a plan for positive health action.

Individuals vary in their ability to sustain attention and avoid disruption of health behaviors. Some individuals may be predisposed developmentally or biologically to be more easily swayed from a course of action. Inhibiting competing preferences requires the exercise of self-regulation and control capabilities. Strong commitment to a plan of action may sustain dedication to complete a behavior in light of competing demands or preferences. In the HPM, immediate competing demands and preferences are proposed to directly affect the probability of occurrence of health behavior as well as moderate the effects of commitment. Wu (1999) tested the effects of competing demands on physical activity behavior among Taiwanese adolescents. However, competing demands were not a significant predictor of physical activity. More sensitive measures of this variable need to be developed prior to its use in subsequent studies.

Health-Promoting Behavior

Health-promoting behavior is the endpoint or action outcome in the HPM. However, health-promoting behavior is ultimately directed toward *attaining positive health outcomes* for the client. Health-promoting behaviors, particularly when integrated into a healthy lifestyle that pervades all aspects of living, results in improved health, enhanced functional ability, and better quality of life at all stages of development.

Interventions for Health Behavior Change

Increasing healthy behaviors and decreasing risky or health-damaging behaviors are the major challenges facing health professionals. Thus, a critical question is, what are the critical interventions based on health-promotion and prevention theories that nurses need to enable them to assist clients to make desired changes in health-related behaviors. Behavior-change strategies based on the theories that have been presented are used to illustrate evidence-based counseling and behavioral interventions.

Raising Consciousness

The transtheoretical model emphasizes the importance of raising consciousness at the point when the client is either not considering behavior change or just beginning to consider a change. Awareness of benefits of adopting a healthy behavior or discontinuing a risky behavior is enhanced through seeking and processing information, observing others, and interpreting information in light of one's personal situation. The client should be provided materials about health-related issues relevant to the target behavior including the short- and long-term consequences for the individual and for significant others. Risk-appraisal and risk-reduction counseling may be used to raise consciousness concerning how behavior change lowers the risk for chronic illness. "Headliners" from national newspapers and magazines that focus on the benefits of change or the negative consequences of not changing may be particularly effective in raising consciousness due to the "eye-catching" format in which the information is presented. The client should be given a list of information resources and encouraged to become an active participant in information gathering (Chen, 1995). The materials used for raising consciousness need to be culturally specific to the client to optimize impact.

Reevaluating the Self

Self-reevaluation, a process identified in social cognitive theory, is based on the premise that change results from the arousal of an affective state of dissatisfaction within the client as a result of recognition of disturbing inconsistencies between self-standards (values, beliefs) and behaviors. The client may ask questions such as: will I like myself better if I am thinner, more physically active, or no longer smoke? A contradiction between the personal values and current behavior is most directly resolved by engaging in behavior change. Further, the more clients perceive that they are the kind of person that engages in a particular behavior, the more likely they are to perform the behavior consistent with self-standards. Adherence to standards that are set for personal behavior will enhance self-concept through feelings of pride and self-satisfaction, whereas violation of self-standards for behavior will result in negative feelings of guilt and self-censure. Strong intentions to meet personal standards will likely lead to increasing performance of the behavior and eventually to permanent behavior change (Prochaska, Norcross, et al., 1994).

The client may also use self-reevaluation to contrast the personal behavioral consequences of continuing a health-damaging behavior with the consequences of discontinuing the behavior. For example, the nurse may ask the client to list several activities that would be possible if smoking were discontinued, then list likely restrictions on activities if smoking behavior were not changed. Also, considering specific differences between self and "models" or important reference groups the client admires is an impetus to make personal changes in behavior consistent with a reorientation in self-standards and values.

Promoting Self-Efficacy

The most powerful input to self-efficacy is successful performance of a behavior. Whenever possible, the nurse facilitates the client to perform the target behavior in the presence of the nurse and provides positive feedback on those aspects of the behavior that were performed appropriately. For example, having the client select low-fat foods from an array of pictures or models of foods and providing immediate feedback on correct choices enhances task self-efficacy. Praise and positive feedback along with persuasion and reassurance are concrete ways to build self-efficacy relevant to a particular behavior. The nurse builds regulatory self-efficacy by providing clients with strategies to overcome barriers to performing the target behavior as well as enhancing confidence that the client can successfully overcome the barriers. Learning from the reported experiences of others or directly observing their coping behaviors increases clients' perceptions of self-efficacy and lowers perceived barriers to successful behavior change.

Observation of others engaging in the desired behavior is important during the action phase to refine clients' performance capabilities and enhance self-efficacy. Modeling of behavior by others is especially helpful when clients are aware of their specific health goal but are uncertain about the exact behaviors that should be developed to move toward the goal. The following considerations are important to effectively use modeling to facilitate self-efficacy and resultant behavior change:

- Models must be available with whom the client can identify (e.g., gender specific, age specific, culture specific).
- Learners must have an actual opportunity to observe the desired behavior and must attend to important aspects of the behavior.
- Clients must have the requisite knowledge and skills to reproduce the behavior.
- Clients must perceive benefits from imitating the target behavior.
- Learners must have the opportunity to rehearse the target behavior.

Enhancing the Benefits of Change

Behavioral beliefs in the TRA and the TPB as well as outcome expectations in social cognitive theory are considered to be necessary conditions for behavior change (Ajzen, 1991; Brownell et al., 1986; Fishbein & Ajzen, 1975; Schwarzer, 1992). Planning for reward or reinforcement is a unique way to expand the benefits or positive outcomes derived from behavior change. The importance of reinforcement is based on the premise that all behaviors are determined by their consequences. If positive consequences result, the probability is high that the behavior will occur again. If negative consequences occur, the probability is low for the behavior to be repeated. Positive reinforcement (reward) rather than negative reinforcement (removal of an aversive condition) or punishment (aversive experience) provides the most effective motivation for behavioral change (Ajzen, 1991). When self-modification is the focus of nursing intervention, clients select the behavior they will change and the rewards they will receive for change. Behaviors that are to be reinforced must be clearly identified and a plan or contract for change negotiated either between the client and the health care provider or between the client and significant others.

If a client wishes to increase the incidence of a specific health-promoting behavior or decrease the incidence of a health-damaging behavior, it is important to obtain an initial frequency count of the target behavior (baseline data) so that extent of progress toward the desired change may be accurately assessed. An example of a daily record of smoking behavior is presented in Figure 2–5.

Benefits are classified as tangible, social, or self-generated and serve to reinforce desired behavior. Tangible benefits include objects or activities, such as purchasing a magazine or going to a movie. Social benefits include telephoning a friend or visiting with a neighbor. Self-generated benefits include self-praise and self-compliments. The time frame for application of reinforcement is critical. Immediate and continuous reinforcement is highly desirable, particularly in the early phases of self-change as it

Behavior to Be Observed:	Smoking	
Observation Categories:	Morning Afternoon Evening	
Method of Coding Behavior:		E = Smoking after or during eating and drinking S = Smoking while nervous in a social situation D = Smoking while driving the car O = Smoking at other times

Smoking Record

Date: Tuesday, August 26

Morning	Afternoon	Evening
E E D O S S S E	O S S D S E E E	E O

Date: Wednesday, August 27

Morning	Afternoon	Evening
E E E D D S S E E	S S S S D D E E E E	S E O

FIGURE 2–5 Self-Observation Sheet

(From Watson Tharp, 1974, *Self-Directed Behavior, Self-Modification for Personal Adjustments* (1st ed.). © 1974 Reprinted with permission of Wadsworth, a division of Thomson Learning: *www.thomsonrights.com.* Fax 800 730-2215.)

promotes rapid learning of the desired behaviors. Intermittent reinforcement applied later stabilizes the behavior and makes it resistant to extinction (Deci & Ryan, 1985).

Many behaviors are too complex to be acquired all at once. Gradually shaping desired behaviors is an effective approach to make permanent changes in lifestyle. An example of shaping is the following:

- Brisk walk for 15 minutes 2 days of first week
- Brisk walk for 20 minutes 3 days of second and third week
- Brisk walk for 30 minutes 3 days of fourth and fifth week
- Brisk walk for 45 minutes 4 days of sixth and seventh week
- Brisk walk for 60 minutes 5 days of eighth and ninth week

Each step toward the final behavior should be mastered before the next step is attempted.

Once the client starts engaging in a desired behavior, the consequences, such as losing weight, feeling more relaxed, or feeling more energetic, have reinforcing properties. When the behavior begins to offer its own reward, the nurse counsels the client that other sources of reward to enhance the benefits of the behavior may no longer be necessary (Deci & Ryan, 1985).

Controlling the Environment

Modifying the environment to support behavior change is an important tenet of social cognitive theory (Levin, 1999). Stimulus control includes structuring multiple environments to elicit the desired behavior. Internal prompts coupled with external prompts encourage action; for example, "feeling good after brisk walking" coupled with "the invitation from spouse to take a walk." Synergistically, this provides powerful stimuli for behavior change. Table 2–3 presents an overview of possible stimulus configurations that prompt health-promoting and prevention behaviors.

Individuals define relevant environmental changes to make based on past knowledge and experience. Reconfiguring environmental stimuli augments conditions for desirable behaviors or decrease conditions for undesirable behaviors. Specific approaches to stimulus reconfiguration include *cue elimination*, *cue restriction*, and *cue expansion*. In *cue elimination* (Montano, 2002), environmental cues for undesired behaviors are decreased. Examples include sitting in no-smoking areas of restaurants or eating meals only with nonsmokers if cessation of smoking is the goal. In successful cue elimination, external stimulation the behavior results.

Frequently, cues cannot be totally eliminated but can be reduced or restricted. In *cue restriction*, for example, eating may be reduced to one room in the house, the kitchen or dining room. By localizing the cues that activate behavior, arrangements limited encounter with the cues are possible. In *cue expansion* (Montano et al.), the number of prompts to desired behaviors is increased. For instance, whereas personal preparation of food in one's own kitchen may prompt small servings of meals, fruits, and vegetables, the environment of a restaurant may prompt selection rich entrées and desserts. In expansion, being given a menu at a restaurant provides cues for looking only at salad and vegetable options as opposed to scanning the

TABLE 2–3 Possible Cues for Health-Promoting and Preventive Actions

Internal Cues

Bodily states; e.g., feeling good, feeling energetic, recognizing aging, fatigue, cyclical discomfort

Affective states; e.g., enthusiasm, motivation for self-preservation, high level of self-esteem, happiness, concern

External Cues

Interactions with significant others; e.g., family, friends, colleagues, nurse, and physician

Impact of communication media; e.g., motivational messages from television, radio, newspapers, advertisements, and special mailings

Visual stimuli from the environment; e.g., passing a diabetic screening clinic, billboards, attendance at a health fair, passing a gym or exercise center, or viewing others participating in target activity dessert section. By expanding the range of cues that elicit specific responses, desirable behaviors may occur more frequently and with greater regularity. Controlling the environment conducive to the behavior through the elimination, restriction, or expansion of cues assists clients in creating internal and external conditions supportive of positive health practices.

Managing Barriers to Change

Barriers to change are central constructs in the Health Belief Model (Strecher & Rosenstock, 2002). The nurse facilitates the preparation, action, and maintenance stages of behavior change by assisting clients in minimizing or eliminating barriers to action. It is futile to encourage clients to take actions that are highly likely to be blocked or cause the client frustration.

Internal barriers to self-modification include:

- Unclear short-term and long-term goals
- Lack of skill to follow through with self-modification
- Perceptions of lack of control over the environment (cues, reinforcements, time)
- Lack of motivation to pursue selected health actions

Barriers such as these often reflect insufficient attention to the preparation stage of behavior change.

The interaction of level of readiness and barriers to action is depicted in Table 2–4. Consequences for the client and appropriate nursing interventions are also presented. When clients have a high level of readiness to engage in health-promoting or preventive behaviors and barriers are low, only a low-intensity cue is needed to activate behavior. A high-intensity cue under these conditions may actually be a negative force. When readiness is high and barriers to action are also formidable, barriers need to be reduced or eliminated. When both readiness and barriers are low, readiness to act should be increased in order to initiate action. When readiness is low and barriers are high, both factors should be addressed, or behavior change is unlikely to occur.

Significant others often serve as barriers to health actions. When family members or other persons disagree or are neutral or apathetic toward health behaviors, the constraints

TABLE 2–4 Interrelationships Among Level of Readiness to Take Health Actions, Barriers, Consequences for Clients, and Nursing Interventions

Level of Readiness	Barriers to Action	Consequences for Client	Nursing Interventions
High	Low	Action	Support and encouragement; provide low-intensity cue
High	High	Conflict	Assist client in lowering barriers to action
Low	Low	Conflict	Provide high-intensity cue
Low	High	No action	Assist client in lowering barriers to action and then provide high-intensity cue

created for the client depend on the following factors:

- Relevance of disagreeing persons
- Attractiveness of disagreeing persons
- Extent of disagreement of relevant persons
- Number of persons relevant to the client who disagree with behavior
- Extent to which client is self-directed rather than other-dependent

Membership in self-help or self-change groups may be critical at this point, because the group often provides input to the client on the process of change, the barriers likely to be encountered in making changes, and various means of overcoming these constraints.

Tailoring Behavior-Change Interventions

Tailoring print and interactive computer communications in health promotion and prevention offers exciting opportunities for nurses to engage in development, testing, and implementation of individualized behavior-change strategies. The computer does not replace the nurse but provides the nurse–client team with more power in information gathering, information processing, collaborative goal setting, and tailoring care strategies to assist individuals and families in achieving important health goals. One-size-fits-all health education materials are rapidly becoming outdated as information technology expands the range of possibilities for using complex, interactive behavior-change strategies that are relevant to clients, practical for providers, and most likely cost-effective for health care systems. The one-size-fits-all approach cannot address the range of details that vary from person to person and influence individuals' health-related decisions and health behaviors. Kreuter and colleagues (1999, 2000) distinguished between generic materials, targeted generic materials, and tailored communications. Generic materials include the same general information for everyone and usually consist of a single communication. Targeted generic materials are aimed at reaching a specific subgroup of the population. Tailored materials are intended to reach one specific person, based on characteristics unique to that person, related to the outcome of interest, and derived from an individual assessment.

Tailored materials for interventions should be theoretically driven (Montgomery, 2003). For example, a tailored intervention using the Theory of Reasoned Action will emphasize attitudes, subjective norms, and intentions. Social cognitive theory tailored interventions will emphasize outcome expectations and efficacy expectations as well as relevant components of the environment. The selected theory provides the conceptual structure for designing the assessment, the message database, and the algorithms to match client characteristics to individually tailored interventions (Rakowski, 1999). Tailored messages may be delivered through many channels: print, interactive computer programs, telephone, audio, video, or the Internet.

Kreuter and Strecher (1996) evaluated the effectiveness of tailored behavior-change messages in comparison to typical messages with minimal feedback or no feedback. They found individuals who received the tailored health risk feedback were 18% more likely to change at least one risk behavior when queried 6 months later than were patients receiving typical or no feedback. The most frequent changes made were obtaining cholesterol screening, decreasing dietary fat consumption, and increasing physical activity. Marcus and colleagues (1998) assessed the effectiveness of an individualized, motivationally tailored physical activity intervention compared to a standardized self-help intervention. The individually tailored intervention used an expert system to assess motivational readiness for physical activity adoption, self-efficacy, decisional balance between pros and cons of change, use of cognitive and behavioral processes of change, and actual physical activity participation. Motivationally matched manuals, according to stage of behavior change, were used. At the end of the intervention, 44% of the tailored group compared to 18% in the standardized group participated in moderate-intensity physical activity at least 5 days per week for a total of 30 minutes each day (Marcus et al., 1998).

Velicer, Prochaska, Fava, Laforge, and Rossi (1999) evaluated whether interactive, individually tailored sequential messages were more effective than simply stage-matched manuals for smoking cessation among adults in a managed-care system. The interactive, tailored intervention outperformed the stage-matched manual intervention in abstinence rates at 6, 12, and 18 months. Although some studies have not found tailored materials to be superior (Brug, Steenhuis, VanAssema, & DeVries, 1996), most studies support continuing to build tailoring capabilities for health counseling and intervention in health care. Skinner, Campbell, Rimer, Curry, and Prochaska (1999) provide an excellent overview of intervention studies using tailored print health communications. Further assessment of tailored interventions is needed to determine when they are likely to be most effective.

Maintaining Behavior Change

Maintenance of health behavior raises special challenges for the client. Changes in behavior that are transient accomplish little in enhancing client health status. The behavior must be sustained in the environment in which it is learned, and the behavior must also be generalized to other situations. Factors that affect continuation of positive health behaviors include:

- Extent of personal skill to carry out the behavior
- Number of personal beliefs and attitudes that support the target behavior, including beliefs about self-efficacy
- Extent of positive emotional response (positive affect) and cognitive commitment (intention) to perform the behavior
- Ease of incorporating behavior into lifestyle
- Absence of environmental constraints to performing the behavior
- Extent to which the behavior is intrinsically rewarding
- Extent to which the decision to take action has been communicated to others and there is social support for the behavior
- Consistency of behavior with self-image
- Personal attractiveness of incompatible action (Fishbein et al., 1991)

The maintenance phase of health behavior extends from beginning stabilization of the new behavior throughout the client's life span. Habit formation facilitates maintenance of behaviors. Habits are behaviors that become automatic and are maintained on a stimulus–response level with little conscious effort. Habit formation results in stable patterns of behavior. The nurse assists clients in habit formation by helping them plan for certain health-promoting behaviors to occur repeatedly in the same setting or context. For example, a client who exercises each noon in the company fitness center, 3 to 5 days a week for a period of time, is likely to continue to exercise as routinely as brushing teeth or showering.

A sixth stage of behavior change is transformation. In Cardinal's study (1999), 16% of participants had well-established patterns of physical activity and were 100% confident that they could maintain regular physical activity for the rest of their life. Transformation appeared to differ from maintenance. Individuals in the transformed stage were active at a higher level of intensity and had a more positive attitude toward role-modeling healthy behavior than did individuals in the maintenance stage. Persons in the transformed stage appeared highly resistant to relapse. Research is needed to determine if there is a stage beyond maintenance in which habit and personal confidence ensure permanent behavior change and transformation of behavioral patterns.

Ethics of Behavior Change

Autonomy and self-determinism of the client are major tenets of professional nursing practice in situations in which autonomous behavior is not a threat to the health and welfare of others. Individuals and families should select their behavioral patterns and lifestyle based on sound information from health professionals and/or other credible information sources. Not all members of society will choose the most healthful behaviors, and this is their right when their actions do not harm others (O'Connell & Price, 1983). Nurses assist all clients who seek help in adopting health-promoting lifestyles and must avoid authoritarian and coercive strategies. Allowing clients to assume leadership in modifying their lifestyles is an ethical, nonmanipulative approach to improving the health of individuals and families.

Directions for Research in Health Behavior

A multitheory approach to intervention is the most productive (Montgomery, 2002; Weinstein, 1993). Models need further exploration and testing that incorporate optimal behavior-change strategies as well as methods to combine change strategies and that are culturally relevant.

Research in the following areas is recommended:

1. Develop and test interventions that are based on a logical integration of multiple theories.
2. Describe developmental patterns that play a role in motivating health behaviors.
3. Develop and test the effectiveness of tailored interventions focused on removal of perceived internal and external barriers to change.
4. Develop and test models that incorporate long-term behavior change.

Research requires collaboration of scientists from multiple disciplines to design and test the effectiveness of behavior-change interventions that are culturally and developmentally sensitive. Information about funding for health-promotion and prevention intervention research is available on the National Institute of Nursing Research web site.

Directions for Practice in Motivating Health Behavior

Knowledge of individual theories of health behavior makes it possible for the nurse to select the theory or theories that are most appropriate for the client and the behavior change anticipated. Choice of theory needs to take into account the needs of the individual client. For example, barriers such as discomfort, travel, or cost may be significant for a woman who needs to obtain mammography. In contrast, self-efficacy may be important to address for individuals who desire to develop healthy food preparation and eating patterns. The emerging availability of interactive information technology augments the efforts of the nurse to assist clients in assessing their health beliefs and health behaviors and in successfully changing their behavior.

Strategies for behavior change are useful nursing interventions at different stages of change. For example, raising consciousness has been shown to be an effective strategy in making clients aware of the benefits of behavior change. This strategy is more effective in the early stages of behavior change such as precontemplation, contemplation, or preparation. Restructuring the environment to achieve stimulus control is more effective in the adoption and maintenance stages of behavior change when cues for behavior need to be abundant to trigger the behavior on a regular basis. Having healthy foods such as fruits and vegetables available in the house serves as a trigger for healthy family eating. Sitting in the smoke-free area of a restaurant is a trigger for tobacco avoidance. Building walking paths in the community creates visible cues for individuals and families to develop regular walking habits.

Existing theories, models, and related strategies enable the nurse to engage in evidence-based counseling and behavioral intervention for health promotion and prevention. The social cognitive theory, Health Belief Model, and Health Promotion Model are leading theories in adolescent health-promotion research that have resulted in practice guidelines (Montgomery, 2002). The flexible use of this knowledge to fit each individual, family, or community will enhance the quality of health-promotion and preventive care for diverse groups. For more information on evidence-based counseling strategies, view the Agency for Health Care Research and Quality web site.

SUMMARY

This chapter presents an overview of models and theories relevant to individual health behaviors. Continuing development of theories that incorporate a wider range of powerful explanatory and predictive variables for effective health-promotion and prevention interventions is imperative. A number of theory-based behavior-change strategies have also been described for nurses to assist individuals, families, and communities to modify health behaviors, promote desired changes, and provide clients with skills for continuing self-change and self-actualization. Learning that has lifelong application empowers clients to engage in a wide array of behavior changes to improve their health and well-being.

LEARNING ACTIVITIES

1. Choose one of the theories described in the chapter and use it to develop an intervention to address a selected behavior change for yourself.
2. Describe issues that you will face in maintaining your behavior change.
3. List the ethical considerations that are important to you in your personal decision to change a behavior.

SELECTED WEB SITES

Agency for Health Care Research and Quality: Guide to Clinical Preventive Services

http://www.ahrq.gov/clinic/prevenix.htm

American Medical Association: Guidelines for Adolescent Preventive Services

http://www.ama-assn.org/adolhlth/recommend/monogrf1.htm

Bureau of Maternal/Child Health: Bright Futures

http://www.brightfutures.org

Healthy People 2010

http://www.health.gov/healthypeople

National Institute of Nursing Research

http://www.nih.gov/ninr

REFERENCES

Abrams, D. B., Orleans, C. T., Niaura, R. S., et al. (1996). Integrating individual and public health perspectives for treatment of tobacco dependence under managed care: A combined stepped-care and matching model. *Annals of Behavioral Medicine, 18*(4), 290–304.

Agazio, J. G., Ephraim, P. M., Flaherty, N. B., & Guerney, C. A. (2002). Health-promotion in active-duty military women with children. *Women and Health, 35*(10), 65–82.

Ajzen, I. (1991). The theory of planned behavior. *Organizational Behavior and Human Decision Processes, 50,* 179–211.

Bandura, A. (1977). Self-efficacy: Toward a unifying theory of behavioral change. *Psychol Rev, 84,* 191–215.

Bandura, A. (1985). *Social foundations of thought and action: A social cognitive theory.* Upper Saddle River, NJ: Prentice Hall, Inc.

Bandura, A. (1997). *Self-efficacy: The exercise of control.* New York: W. H. Freeman.

Becker, M. H., Haefner, D. P., & Kasl, S. V., et al. Selected psychosocial models and correlates of individual health-related behaviors. *Med Care, 15,* 27–46.

Bolio, S. M. (1999). Reported health-promoting behaviors of incarcerated males (prisoner health, family support). University of Massachusetts. *Dissertation Abstracts International.* University Microfilms No. AAG9920586.

Brewer, J. L., Blake, A. J., & Rankin, S. A. (1999). Theory of reasoned action predicts milk consumption in women. *Journal of the American Diabetes Association, 99*(1), 39–44.

Brown, A. D., & Garber, A. M. (1998). Cost effectiveness of coronary heart prevention strategies in adults. *Pharmacoeconomics, 12,* 27–48.

Brownell, K. D., Marlatt, G. A., Lichtenstein, E., et al. (1986). Understanding and preventing relapse. *Am Psychol, 41,* 765–782.

Brug, J., Steenhuis, I., VanAssema, P., & DeVries, H. (1996). The impact of a computer-tailored nutrition intervention. *Prev Med, 25,* 236–242.

Cardinal, B. J. (1999). Extended stage model of physical activity behavior. *J Human Movement Studies, 37,* 37–54.

Champion, V. (1999). Revised susceptibility, benefits and barriers scale for mammography screening. *Res Nurs Health, 22,* 341–348.

Chen, C. H. (1995). Physical exercise and sense of well-being among Chinese elderly in Taiwan. University of Texas at Austin. *Dissertation Abstracts International.* University Microfilms No. AAI9603814.

Cox, C. (1982). An interaction model of client health behavior: Theoretical prescription for nursing. *Adv Nurs Sci, 5,* 41–56.

Cox, C. (1985). The health self-determinism index. *Nurs Res, 34*(3), 177–183.

Cox, C. L., Cowell, J. M., Marion, L. N., et al. (1990). The health self-determinism index for children. *Res Nurs Health, 13*(4), 237–246.

Craig, S., Goldberg, J., & Dietz, W. H. (1996). Psychosocial correlates of physical activity among fifth and eighth graders. *Prev Med, 25*(5), 506–514.

Deci, E. L., & Ryan, R. M. (1985). *Intrinsic motivation and self-determination in human behavior.* New York: Plenum Press.

Dennis, C. L., & Faux, S. (1999). Development and psychometric testing of the breastfeeding self-efficacy scale. *Res Nurs Health, 22,* 399–409.

Dunn, H. L. (1959a). High-level wellness for men and society. *Am J Public Health, 49*(6), 786–792.

Dunn, H. L. (1959b, November). What high-level wellness means. *Can J Public Health, 50*(11), 447–457.

Elder, J. P., Ayala, G. X., & Harris, S. (1999). Theories and intervention approaches to health-behavior change in primary care. *Am J Prev Med, 17*(4), 275–284.

Farrand, L. L., & Cox, C. L. (1993). Determinants of positive health behavior in middle childhood. *Nurs Res, 42*(4), 208–213.

Feather, N. T. (Ed.). (1982). *Expectations and actions: Expectancy-value models in psychology.* Hillsdale, NJ: Lawrence Erlbaum Associates, Inc.

Fishbein, M., & Ajzen, I. (1975). *Belief, attitude, intention and behavior: An introduction to theory and research.* Boston, MA: Addison-Wesley Publishing Co., Inc.

Fishbein, M., Bandura, A., Triandis, H. C., et al. (1991). *Factors influencing behavior and behavior change: Final report of a theorists' workshop on AIDS-related behaviors.* Washington, DC: National Institute of Mental Health, National Institutes of Health.

Gauvin, L., & Rejeski, W. J. (1993). The exercise-induced feeling inventory: Development and initial validation. *J Sport Exerc Psychol, 15,* 403–423.

Gillis, A. J. (1993). The relationship of definition of health, perceived health status, self-efficacy, parental health-promoting lifestyle, and selected demographics to health-promoting lifestyle in adolescent females. University of Texas at Austin. *Dissertation Abstracts International.* University Microfilms No. AAG9323405.

Godin, G. (1987). Importance of the emotional aspect of attitude to predict intention. *Psychol Rep, 61,* 719–723.

Hardy, C. J., & Rejeski, W. J. (1989). Now what, but how one feels: The measurement of affect during exercise. *J Sport Exerc Psychol, 11,* 304–317.

Harrison, R. L. (1993). The relationship among hope, perceived health status and health-promoting lifestyle among HIV seropositive mean (immune deficiency). New York University. *Dissertation Abstracts International.* University Microfilms No. AAG9317666.

Hausenblas, H. A., Carron, A. V., & Mack, D. E. (1997). Application of the theories of reasoned action and planned behavior to exercise behavior: A meta-analysis. *J Sport Exerc Psychol, 19,* 36–51.

Horan, M. L., Kim, K. K., Gendler, P., Froman, R. D., & Patel, M. D. (1998). Development and evaluation of the osteoporosis self-efficacy scale. *Res Nurs Health, 21,* 395–403.

Hulme, P. A., Walker, S. N., Effle, K. J., Jorgensen, L., McGowan, M. G., Nelson, J., & Pratt, E. N. (2003). Health-promoting lifestyle behaviors of Spanish-speaking Hispanic adults. *J Transcult Nurs, 14*(3), 244–254.

Hutchinson, K. C. (1996). Factors that predict health-promoting lifestyle behaviors among African-American university students. Northern Illinois University. *Dissertation Abstracts International.* University Microfilms No. AAG9639920.

Janis, I. L., & Mann, L. (1985). *Decision-making: A psychological analysis of conflict, choice, and commitment.* London, England: Free Press.

Jeffries, P. R. (1996). Predictor variables of exercise and nutrition for expatriates in Indonesia utilizing Pender's Health Promotion Model. Indiana University School of Nursing. *Dissertation Abstracts International.* University Microfilms No. AAG9639877.

Jemmott, J. B., III, & Jemmott, L. S. (2000). HIV behavioral interventions for adolescents in community settings. In J. L. Peterson & R. J. DiClemente (Eds.), *Handbook of HIV prevention* (pp. 103–127). New York: Kluwer/Plenum.

Kaplan, R. M. (2000). Two pathways to prevention. *American Psychol., 55*(4), 382–396.

Kaplan, R., & Kalpan, S. (1989). *The experience of nature: A psychological perspective.* Cambridge, England: Cambridge University Press.

Kerr, M. J., Lusk, S. L., & Ronis, D. (2002). Explaining Mexican American workers' hearing protection use with the health promotion model. *Nurs Res, 51*(2), 100–109.

Klar, Y., Nader, A., & Mallor, T. E. (1992). Opting to change: Student's informal self-change endeavors. In Y. Klar, J. D. Fisher, J. M. Chinsky, et al. (Eds.), *Self-change: Social and psychological perspectives* (pp. 63–83). New York: Springer-Verlag.

Kreuter, M. W., Farrell, D., Olevitch, L., & Brennan, L. (2000). *Tailoring health messages: Customizing communication using computer technology.* Mahwah, NJ: Lawrence Erlbaum Associates, Inc.

Kreuter, M. V., & Strecher, V. J. (1996). Do tailored behavior change messages enhance the effectiveness of health risk appraisal? Results from a randomized trial. *Health Educ Res, 11*(1), 97–105.

Kreuter, M. W., Strecher, V. J., & Glassman, B. (1999). One size does not fit all: The case for tailoring print materials. *Annals of Behavioral Medicine, 21*(4), 276–283.

Levin, P. F. (1999). Test of the Fishbein and Ajzen models as predictors of health care workers' glove use. *Res Nurs Health, 22*, 295–307.

Lewin, K., Dembo, T., Festinger, L., et al. (1994). Level of aspiration. In J. Hunt (Ed.), *Personality and the behavioral disorders: A handbook based on experimental and clinical research* (pp. 333–378). New York: Ronald Press.

Lohse, J. L. (2003). A bicycle safety education program for parents of young children. *J Sch Nurs, 19*(2), 100–110.

Lucas, J. A., Orshan, S. A., & Cook, F. (2000). Determinants of health-promotion behavior among women ages 65 and above living in the community. *Sch Inq Nurs Pract, 14*(1), 77–100.

Lusk, S. L., Kerr, M. L., Ronis, D. L., & Eakin, B. L. (1999). Applying the Health Promotion Model to development of a worksite intervention. *Am J Health Prom, 13*(4), 219–226.

Marcus, B. H., Bock, B. C., Pinto, B. M., Forsyth, L. A., Roberts, M. B., & Traficante, R. M. (1998). Efficacy of an individualized, motivationally tailored physical activity intervention. *Annals of Behavioral Medicine, 20*(3), 174–180.

Marcus, B. H., Selby, V. C., Niaura, R. S., et al. (1992). Self-efficacy and the stages of exercise behavior change. *Res Q Exerc Sport, 63*(1), 60–66.

Marlatt, G. A., & Gordon, J. R. (1985). *Relapse prevention: Maintenance strategies in the treatment of addictive behaviors.* New York: Guilford Press.

Martinelli, A. M. (1996). A study of health locus of control, self-efficacy, health promotion behaviors, and environmental factors related to the self-report of the avoidance of environmental tobacco smoke in young adults. University of Michigan. *Dissertation Abstracts International.* University Microfilms No. AAG9633458.

McAuley, E., & Courneya, K. S. (1992). Self-efficacy relationships with affective and exertion responses to exercise. *J Appl Soc Psychol, 22*, 312–326.

McAuley, E., & Mihalko, S. L. (1998). Measuring exercise-related self-efficacy. In J. L. Duda (Ed.), *Advances in sport and exercise psychology measurement* (pp. 371–390). Morgantown, WV: Fitness Information Technology.

McCullagh, M., Lusk, S. L., & Ronis, D. (2002). Factors influencing use of hearing protection among farmers: a test of the Pender Health Promotion Model. *Nurs Res, 51*(1), 33–39.

McCullagh, M. C. (1999). Factors affecting hearing protector use among farmers. *Dissertation Abstracts International, 61*(02). University Microfilms No. AAT9959819.

McKinlay, J. B. (1993). The promotion of health through planned sociopolitical change: Challenges for research and policy. *Social Science and Medicine, 36*, 109–117.

Millard, S. R. (1998). Factors related to health-promoting behaviors in Seventh-Day Adventist older adults (quality of life). University of Texas at Austin. *Dissertation Abstracts International.* University Microfilms No. AAG9838052.

Montano, D. E., Kasprzyk, D., & Taplin, S. H. (2002). The theory of reasoned action and the theory of planned behavior. In K. Glanz, F. M. Lewis, & B. K. Rimer (Eds.), *Health behavior and health education theory, research and practice* (3rd ed., pp. 85–112). San Francisco: Jossey-Bass.

Montgomery, K. S. (2002, Summer). Health promotion with adolescents: Examining theoretical perspectives to guide research. *Research and Theory for Nursing Practice, 16*(2), 119–134.

Montgomery, K. S. (2003). Health promotion for pregnant adolescents. *AWHONN Lifelines, 7*(5), 434–444.

Moore, E. J. (1992). The relationship among self-efficacy, health knowledge, self-rated health status, and selected demographics as determinants of health-promoting behavior in older adults. University of Akron. *Dissertation Abstracts International.* University Microfilms No. AAG9225233.

Nikulich-Barrett, M. J. (1997). Impact of perceived general health status, physical functioning, and self-efficacy on health promoting lifestyles of rural older black and white women (women elderly). State University of New York at Buffalo. *Dissertation Abstracts International.* University Microfilms No. AAG9807369.

O'Connell, J. K., & Price, J. H. (1983). Ethical theories for promoting health through behavior change. *J School Health, 53*, 476–479.

Pender, N. J. (1982). *Health promotion in nursing practice.* Norwalk, CT: Appleton-Century-Crofts.

Pender, N. J. (1987). *Health promotion in nursing practice* (2nd ed.). Norwalk, CT: Appleton & Lange.

Pender, N. J. (1996). *Health promotion in nursing practice* (3rd ed.). Stamford, CT: Appleton & Lange.

Pender, N. J., Murdaugh, C. L., & Parsons, M. A. (2002). *Health promotion in nursing practice* (4th ed.). Prentice Hall.

Pender, N. J., Walker, S. N., Frank-Stromborg, M., Sechrist, K. R., et al. (1990). *The health promotion model: Refinement and validation.* Final report to the National Center for Nursing Research, National Institutes of Health (Grant no. NR01121). Dekalb, IL: Northern Illinois University Press.

Pender, N. J., Walker, S. N., Sechrist, K. R., et al. (1990). Predicting health-promoting lifestyles in the workplace. *Nurs Res, 39*(6), 326–332.

Peterson, T. R., & Aldana, S. G. (1999). Improving exercise behavior: An application of the stages of change model in a worksite setting. *Am J Health Prom, 13*(4), 229–232.

Piazza, J., Conrad, K., & Wilbur, J. (2001). Exercise behavior among female occupational health nurses: Influence of self-efficacy, perceived health, control, and age. *AAOHN, 49*(2), 79–86.

Poss, J. E. (1999). Developing an instrument to study the tuberculosis screening behaviors of Mexican migrant farm workers. *Journal of Transcultural Nursing, 10*(4), 306–319.

Prochaska, J. O. (1994). Strong and weak principles for progressing from precontemplation to action on the basis of twelve problem behaviors. *Health Psychol, 13*, 47–51.

Prochaska, J. O., & DiClemente, C. C. (1984). *The transtheoretical approach: Crossing traditional boundaries of change.* Homewood, NJ: Dow Jones-Irwin.

Prochaska, J. O., DiClemente, C. C., & Norcross, J. C. (1992). In search of the structure of change. In Y. Klar, J. D. Fisher, J. M. Chinsky, et al. (Eds.), *Self-change: Social psychological and clinical perspectives* (pp. 87–114). New York: Springer-Verlag.

Prochaska, J. O., Norcross, J. C., & DiClemente, C. C. (1994). *Changing for good: A revolutionary six-stage program for overcoming bad habits and moving your life positively forward.* New York: Avon.

Prochaska, J. O., Velicer, W. F., Rossi, J. S., et al. (1994). Stages of change and decisional balance for 12 problem behaviors. *Health Psychol, 13*(1), 39–46.

Rakowski, W. (1999). The potential variances of tailoring in health behavior interventions. *Annals of Behavioral Medicine, 21*(4), 284–289.

Rejeski, W. J., Gauvin, L., Hobson, M. L., et al. (1995). Effects of baseline responses, in-task feelings, and duration of activity on exercise-induced feeling states in women. *Health Psychol, 14,* 350–359.

Rosenstock, I. M. (1960). What research in maturation suggests for public health. *American Journal of Public Health, 50,* 295–301.

Rosenstock, I. M., Strecher, V. J., & Becker, M. H. (1988). Social learning theory and the health belief model. *Health Educ Q, 15*(2), 175–183.

Sample, D. A., Sinicrope, P. S., Wargovich, M. J., & Sinicrope, F. A. (2002). Post-study aspirin intake and factors motivating participants in a colorectal cancer prevention trial. *Cancer Epidemiol Biomarkers, 11*(3), 281–285.

Sapp, S. G., & Jensen, H. H. (1998). An evaluation of the health belief model for predicting perceived and actual dietary quality. *J Appl Soc Psychol, 28*(3), 235–248.

Schwarzer, R. (Ed.). (1992). *Self-efficacy: Thought control of action.* Washington, DC: Hemisphere Publishing Corp.

Shiffman, S., Hickcox, M., Paty, J., Gnys, M., Kassel, J., & Richards, T. (1997). The abstinence violation effect following smoking lapses and temptations. *Cognitive Therapy and Research, 21,* 497–523.

Siela, D., & Wieseke, A. W. (2000). Stress, self-efficacy, and health. In V. H. Rice (Ed.), *Handbook of stress, coping and health: Implications for nursing research, theory, and practice* (pp. 496–498). Thousand Oaks: Sage Publications, Inc.

Skinner, C. S., Campbell, M. K., Rimer, B. K., Curry, S., & Prochaska, J. O. (1999). How effective is tailored print communication? *Annals of Behavioral Medicine, 21*(4), 290–298.

Strecher, V. J., & Rosenstock, I. M. (2002). The health belief model. In K. Glanz, F. M. Lewis, & B. K. Rimer (Eds.), *Health behavior and health education: Theory, research and practice* (3rd ed.). San Francisco: Jossey-Bass.

Stutts, W. C. (1997). Use of the Health Promotion Model to predict physical activity in adults (weight control, self-efficacy). University of North Carolina at Chapel Hill. *Dissertation Abstracts International.* University Microfilms No. AAG9730610.

Suwonnaroop, N. (1999). Health-promoting behaviors in older adults: The effect of social support, perceived health status, and personal factors. Case Western Reserve. *Dissertation Abstracts International.* University Microfilms No. AAG9941265.

Tober, J. A. (1996). Investigation of predictors of successful weight loss in a morbidly obese population (optifast). University of Waterloo (Canada). *Dissertation Abstracts International.* University Microfilms No. AAGNN15346.

Troumbley, P. F., & Lenz, E. R. (1992). Application of Cox's interaction model of client health behavior in a weight control program for military personnel: A preintervention baseline. *Adv Nurs Sci, 14*(4), 65–78.

Vara, L. S., & Epstein, L. (1995). Laboratory assessment of choice between exercise or sedentary behaviors. *Res Q Exerc Sport, 64,* 356–360.

Velicer, W. F., DiClemente, C. D., Rossi, J. S., et al. (1990). Relapse situations and self-efficacy: An integrative model. *Addict Behav, 15,* 271–283.

Velicer, W. F., Prochaska, J. O., Fava, J. L., Laforge, R. G., & Rossi, J. S. (1999). Interactive versus noninteractive interventions and dose-response relationships for stage-matched smoking cessation programs in a managed care setting. *Health Psychol, 18*(1), 21–28.

Warren, M. T. (1993). The relationships of self-motivation and perceived personal competence to engaging in a health-promoting lifestyle for men in cardiac rehabilitation programs. New York University. *Dissertation Abstracts International.* University Microfilms No. AAG9333943.

Weinstein, N. D. (1993). Testing four competing theories of health-protective behavior. *Health Psychol, 12*, 324–333.

Wu, T. (1999). Determinants of physical activity among Taiwanese adolescents: An application of the Health-Promotion Model. University of Michigan. *Dissertation Abstracts International.* University Microfilms No. AAG9938572.

Wu, T. Y., & Pender, N. (2002). Determinants of physical activity among Taiwanese adolescents: an application of the health promotion model. *Res Nurs Health, 25*(1), 25–36.

3

Community Models to Promote Health

OBJECTIVES

1. Describe commonalities and differences in the various definitions of communities.
2. Discuss the key concepts and features of social-ecological models of health-promotion.
3. Describe the characteristics of social capital and the role of social support in this approach.
4. Define the steps in the PRECEDE-PROCEED Model in planning health-promotion programs.
5. Compare and contrast the Diffusion of Innovation and social marketing models.

OUTLINE

- The Concept of Community
- Community Assessment Interventions and Health Promotion
- Community Ecological Models and Theories
  A. Social-Ecological Models
  B. Social Capital Theory
- Community Planning Models for Health Promotion
  A. The PRECEDE-PROCEED Model
- Community Diffusion Models to Promote Health
  A. Diffusion of Innovations Model
  B. Social Marketing Model

Attention to community-based approaches to promote health and prevent disease by health professionals has dramatically increased in recent years. The increased emphasis is due to many factors, including a greater understanding of the complex etiologies of health problems, an appreciation of the relationship of individuals with their environment, and recognition of the limits of focusing only on individual behaviors to promote health (Norton, McLeroy, Burdine, Felix, & Dorsey, 2002). A greater appreciation of the role of the environment in the achievement of health has resulted in multiple approaches to promoting wellness. Individual approaches to health promotion identify a finite number of lifestyle areas that can be quantified and targeted for intervention. Community-based models move beyond individual lifestyles to distal factors that influence health, such as social conditions. Within a community-based view, the social, political, institutional, legislative, and physical environments in which behavior occurs can be targeted for change to promote health. Community approaches place an emphasis on populations and communities as clients, as opposed to individual health, and acknowledge that the greater environment influences individual health behaviors.

While it is now recognized that attention to the environment is necessary for health promotion, community-based models are not intended to neglect the individual. Individuals make up communities, so while the community may be targeted, individuals play a critical role in providing leadership. Community-based strategies for health promotion place control with individuals who reside in the community. The focus of this chapter is to introduce the concepts in community models as well as provide an overview of the major community models and theories in the literature.

The Concept of Community

Community has been defined in multiple ways. It is commonly defined as a collective body of individuals identified by geography, common interests, concerns, characteristics, or values (WHO, 1974). A community may be considered to be an association, a self-generated gathering of common people or citizens who have the creativity and capacity to solve problems (McKnight, 2002). The definition has evolved from a structural focus on geographic boundaries to a functional focus of people interacting in social units and sharing common interests. Whatever the definition of community, residents must share values and are linked together for common goals or other purposes. Members must also have a sense of community, or a sense of identity, shared values, norms, communications, and helping patterns and identify themselves as members of the same community.

The community in which individuals live, work, and play is critical to health promotion and prevention. The community context refers to the interdependence that exists between selected aspects of a given environment or setting. The context includes personal, physical, cultural, and social aspects of environments and the relationship between them that may influence an individual's mental and physical health, opportunities, achievement, and developmental outcomes (Clitheroe & Stokols, 1998). The relationship between individuals and the context or social system in which they interact is reciprocal, as individuals may work to change their neighborhood context, just as the context influences the individual. For example, lack of street lighting may limit persons from walking later in the evening. However, individuals may work to have appropriate lighting installed in their community to facilitate safe walking.

The context encompasses social institutions within a community, surroundings, and social relationships (Anderson, Scrimshaw, Fullilove, & Fielding, 2003). Social institutions include cultural and religious organizations, economic systems, and political structures. Surroundings include neighborhoods, workplaces, towns, and cities; social relationships include position in the social hierarchy, social group, and social networks. All of these aspects represent resources needed to sustain health. Lack of access to these resources is a potential stressor that may increase health risks.

A risk environment is an example of a context in which factors interact to increase the chances of risk behaviors and harm. Risk environments have two key dimensions: the type of environmental influence (physical, social, economic, and policy) and level of environmental influence (micro and macro; Rhodes, 2003). Aspects of the physical environment that may increase risks or decrease health-promotion efforts include lack of running water, poor transportation, heavy street traffic with noise, and air pollution. Micro level influences that may increase risk and decrease health-promoting efforts include social networks, social norms, values and rules, peer and social influence, and the social setting where one resides. Macro level influences take into account one's economics, gender, ethnicity, and culture, as well as the legal and policy environment, including state and federal laws. Micro and macro level influences intersect with the environment to either increase risks or enable individuals to promote health. Knowledge of the environmental context is useful for creating an enabling environmental context in which potential risks are reduced in order to maximize healthy behavior change.

The client becomes the community when the focus is on the collective of the population's common good instead of the individual's level (Shuster & Goeppinger, 2004). In the community models discussed in this chapter, the nurse works with individuals and groups. However, the outcomes of health-promotion programs are expected to affect the entire community. For example, the nurse may work with parents to get safe walking tracks for adults and recreational parks for children. These changes improve the health of the community. In community health promotion, change has to occur at multiple levels, beginning with the individuals and moving to the community as a whole (Shuster & Goeppinger, 2004). Policy changes may need to occur at the societal level for community-wide change to occur. When the community is the client focus, the nurse and the community work together to achieve mutual goals, as community members are actively involved in all steps of the process.

Community Assessment Interventions and Health Promotion

Community interventions differ from interventions within a community (Green & Kreuter, 1999). Community interventions target either the majority of the population in a community or the community as a whole, as the goal is to change the entire setting. Community interventions have multiple advantages. First, they have the potential to make population changes. Interventions based on community models focus both on high-risk persons and the larger community to promote health, and the interventions are relevant for the population in the community (Eriksson, 2002). Other benefits include a high level of exposure to the intervention and increased generalizability of the intervention to other communities. In addition, the interventions are likely to be valuable in the development of public health policies. Community changes are integrated into existing structures within the community, thereby changing the system that influences health behaviors.

Community models are based on four underlying assumptions (Minkler & Wallerstein, 2002). First, communities shape individual behaviors through community values and norms. Second, communities can be mobilized to change individual behaviors by legitimizing the desirable behaviors and changing environments to facilitate the new behaviors. The third assumption is that participation of community leaders is crucial for community ownership; and last, members of the community must have a sense of responsibility and control over the planned change. In other words, they must own the planned change for it to be successful. People are more likely to commit to and sustain change if they participate in identifying the problem, and developing and implementing the program to address the problem (Green & Kreuter, 1999). Community interventions must engage participants to promote successful behavior change. Members must be involved early in the planning process to identify needs, develop priorities, and plan programs to promote change. Community-based models take into consideration individuals in interaction with their families, cultures, and social structures, as well as the actual physical environment. The "twin pillars" of community-based health promotion programs are *empowerment* and *community participation* (Robertson & Minkler, 1995).

Community empowerment is a social action process by which people and communities are enabled to participate and act to transform their lives and their environments (Minkler, 2000). The concept of empowerment refers to a process by which people and communities gain mastery over their lives. Empowerment principles are essential components of participatory research in health promotion. Empowered communities are visible when people within the community participate in equal partnership with health professionals in defining their problems and developing solutions. In addition community members receive the benefits of the interventions and are partners in evaluation of the effectiveness of the intervention. Community empowerment is not new in public health, as public health practitioners have long recognized the need for community members to take control of the health of their community.

Community participation is the process of taking part in activities, programs, or discussions to promote planned change or improve the community. Community participation is a basic principle in health education and has been the major focus of chronic disease prevention. Community participation is expected to empower individuals and communities through group decision making and knowledge of resources, as well as creating new networks and opportunities. Participation of community members results in greater buy-in, greater participation, and greater sustainability. Empowerment and community participation go hand in hand, as empowered members participate in the health agenda for the community.

Community Ecological Models and Theories

An overview of systems theory is helpful to understand ecological models. Systems theory was originally described in the biological sciences as a complex of elements mutually interacting (Joos, Nelson, & Lyness, 1985; Von Bertalanffy, 1975). Some of the major terms used in systems theory include *boundary*, *adaptation*, *entropy*, *negentropy*, *equifinality*, and *feedback*. In social ecological models, communities are open systems in which there are interactions within a community among its members, as well as between community members and their environment. A community is made of many interrelated and independent parts that are organized to function for the good of the community (Lowry & Martin, 2004; Shuster & Goeppinger, 2004). These parts include school systems, health care, churches, welfare systems, law enforcement, economics, and recreational areas. The functions of these parts are interrelated, as a change in one part affects other parts of the community. Functions require energy to carry out their activities. Communities have geographical boundaries that determine the external borders as well as internal boundaries within the community, such as isolated neighborhoods of poverty or wealth. Communities experience change within their environments, which is managed through the process of adaptation. Adaptation occurs when members of the community make changes, or changes occur within the community environment. Negentropy refers to energy used by the system for maintenance or growth. Negentropy is the positive aspect of a community that promotes well-being, such as adequate social support systems, jobs, and good health. Entropy is the tendency of the system to break down or a measure of disorder in the system. Entropy refers to negative aspects that do not contribute to the well-being of a community, such as deteriorating conditions seen in communities of poverty. As open systems, communities have inputs, throughputs, and outputs. Inputs take energy into the system. Inputs come from sources outside the system as well as members within the community. Throughput refers to the process of using inputs, such as community activities; outputs are the results of these activities. Feedback occurs through communication of the community's subparts as they interact to facilitate effective functioning of the whole.

The term *ecology* has its roots in biology and refers to the interrelations between organisms and their environments. The concept has evolved to provide an understanding of the interactions of people with their physical and sociocultural environments (Stokols, 2000). Ecological models emphasize the social, institutional, and cultural contexts of people-environment relations.

Social-Ecological Models

Stokols (2000) expanded the concept of an ecology model to a social-ecological approach to health promotion. He described certain core assumptions about human health and the development of strategies to promote personal and collective well-being. First, the healthfulness of a situation and the well-being of its individuals are assumed to be influenced by both the physical and social environments as well as personal attributes of the individual. Second, environments are multidimensional and complex and can be described in physical and social terms, objective or subjective (perceived), proximal or distal, and other attributes, such as noise, group size, and so forth, or as constructs, such as social climate. Third, individuals within an environment can be described at multiple levels, such as individuals, families, groups, organizations, (such as schools), and populations. Last, systems theory concepts, including interdependence, homeostasis, and feedback, help to understand the interrelationships between people and their environments. Environments are viewed as complex systems, and efforts to promote well-being must take into account the interdependence among all components and levels of the environment.

In an ecological perspective, health-promotion interventions target environmental factors that either facilitate or block health behaviors as well as individual behaviors (von Bertalanffy, 1975). This approach suggests that the effectiveness of health-promotion interventions can be increased through multilevel interventions, which combine behavioral and environmental strategies. In a social ecological approach to health-promotion the interplay between environmental resources and the health habits and lifestyles of individuals within that environment are analyzed to identify features of the environment that promote or hinder well-being. Identifying these interdependent links helps to define both environmental components and individual characteristics that need to be targeted to promote healthy lifestyles.

A key feature of social ecological models is analysis of the physical and sociocultural environments. Identifying health-promoting environments extends the narrow focus on individual behaviors to promote health. However, ecological models go beyond a focus solely on environmental factors to include transactions of the individual and groups with the environment. This is a major strength as strategies for behavior change are integrated with environmental change strategies.

Sallis and Owen (2002) formulated seven principles to guide social-ecological approaches for interventions and research. These principles were developed after a review of ecological concepts and are listed in Table 3–1. Ecological models have been applied for obesity prevention, physical activity promotion, and tobacco cessation (Corbett, 2001; Sallis et al., 2003; Spence & Lee, 2003).

Evidence to date indicates a multilevel ecological approach that incorporates intrapersonal, sociocultural, and environmental policy components is promising for health promotion. Further development and testing of ecological models is a high priority for nurse researchers, as these models have only recently begun to receive serious attention and the limited results are positive for promoting health.

Social Capital Theory

The theory of social capital focuses on resources embedded in one's community network and how access to and use of such resources benefit the actions of individuals within the

TABLE 3-1 Principles of Ecological Approaches for Health-Behavior Change

1. Multiple levels of factors have an influence on health behaviors.
2. Multiple types of environment have an influence on health behaviors.
3. Behavior-specific ecological models can guide interventions to target specific health behaviors.
4. Multilevel interventions that combine individual, community, and environmental components are more effective.
5. A multidisciplinary approach is more effective to implement multilevel interventions.
6. Ongoing process evaluations are needed to monitor implementation of multilevel interventions.
7. Ecological interventions can be hindered by political agendas.

community (Lin, 2001). Resources are defined as valued goods in a society. The theory focuses on actions taken to either maintain or gain valued resources.

Social capital as a determinant of health behavior has been defined in many ways. Although there is a lack of consensus for a definition of social capital, in all definitions trust and reciprocity are central components (Kreuter & Lezin, 2002). A recent definition of social capital is the specific processes among people and organizations working collaboratively in an atmosphere of trust that lead to accomplishing mutual social goals (Kreuter & Lezin, 2002). Green and Kreuter (1999) add two additional components, cooperation and civic engagement. Putnam's classic research on the efficiency of local governments in Italy (2000) popularized the social capital concept. He suggested the core elements of social capital, trust and cooperation, are learned behaviors, indicating that social capital can be created. Putnam defined the characteristics of social capital, which include (a) measures of community organizational life or human interactions, such as clubs, churches, and other group organizations; (b) measures of engagement in civic affairs such as participation of people in presidential elections; (c) measures of community voluntarism; (d) measures of reciprocity or mutual help among members of a community; and (e) measures of social trust. Putnam also distinguished between bonding (within groups) social capital and bridging (across groups) social capital. Bonding social capital refers to the reinforcement of links between similar people. It builds strong ties, but can also build higher walls to exclude those who are different. Bonding social capital is assumed to be a critical factor in creating and nurturing group solidarity seen in close neighborhoods and ethnic groups. Bridging social capital refers to building connections between heterogeneous groups. Bridging social capital facilitates linkages among different agencies and organizations in a community around a common purpose. A weakness is that measures of these types of social capital do not exist. Social capital functions as invested financial capital, as it generates further production (Putnam, 2000). The property that distinguishes social capital from other forms of capital is a commitment to public good.

A key ingredient of social capital is social support, as this is the initial informal link among individuals. It is important to note the difference between social support, an ingredient of social capital, and social capital, as some authors believe they are the same (Kritsotakis & Gamarnikow, 2004). Social capital is a property of communities, and social support is a property of individuals. Clearly more work is needed to differentiate the two concepts and their influence on the community's health.

The social support component of social capital draws attention to the significant role of the family as a builder and source of social capital through its nurturance, care giving, socialization, values, attitudes, expectations, and habitual patterns of behavior (Bulboz, 2001). Building trust, a component of social capital, begins with the attachment process in infancy and continues throughout early life. Family relationships and behavior also help to establish the principle of reciprocity, the idea of receiving and giving in return, which is another major component of social capital.

Research to test the relationship between social capital and community health promotion has been limited due to the criticism that the social capital concept is too broad and, therefore, not measurable. Descriptive studies provide evidence for a link between social capital and physical and emotional health, rates of violent crime, and children's quality of life (Bolin, Lindgren, Lindstrom, & Nystedt, 2003; Drukker, Kaplan, Feron, & van Os, 2003; Kawachi, Kennedy, & Glass, 1999; Rose, 2000). Contrary findings have also been reported. However, a major issue with these reports is the lack of consistency and limited measures of social capital. Clear definitions and accurate and valid measures are needed to test the theory. Once the link between social capital and health behaviors is clearly established, the next step will be to develop and implement interventions to maintain or promote social capital.

Community Planning Models for Health Promotion

The PRECEDE-PROCEED Model

The PRECEDE-PROCEED Model was designed by Green and colleagues (1999) as a planning model to guide the development of health education programs. The model, which is shown in Figure 3–1, provides a structure to identify and implement the most appropriate intervention strategies. It can be thought of as a road map that provides all possible routes, while theories suggest which avenues to follow. Two fundamental propositions of the model are (a) health and health risks have multiple determinants, and (b) efforts to change the behavioral, environmental, and social environment must be multidimensional. The PRECEDE framework was initially developed in the 1970s. The acronym stands for Predisposing, Reinforcing, and Enabling Constructs in Educational/Ecological Diagnosis and Evaluation. The PRECEDE model is based on the premise that an educational diagnosis should precede an intervention plan. PROCEED was added to the framework to account for the role of environmental factors in health. PROCEED recognizes forces outside the individual that may influence lifestyle behaviors. The acronym stands for Policy, Regulatory, and Organizational Constructs in Educational and Environmental Development. Nine steps make up the planning process. Planning begins with a social assessment to learn people's perceptions of their own needs and life quality. This step involves a community assessment, including problem solving capacity, strengths, and readiness for change. In step 2 an epidemiologic assessment is performed to identify health problems that are most important. Secondary sources of data can be used, such as state and national surveys, to identify major health problems in the community. A behavioral and environmental assessment is performed in step 3 to identify factors that may contribute to

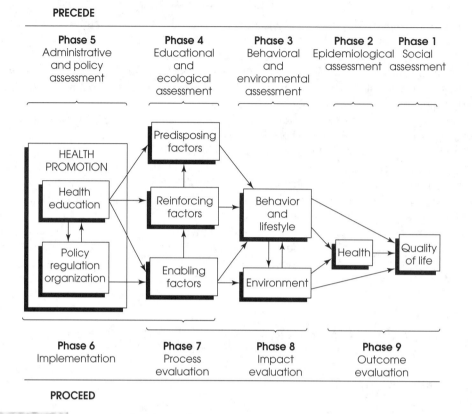

PRECEDE

Phase 5	Phase 4	Phase 3	Phase 2	Phase 1
Administrative and policy assessment	Educational and ecological assessment	Behavioral and environmental assessment	Epidemiological assessment	Social assessment

Phase 6	Phase 7	Phase 8	Phase 9
Implementation	Process evaluation	Impact evaluation	Outcome evaluation

PROCEED

FIGURE 3–1 **The PRECEDE-PROCEED Model for Health Promotion Planning and Evaluation**

(From L. W. Green and M. W. Kreuter, 1999, *Health Promotion Planning: An Educational and Ecological Approach* (3rd ed.), Boston: McGraw Hill. Used with permission.)

the health problem. Behavioral factors include lifestyle behaviors of individuals at risk for the problem, while physical, social, and environmental factors may influence lifestyle behaviors. The community then ranks the identified factors that are amenable to change to prioritize their importance and changeability. At this time individual level as well as community level theories that may be useful are identified to guide interventions for the priority health problems. Step 4 consists of an educational and ecological assessment to identify the predisposing, reinforcing, and enabling factors that must be in place to initiate and sustain the proposed change. Predisposing and reinforcing factors target individual level factors, while enabling factors focus on community level factors such as programs, services, and resources needed. These factors are also prioritized for interventions as in step 3. As in the prior stage, individual and community level interventions are also relevant to guide appropriate interventions. In step 5, administration and policy assessment intervention strategies and planning for implementation occurs. Policies and resources are identified that may facilitate or hinder program implementation. Resources needed, barriers to implementation, and organization policies that may affect implementation are assessed. In step 6 implementation of the planned intervention takes place and both process and outcome evaluations are performed in steps 7 through 9. Objectives, which are written at each step, are the basis for evaluating accomplishments.

The PRECEDE-PROCEED Model has been widely used to plan health promotion programs. Despite its success, several weaknesses have been identified (Gielen & McDonald, 2002). Application of the model requires significant human and financial resources, as the model is data driven. The planning process is time intensive, which may dampen enthusiasm by community members who want to quickly implement change strategies. The model also does not focus on intervention development, so additional guidance may be needed. However, the model is comprehensive, as it incorporates both an individual and community perspective and can be used in a variety of settings. A bibliography of over 700 published papers reporting application of the model is available. (See web site at the end of the chapter.) Application manuals are also available to facilitate its use by practitioners.

Community Dissemination Models to Promote Health

Diffusion of Innovations Model

The Diffusion of Innovations Model was developed to help disseminate health behavior interventions that have been successfully tested into the mainstream for practical use (Rogers, 2003). The framework enables one to understand the process of innovation and the various stages involved in adopting a new idea, thereby narrowing the gap between what is known and what is put to use.

Diffusion has been defined as the process through which an innovation is communicated through certain channels, over time, among members of a social system (Rogers, 2003). It is a special kind of communication to spread messages about new ideas that might represent a certain degree of uncertainty to the individual or organization. Diffusion is a type of social change, as social changes may occur when new ideas are adopted. The terms *dissemination* and *diffusion* are used interchangeably in the Diffusion of Innovations Model.

Four main elements of the diffusion of new ideas are (a) innovation, (b) communication channels, (c) time, and (d) social system. These elements, shown in Figure 3–2, are found in every diffusion program. An innovation is an idea or practice that is thought to be new. It does not matter if the idea is not new, as it is the perceived newness that decides how individuals will react to it. Characteristics that help explain the rate of adoption of an innovation include relative advantage, compatibility, complexity, trialability, and observability. *Relative advantage* is the degree to which the innovation is perceived better than the current, older idea. It does not matter if the innovation has no true advantage. What matters is whether an individual thinks the innovation will be better. *Compatibility* is the degree to which an innovation is perceived to fit with existing values and past experiences. Innovations that are consistent with the prevalent values and norms of the social system are more likely to be adopted. For example, an incompatible

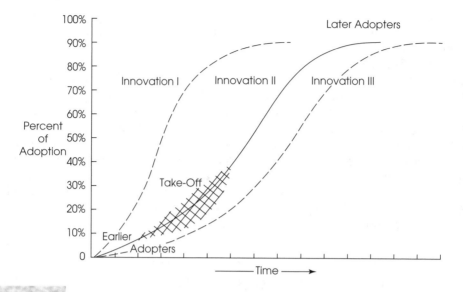

(From G. M. Rogers, 1971)

FIGURE 3–2 **The Diffusion Process**

innovation is the use of contraceptives in a traditionally Catholic country, as it is unlikely that the majority would adopt it. *Complexity* is the degree to which the innovation is thought to be difficult to understand or use. In general new ideas that are simple to understand are more easily adopted than complex ones. *Trialability* is the extent to which the innovation may be considered tentative for a limited time period. Ideas that can be tried in installments are usually adopted more quickly than ones that cannot be divided. Last, *observability* is the degree to which the results of the innovation are visible to others. The easier it is to see results, the more likely the idea will be adopted. These five characteristics are not the only ones that influence the diffusion of innovations. However, they are the most important ones for adoption. Additional characteristics include the influence of the innovation on social relationships, the ability to reverse the innovation, the ability to easily communicate the innovation, the time needed to adopt the innovation, the commitment needed to adopt the innovation, and the ability to modify the innovation over time (Olderburg & Parcel, 2002).

Communication must take place for an innovation to spread. Mass media channels are used to reach large audiences to provide initial information of the innovation. Since diffusion is a process of people talking to people, interpersonal, or face-to-face, communication channels are more effective in forming and changing attitudes toward a new idea.

Innovativeness refers to the degree to which individuals, organizations, or systems adopt new ideas or practices. Five adopter categories have been described: innovators, early adopters, early majority, late majority, and laggards. These patterns of adoption have been shown to be predictable in a variety of populations and settings. *Innovators* are active information seekers and are able to cope with high levels of uncertainty about a new idea. They are the first to adopt a new idea and are role models for others in the social system. *Early adopters* have the greatest degree of opinion leadership in most social systems and are considered the person to check with before adopting the innovation. The *early majority* may deliberate before adopting, so they seldom lead in adoption of the idea. The *late majority* view innovations with skepticism and may only adopt because of increasing pressure from peers, or they feel it is safe to adopt. Needless to say, the *laggards* tend to be suspicious of innovations and change. They must be sure that the innovation will not fail before they will adopt and often slow down the innovation diffusion process. Identification of adopter categories facilitates implementing new health-behavior programs or behaviors, as it is important to know that everyone will not accept the change in the same time frame. Laggards, for example, will need more time and evidence that the change is effective and safe. Identification of early adopters will facilitate change, as these are the opinion leaders in a social system who can influence others.

Preventive innovations are defined as new ideas that require action at one point in time in order to avoid unwanted consequences at a future point in time (Rogers, 2002). The rewards of adopting a preventive innovation are delayed, intangible, and unwanted consequences may never occur, resulting in a low relative advantage of the innovation. Relative advantage is the most important predictor of the rate of adoption of an innovation, so it is understandable why preventive innovations may be slow or may fail to be adopted. To increase the rate of adoption of a preventive innovation, perceived relative advantages of the preventive innovation need to be identified and made visible as much as possible. For example, the relative advantage of dietary changes for those at risk for hypertension is low, as hypertension does not have immediate or obvious symptoms.

Strategies to speed up the adoption of preventive innovations include increasing the relative advantage of the innovation; using role models to devote their personal influence to promote the innovation; changing the system norms through peer support; placing educational ideas in entertainment messages; and activating peer communication networks.

Diffusion of an innovation is a complex multilevel change process, as change must occur at multiple levels across different settings, using multiple change strategies. A multilevel change process is needed to promote widespread behavior change. Application of the diffusion model has resulted in a decrease in the rate of smoking in many countries (Warner, 2000). Diffusion of Innovation Models have also been successful in promoting safe sexual practices in the general population (De Vroome, Paalman, Dingelstad, Kolker, & Sandfort, 1994). Understanding the diffusion process enables health care practitioners to implement behavior changes at multiple levels. The theory is based on many years of research in diffusion of innovations to change behaviors, programs, and policies to promote health. The theory incorporates strategies to promote widespread, long-term change. The theory also takes into account social structures and communication systems, as well as characteristics of the innovation to promote successful behavior change.

Social Marketing Model

In a social marketing model, commercial marketing technologies are applied to plan, implement, and evaluate programs to influence voluntary behavior change of target audiences to improve health (Anderson, 1995). Marketing practices that have traditionally been used in business advertising are applied to social purposes to adopt an idea, product, or behavior. Six principles are adhered to in social marketing (Bryant, 2000). These include (a) a consumer orientation, (b) the use of a marketing framework to design behavior change interventions, (c) recognition of competition, (d) reliance on research to understand consumer needs and desires, (e) segmentation of populations and careful selection of target audiences, and (f) continuous monitoring and revision of program tactics to achieve positive health outcomes. A marketing approach goes beyond education to change behavior, as social marketers attempt to increase the attractiveness of the desired behavior, so that consumers will desire the new behavior. Efforts are made to provide immediate effects, as immediate reinforcement has a greater potential to shape behavior (Maibach, Rothschild, & Novelli, 2002).

The social marketing framework considers the "Four P's": product, price, place, and promotion (Kotler & Roberto, 1989). The product is the health-promotion program or desired health behavior. Price refers to the social, emotional, and monetary costs associated with adoption of the program or behavior. Place is the distribution point or location of the intervention program, and promotion refers to the behavior being promoted and strategies used to persuade adoption of the desired behavior. An additional concept is the product's competition, or the risk behavior currently practiced.

The five interrelated components and basic principles previously described serve as guides to design implementation strategies for target populations. The product must provide a solution to problems that consumers believe is important to them. Competition means that consumers are confronted with making a choice between the new behavior and the current risk behavior. Thus, the new behavior (product) must offer benefits to the consumer. Price, from the consumer's perspective, is the cost, such as the cost of joining a health club to exercise. Costs may also be time, effort, and emotional discomfort in changing behaviors such as smoking cessation. Place is also an important component for consumers, and social marketers try to assess when and where the target audience will be most receptive to messages, or where and when they are ready to purchase products. Promotion uses strategies, such as communication objectives for the target audience, strategies for designing attention getting, effective messages, and credible, trustworthy spokespersons. Strategies may include mass communication, public information, consumer education, direct mail, public relations, and printed materials. Additional promotion strategies that may be implemented include service delivery enhancements, policy changes, and use of coupons to attract consumers.

The consumer orientation in social marketing distinguishes it from other approaches in health promotion. In a consumer orientation, one must understand the consumer's perception of product benefits, price, the competition's benefits and costs, and other factors that may influence consumer behavior. Research findings are used to identify recommendations for health-promotion programs. Recommendations, based on research defining what works best, assist in planning marketing strategies.

Social marketing uses audience segmentation to select target audiences, a process of dividing the population into distinct segments based on characteristics that might influence their response to the marketing program (Bryant, 2000). Segments identify smaller groups that can be reached with available resources. Group profiles help decide who to target and the best way to reach the targeted segment.

In social marketing, programs are monitored continuously to evaluate their effectiveness in promoting change. Continuous monitoring also enables one to identify activities that need to be revised as well as activities that are most effective. The target audience is constantly checked for their responsiveness to the intervention.

Social marketing models of dissemination have been successfully combined with the PRECEDE-PROCEED Model to plan the proposed intervention (Guidotti, Ford, & Wheeler, 2000). In the Fort McMurray Project, which promoted community health and safety, marketing strategies included use of a mascot for visual identity for the project, cable television public service announcements, programs in local schools, and consumer safety audits. An older example of the application of social marketing strategies to cardiovascular disease prevention is the Pawtucket Heart Health Project (Lefebure, Harder, & Zampa, 1998). The project combined a social marketing model with a social-ecological approach and social learning theory. Social marketing was used to promote and deliver the program for segments of the community. Channels of communication included personal contact by peers and mass media. The community was a valuable partner throughout the project. Social marketing models have also been implemented to promote fruit and vegetable consumption, safe sex practices, physical activity, prenatal care, and family planning.

The social marketing model is a valuable model to assist in disseminating results of health-promotion programs. As with other models, it requires time and resources. However, a consumer orientation is worth the effort as it has the potential to promote healthy communities by promoting such activities as physical activity in communities, and healthy choices when eating out, as well as larger scale environmental changes, including decreasing single occupancy vehicles and increasing public transportation use (Maibach, 2003).

Directions for Research in Community-Based Models

Limited success of individual level theories and models to achieve long-term changes in health behavior has led to an exploration of the role of community theories and models in health promotion. Community level theories and models are not new. However, these models have only recently been used to guide health-promotion interventions to promote community change, so many questions still need to be answered. Research is needed to test and refine these theories. Application of these models will open avenues to develop new theories and models to guide behavior change for communities. Since the individual, group, and community are of interest in community health promotion, models that include all three levels are needed. Multilevel models are complex and need further development and testing. Additional research in the following areas is recommended.

1. Identify and describe the critical sociocultural and environmental influences on health behavior.
2. Develop and test reliable and valid measures of social capital.
3. Identify sensitive and measurable community outcomes of health promotion.
4. Develop and test programs that target community change.
5. Test the effectiveness of the diffusion models to produce community-level changes in health behaviors.

Directions for Practice Using Community Models of Health

Although community models of health promotion have been limited in their application, the concepts are important for practice. Individuals as well as communities in which they live need to be assessed prior to implementing health-promotion programs. For example, assessment of an individual's physical and social environment as well as social capital will provide helpful information about facilitators and barriers to healthy lifestyle practices in the community. Knowledge of the physical environment will shed light on the resources (or lack thereof) in a neighborhood, such as walking areas and access to grocery stores or transportation, that influence one's ability to implement the proposed change. The Diffusion of Innovations Model, as well as social marketing approaches, can be used to facilitate change within a community. Learning to identify characteristics of adopters will enable the nurse to choose specific strategies that need to be stressed for successful change, depending, for example, on whether one is an innovator or laggard. As the nurse gains a broader understanding of the role of the community and greater social system in promoting health, interventions can be developed to target changes that are realistic, feasible, and likely to be successful for individuals and communities.

SUMMARY

The increased interest in community-based models to promote healthy behaviors has occurred because of a greater need to understand the complex etiologies of health problems, an appreciation of the interrelationship between individuals and their social and physical environment, and recognition of the limits of individual models to promote health. Community-based models focus on contextual factors that influence health, such as social conditions, and the political, institutional, legislative, and physical environments in which behavior occurs. Community models are in the early stages of testing, so additional research is needed before the most effective models are identified to guide health promotion interventions. Last, diffusion of innovations and social marketing models have the potential to promote widespread change.

LEARNING ACTIVITIES

1. Describe three ways in which people in communities can be empowered to participate in their health.
2. What elements in a community would you assess using a social-ecological model for health behavior?
3. Apply the nine steps in the PRECEDE-PROCEED Model to design a program to improve a specific health behavior such as physical activity for adolescents. Which individual and community theories would you choose to implement the program?

4. Using the "Four P's" of the social marketing framework, choose and design a behavior change intervention for a specific segment of the population, such as women between the ages of 25 and 40 years or men over the age of 50 years. How would you evaluate the effectiveness of the change?

SELECTED WEB SITES

Diffusion of Innovation Model

http://www.ksu.edu/humec/atid/UDF/diffusion_model.htm

PRECEDE-PROCEED Model

http://www.ihpr.ubc.ca.

http://www.med.usf.edu/~kmbrown/PRECEDE_PROCEED_Overview.htm

REFERENCES

Anderson, A. (1995). *Marketing social change: Changing behavior to promote health, social development and the environment.* San Francisco: Jossey-Bass.

Anderson, L. M., Scrimshaw, S. C., Fullilove, M. T., & Fielding, J. E. (2003). Task force on community preventive services. The community guide's model for linking the social environment to health. *American Journal of Preventive Medicine, 24*(suppl 1), 12–20.

Bolin, K., Lindgren, B., Lindstrom, M., & Nystedt, P. (2003). Investment in social capital: Implications of social interactions for the production of health. *Social Science & Medicine, 6,* 2379–2390.

Bryant, C. (2000). Social marketing: A new approach to improved patient care. *Primary Care Update OB/Gyns, 7,* 161–167.

Bulboz, M. M. (2001). Family as source, user and builder of social capital. *Journal of Socio-Economics, 30,* 29–131.

Clitheroe, H. C., & Stokols, D. (1998). Conceptualizing the context of environment and behavior. *Journal of Environmental Psychology, 18,* 3–12.

Corbett, K. K. (2001). Susceptibility of youth to tobacco: A social ecological framework for prevention. *Respiratory Physiology, 128,* 3–118.

De Vroome, E. M., Paalman, M. E., Dingelstad, A. A., Kolker, L., & Sandfort, T. G. (1994). Increase in safe sex among the young and non-monogamous: Knowledge, attitudes and behaviors regarding safe sex and condom use in the Netherlands from 1987–1993. *Patient Education and Counseling, 24,* 79–288.

Drukker, M., Kaplan, C., Feron, F., & van Os, J. (2003). Children's health-related quality of life, neighborhood socio-economic deprivation and social capital. A contextual analysis. *Social Science & Medicine, 57*(5), 825–841.

Eriksson, C. (2002). Learning and knowledge production for public health: A review of approaches to evidenced-based health. *Scand J Public Health, 28,* 298–308.

Gielen, A. C., & McDonald, E. M. (2002). Using PRECEDE-PROCEED planning model to apply health behavior theories. In K. Glanz, B. K. Rimer, & F. M. Lewis (Eds.), *Health behavior and health education theory, research and practice* (3rd ed., pp. 409–436). San Francisco: Jossey-Bass.

Green, L. W., & Kreuter, M. W. (1999). *Health promotion planning: An educational and ecological approach* (3rd ed.). Boston: McGraw Hill.

Guidotti, T. L., Ford, L., & Wheeler, M. (2000). The Fort McMurray demonstration project in social marketing: Theory, design and evaluation. *American Journal of Preventive Medicine, 18,* 163–169.

Joos, I. M., Nelson, R., & Lyness, A. (1985). Systems theory. In *Man, health and nursing* (pp. 79–91). Reston, VA: Prentice Hall.

Kawachi, I., Kennedy, R., & Glass, R. (1999). Social capital and self-rated health: A contextual analysis. *American Journal of Public Health, 89,* 1187–1193.

Kotler, P., & Roberto, E. (1989). *Social marketing strategies for changing public behavior.* New York: Free Press.

Kreuter, M. W., & Lezin, N. (2002). Social capital theory: Implications for community based health promotion. In R. J. DiClemente, R. A. Crosby, & M. C. Kegler (Eds.), *Emerging theories in health promotion practice and research* (pp. 228–254). San Francisco: Jossey-Bass.

Kritsotakis, G., & Gamarnikow, E. (2004). What is social capital and how does it relate to health? *International Journal of Nursing Studies, 41,* 43–50.

Lefebure, R. C., Harder, E. A., & Zampa, B. (1998). The Pawtucket Heart program III: Social marketing strategies to promote community health. *Rhode Island Medical Journal, 71,* 27–30.

Lin, N. (2001). The theory and theoretical propositions. In N. Lin, *Social capital: A theory of social structure and action* (pp. 55–77). Cambridge, United Kingdom: Cambridge University Press.

Lowry, L. W., & Martin, K. S. (2004). Organizing frameworks applied to community health nursing. In M. Stanhope & J. Lancaster (Eds.), *Community and public health nursing* (pp. 194–219). St. Louis: Mosby.

Maibach, E. W. (2003). Recreating communities to support active living: A new role for social marketing. *American Journal of Health Promotion, 18*(1), 114–119.

Maibach, E. W., Rothschild, M. L., & Novelli, W. D. (2002). Social marketing. In K. Glanz, B. K. Rimer, & F. M. Lewis (Eds.), *Health behavior and health education theory, research and practice* (3rd ed., pp. 437–461). San Francisco: Jossey-Bass.

McKnight, J. L. (2002). Two tools for well-being: Health systems. In M. Minkler (Ed.), *Community organizing & community building for health* (pp. 20–29). New Brunswick, NJ: Rutgers University Press.

Minkler, M. (2000). Health promotion at the dawn of the 21st century: Challenges and dilemma. In M. S. Jamner & D. Stokols (Eds.), *Promoting human wellness* (pp. 349–377). Berkeley: University of California Press.

Minkler, M., & Wallerstein, N. B. (2002). Improving health through community organization and community building. In K. Glanz, B. K. Rimer, & F. M. Lewis (Eds.), *Health behavior and health education theory, research and practice* (3rd ed., pp. 279–311). San Francisco: Jossey-Bass.

Norton, B. L., McLeroy, K. R., Burdine, J. N., Felix, M. R., & Dorsey, A. M. (2002). Community capacity: Concept, theory, and methods. In R. J. DiClemente, R. A. Crosby, and M. C. Kegler (Eds.), *Emerging theories in health promotion practice and research* (pp. 194–227). San Francisco: Jossey-Bass.

Olderburg, B., & Parcel, G. S. (2002). Diffusion of innovations. In K. Glanz, B. K. Rimer, & F. M. Lewis (Eds.), *Health behavior and health education theory, research and practice* (3rd ed., 312–334). San Francisco: Jossey-Bass.

Putnam, R. (2000). *Bowling alone: The collapse and revival of American community.* New York: Simon & Schuster.

Rhodes, T. (2003). The "risk environment": A framework for understanding and reducing drug-related harm. *International Journal of Drug Policy, 13,* 85–94.

Robertson, A., & Minkler, M. (1995). The new health promotion movement: A critical examination. *Health Education Quarterly, 21*(3), 295–312.

Rogers, E. M. (2002). Diffusion of preventive innovations. *Addictive Behaviors, 27,* 989–993.

Rogers, E. M. (2003). *Diffusions of innovations* (5th ed.). New York: Free Press.

Rose, R. (2000). How much does social capital add to individual health? A survey study of Russians. *Social Science & Medicine, 51,* 421–435.

Sallis, J., McKenzie, T. L., Conway, T. I., et al. (2003). Environmental interventions for eating and physical activity: A randomized controlled trial in middle schools. *American Journal of Preventive Medicine, 24*(3), 209–217.

Sallis, J. F., & Owen, N. (2002). Ecological models of health behavior. In K. Glanz, B. K. Rimer, & F. M. Lewis (Eds.), *Health behavior and health education theory, research and practice* (3rd ed., pp. 464–484). San Francisco: Jossey-Bass.

Shuster, G. F., & Goeppinger, J. (2004). Community as client: Assessment and analysis. In M. Stanhope & J. Lancaster (Eds.), *Community and public health nursing* (pp. 342–375). St. Louis: Mosby.

Spence, J. C., & Lee, R. E. (2003). Toward a comprehensive model of physical activity. *Psychology of Sport and Exercise, 4,* 7–24.

Stokols, D. (2000). The social ecological paradigm of wellness promotion. In M. S. Jamner & D. Stokols (Eds.), *Promoting human wellness* (pp. 21–37). Berkeley: University of California Press.

Von Bertalanffy, L. (1975). General systems theory. In B. D. Ruben & J. Y. Kim (Eds.), *General systems theory and human communication.* Rochelle Park, NJ: Hayden Book Co.

Warner, K. (2000). The need for and value for a multi-level approach to disease prevention: The case of tobacco control. In D. B. Smedley & S. L. Syme (Eds.), *Promoting health intervention strategies from social and behavioral research.* Washington, DC: National Academy Press.

World Health Organization. (1974). *Community health nursing: Report of a WHO expert committee.* Report No. 559. Geneva, Switzerland: WHO.

Part 2

Planning for Health Promotion and Prevention

4

Assessing Health and Health Behaviors

OBJECTIVES

1. Describe the expected outcomes of a nursing health assessment.
2. Identify the components of a nursing health assessment conducted for an individual client.
3. Describe age-appropriate and culturally appropriate nursing health assessment tools for children, adults, and older adults.
4. Discuss the similarities and differences among the various approaches to assessing the family.
5. Discuss the similarities and differences among the various approaches to assessing the community.

OUTLINE

- Nursing Frameworks for Health Assessment
- Assessment of the Individual Client
  A. Physical Fitness
  B. Nutrition
  C. Life Stress
  D. Spiritual Health
  E. Social Support Systems
  F. Lifestyle
- Assessment of the Family

- Assessment of the Community
- Directions for Research in Health Assessment
- Directions for Practice in Health Assessment
- Summary
- Learning Activities
- Selected Web Sites
- References

A thorough assessment of health and health behaviors is the foundation for tailoring a health promotion-prevention plan to a given client. Assessment provides the database for making clinical judgments about the client's health strengths, health problems, nursing diagnoses, and desired health or behavioral outcomes, as well as the interventions likely to be effective. This information determines the nature of the client–health professional encounter. The portfolio of assessment measures used depends on characteristics of the client, including developmental stage and cultural orientation. The nurse should assess the cultural appropriateness of the various tools for target populations. The nurse also needs to understand her own culture and the client's culture, as well as recognize that diversity exists in all cultures based on educational level, socioeconomic status, religion, rural/urban, and individual and family characteristics. All of these components must be considered in determining the cultural appropriateness of the selected measure. National Standards for Culturally and Linguistically Appropriate Services in Health Care (2004) provide a practical guide for nurses to offer culturally and linguistically sensitive care.

Nursing clinics, community health centers, and primary care centers should maintain an up-to-date resource file of assessment tools so that the portfolio for any given client may be customized. In this chapter, the primary focus is on assessment of the individual. Approaches for assessing families and communities are also discussed.

Nursing Frameworks for Health Assessment

Health assessment performed by the nurse (nursing assessment) is a collaborative process with the client that promotes mutual input into decision making and planning to improve the client's health and well-being. The desired outcomes of a nursing assessment are to determine (a) health assets, (b) health problems (c) health-related lifestyle strengths, (d) key health-related beliefs, (e) health behaviors that put the client at risk, and (f) how desired changes would improve quality of life. The initial assessment provides a valuable baseline against which subsequent assessments may be compared.

Several frameworks for nursing assessment and diagnosis are available. At this point, it is important to differentiate between nursing assessment and nursing diagnosis as they are used in this book. **Nursing assessment** is systematic collection of data about the client's health status, beliefs, and behaviors relevant to developing a health promotion-prevention plan. **Nursing diagnosis** is the identification of areas that may be enhanced to maximize health status.

A number of nursing diagnostic classification systems (taxonomies) have been developed by nursing groups to guide clinical decisions. These taxonomies focus primarily on the individual and aspects of illness. Positive health states or strengths of the individual, family, or community are not adequately addressed in these taxonomies. Some of the taxonomies have been expanded to include diagnoses appropriate to aspects of wellness and family and community-focused needs. Nursing must continue to expand its taxonomies to further classify wellness activities as the knowledge about health promotion and prevention continues to expand.

The North American Nursing Diagnosis Association (NANDA) provides a nursing diagnosis taxonomy structured around the nine human response patterns of exchanging, communicating, relating, valuing, choosing, moving, perceiving, knowing, and feeling. The NANDA defining characteristics of each diagnosis, as well as related factors and risk factors, provide guidance about the critical assessment areas for the diagnosis. Following health assessment, the NANDA classification provides one way to clearly label some of the issues and problems identified. A limited number of diagnoses that address family and wellness have been added to the NANDA classification of 161 nursing diagnoses (Carpenito, 2004). For example, physical activity deficit has been proposed as a diagnosis to encourage nurses to assess exercise habits in the assessment of their clients (Barnett-Damewood & Carlson-Catalano, 2000).

Gordon (2002) grouped the NANDA diagnoses under 11 functional health patterns to assist in classifying nursing diagnoses. The functional health patterns are: health perception–health management, nutritional–metabolic, elimination, activity–exercise, sleep–rest, cognitive–perceptual, self-perception–self-concept, role–relationship, sexuality–reproductive, coping–stress tolerance, and value–belief. A major strength of Gordon's work is the provision of guidelines to conduct a nursing history and examination to assess clients' functional health patterns. As assessment proceeds, diagnostic hypotheses are generated to direct targeted or more detailed data collection. The reader is referred to the *Manual of Nursing Diagnoses* for the recommended formats for assessment of functional health patterns in infants and young children, adults, families, and communities (Gordon, 2002).

An attempt to develop diagnoses related to community nursing resulted in the Omaha Visiting Nurse Association System (Martin & Norris, 1996). The Omaha System incorporates the needs of individuals and families in categories of environment, psychosocial, physiological, and health behavior needs. These categories are referenced by key words such as *individual*, or *family*, or *health promotion*. Health promotion is addressed in the individual and family (Kaiser, Hays, Cho, & Agrawal, 2002). Nurse researchers have shown its usefulness in quantifying nursing practice in home care, nursing centers, and school health programs (Bednarz, 1998; Marek, 1996; Martin & Norris, 1996). The Omaha System does not apply to the health behavior needs of groups and is of limited use in assessing communities, but is useful for target populations (i.e., at risk for heart disease, obesity). One of the difficulties of developing nursing diagnoses for communities is that nursing diagnoses focus on nursing practice whereas community diagnoses must be more interdisciplinary in nature (Ervin, 2002). The Nursing Interventions Classification (NIC) system is relevant for community health because nursing services are categorized and linked to direct reimbursement (Clark, 2003). However, NIC does not have categories for the health behavior of communities.

Assessment of client strengths related to health promotion is the focus of the published guide, *Nursing Diagnosis for Wellness: Supporting Strengths*. This guide incorporates some of the NANDA diagnostic categories but has been expanded to include wellness diagnoses organized according to the functional health patterns proposed by Gordon.

Examples of wellness nursing diagnoses (client strengths) include nutrition, adequate to meet or maintain body requirements (nutrition–metabolic); exercise level, appropriate to maintain wellness state (activity–exercise); and spiritual strength (value–belief). Case studies and sample care plans illustrate how diagnostic statements provide direction for health promotion-prevention care planning (Houldin, Saltstein, & Ganley, 1987).

Assessment of the Individual Client

Assessment of the individual client in the context of health promotion expands beyond physical assessment to also include a comprehensive examination of other health parameters and health behaviors. The components of health assessment focusing on individual clients are (a) functional health patterns (b) physical fitness, (c) nutrition, (d) life stress, (e) spiritual health, (f) social support systems, (g) health beliefs, and (h) lifestyle. Components are addressed based on the purpose of the assessment, setting, functional health, and age of the client. Functional health assessment for patterns includes a health history and physical assessment conducted by the nurse. Other assessment components that focus on individual clients and have particular relevance for health promotion-prevention are described here.

Physical Fitness

Physical activity is an important part of personal health status and is discussed in detail in Chapter 6. Evaluation of physical fitness is a critical part of any nursing assessment because a sedentary lifestyle, for many individuals, begins early in childhood and continues into adulthood. The assessment is applicable to clients of all ages, with restrictions on some areas for individuals who are physically compromised. It is important to differentiate between skill-related physical fitness and health-related physical fitness. Skill-related fitness is defined by qualities that contribute to successful athletic performance: agility, speed, power, and reaction time. Health-related fitness includes qualities found to contribute to one's general health, including cardio-respiratory endurance, muscular endurance, body composition, and flexibility (American College of Sports Medicine [ACSM], 1995). Health-related physical fitness qualities are briefly discussed in the following sections.

Cardio-Respiratory Endurance Fitness reflects the ability of the circulatory and respiratory (CR) systems to efficiently adjust to and recover from exercise. A number of approaches are used to assess CR endurance. For example, the President's Challenge Physical Fitness test, the 1-mile walk/run, may be used for children and adolescents between 6 and 17. The individual is asked to walk or run 1 mile at a steady pace over the entire distance. One mile can be measured on either an outdoor or indoor track. Youths are encouraged to practice the day before and warm up just before the walk or run. Health fitness standards for a 10-year-old boy range from 9 to 11:30 minutes and for a 16-year-old boy, 7 to 8:30 minutes. The range for girls of the same ages is 30 seconds to 1 minute more in each category (Cooper, 1999; Freedson, Cureton, & Heath, 2000).

Another assessment approach is the step test that is a field version of the laboratory stress test for adults. If the step test is conducted in a clinic setting, the electrocardiogram may be monitored. A physician should be available for emergency backup if the client is over 40 years of age, obese, or has a history of cardiovascular problems. The step test is not as physiologically stressful as the laboratory stress test, but caution must be taken in individuals with high-risk profiles for cardiovascular disease. For the step test, a step 16 to 17 inches high is recommended. The step rate should be 24 steps per minute for men and 22 steps per minute for women. Each step consists of the following sequence: left foot up; right foot up; left foot down; right foot down. Apical or carotid pulse rates are measured after stepping for 3 minutes at the prescribed cadence. With the client comfortably seated in a chair following step testing, pulse rates are counted for 15 seconds in immediate recovery (5 to 20 seconds) and multiplied by 4 to obtain recovery heart rate. Recovery rate of 140 for women and 124 for men is in the low-risk range of recovery while a recovery rate of 184 for women and 178 for men is in the high-risk range of recovery (American College of Sports Medicine, 2001).

Muscular Endurance   Bent-knee sit-ups are used as a test of muscular endurance, for children, youths, and adults (Figure 4–1). The number of sit-ups per minute is counted. The fitness standard for 10- to 17-year-olds is 9 to 12 sit-ups in 1 minute (ACSM, 2001). Adults 50 years of age and older and those with cardiovascular disorders must be observed carefully for fatigue during endurance testing. Sit-ups should be terminated if signs of distress occur. Men ages 36 to 45 years are rated as excellent if they can perform 42 or more sit-ups, and women if they can perform 39 or more sit-ups. Men and women in this age range are below average if they can only perform 21 and 12, respectively. Men ages 46 years and older are rated excellent if they can perform 38 or more sit-ups, and women if they can perform 24 or more sit-ups. Men and women are below average if they can perform only 18 and 11, respectively (ACSM, 2001). Sit-ups must be performed accurately to prevent injury.

Timed sit-ups may not adequately measure abdominal strength or endurance because the hip flexor muscles are involved in addition to the abdominal muscles (Cooper, 1999). The push-up muscular endurance test and the bench press test are also used to evaluate muscle endurance. Procedures for conducting these endurance tests are found in the

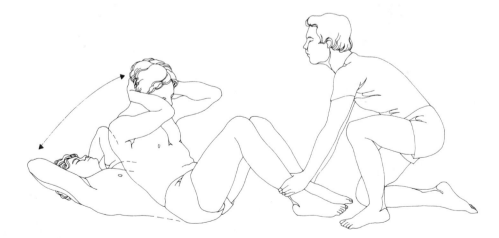

FIGURE 4–1   **Bent-Knee Sit-Ups**

American College of Sports Medicine's (ACSM)'s *Guidelines for Exercise Testing and Prescription* (2001), and Freedson et al.'s (2000) article on fitness testing in children and youth. The nurse must decide which muscular endurance test to use based on the client's health history and current field-testing reports.

Body Composition Estimates of body fat may be done several ways. Hydrostatic underwater weighing is considered the gold standard or most accurate estimate of indirect body fat. However, it is seldom used in the clinical setting because of the complex and expensive equipment required and the time and potential anxiety involved. Skin-fold measurement is used most frequently to assess body composition. Since approximately half of the body fat is subcutaneous, total body fat may be estimated by this method. A pair of skin-fold calipers is used to take measures at the chest, midaxillary, triceps, sub scapular, abdomen, supprailic, and thigh sites (Figure 4–2). Duplicative measures are taken at each of the sites to ensure accuracy. All measurements should be taken on the right side to conform to standard measurement technique. The sum of the sub scapula and the triceps skin folds or the calf and triceps skin folds are used to obtain a measure of body fat in children and youth. For boys between 5 and 18 years of age, a sum of skin folds between 10 and 25 is a measure of normal body fat (10 to 20%). Skin-fold sums between 16 and 30 are measures of normal body fat (14 to 25%) for young girls. High blood pressure and high cholesterol are associated with estimated body fat greater than 30% in girls and 25% in boys (Freedson et al., 2000). For young men 25 years old a triceps skin-fold sum less than 20 is indicative of normal body composition; for 25-year-old women a triceps skin fold of less than 28 represents normal body composition (Table 4–1). Results above or below these values should alert the health care provider to assess for either too much or too little nutrient intake for body requirements. Skin-fold estimates have been shown to have an error rate as high as 21% in young adult males because of the inherent variability in the ratio of subcutaneous to total body fat (Beddoe, 1998). In the absence of a more accurate and

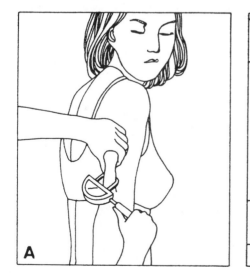
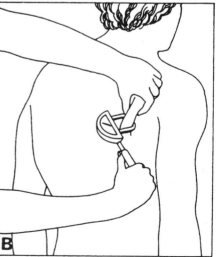

FIGURE 4–2 **Skin-Fold Sites A Triceps. B Sub scapula**

TABLE 4–1	Triceps Skin-Fold Thickness Indicating Obesity (mm)	
Age (yr)	Males	Females
5	≥12	≥15
10	≥13	≥17
15	≥15	≥20
20	≥16	≥28
25	≥20	≥29
30 and above	≥23	≥30

affordable field test to measure body fat, skin-fold measurement must be performed with an appreciation of its limitation. Error may be reduced by adhering to standards related to the location and measurement of the correct sites, use of quality skin-fold calipers, and recognition that body types are different.

Flexibility Flexibility, the ability to move muscles and joints through their maximum range of motion, is also an important component of physical fitness. Flexibility may decrease with age or as a result of chronic illness. The lack of ability to flex or extend muscles or joints often reflects poor health habits, such as sedentary lifestyle, poor posture, or faulty body mechanics. Loss of flexibility greatly decreases one's ability to move about with ease and comfort.

Trunk flexion measures the ability to stretch the low back and thigh or hamstring muscles. The sit-and-reach test is the most commonly used test to measure flexion. The client sits on a floor mat or flat examining table with legs fully extended and feet flat against a box (Figure 4–3). Arms and hands are extended forward as far as possible and held for a count of three. With a ruler, the distance that the client can reach beyond the proximal edge of the box is measured in inches. If the client cannot reach the edge, the distance of the fingertips from the edge is measured and reported as a negative number. Norms for trunk flexion vary among men and women. The desired range for men is + 1 to + 5 inches; for women, + 2 to + 6 (Cooper, 1999). The validity of this test has been challenged by some researchers because one's arm-to-leg length ratio may influence one's reach (Freedson et al., 2000). Individual differences must be taken into consideration; however, despite the limitations of the sit-and-reach test, it does provide a reasonably accurate measure of flexibility.

A physical fitness evaluation will assist the client to plan an appropriate exercise or physical activity program. Careful attention to assessment will optimize the fit of the exercise prescription to the physical capabilities of the client.

Nutrition

Effective planning for health promotion requires evaluation of the nutritional status of clients. Anthropometrical variables, laboratory values, and dietary habits are all important measures to use to establish a base line (McVay-Smith, 2001). Anthropometric assessment measures include height and weight, circumference of various areas of the body, and skinfold thickness. Height is measured wearing 1-inch heels. Weight is taken with lightweight clothing. Body mass index (BMI) is the best method to assess healthy weight (ACSM, 2001).

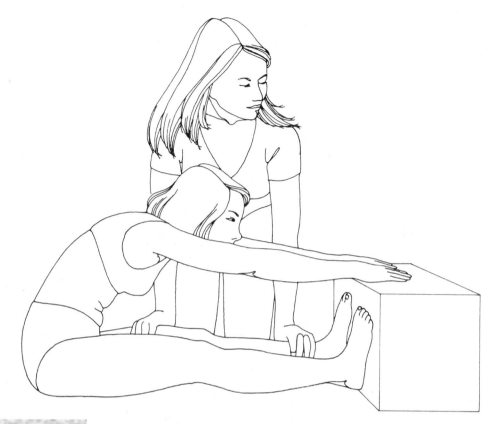

FIGURE 4–3 Trunk Flexion

BMI does not assess body fat distribution, but it is a useful screening tool for overweight or obesity. The BMI table for adults is shown in Table 4–2 and the classification standards for adults are in Table 4–3. A quick measure to assess healthy weight, overweight, and obese categories is found in Table 4–4. In addition to BMI, skin-fold measurements provide a simple criterion for obesity. Triceps skin-fold thickness indicative of obesity for children, adolescents, men, and women of differing age groups are presented in Table 4–1. Deviations from any of the norms on the measurements are recorded in the nutritional assessment. The waist-to-hip ratio is used to assess the amount of fat distributed in the abdomen versus fat distributed below the waist. The ratio is the waist circumference over the hip circumference. The higher the value of the waist-to-hip ratio, the greater the risk of health problems for the client (ACSM, 2001).

Biochemical analyses of blood and urine are used to identify nutritional deficiencies. In addition to laboratory tests for cholesterol, triglycerides, glucose, and high-density lipoproteins, tests for protein (creatinine index, serum protein, serum albumin, total lymphocyte count, blood urea nitrogen, and uric acid), serum or plasma vitamin levels (water-soluble, fat-soluble) and minerals (calcium, sodium, potassium, iron, phosphorus, and magnesium) are used to assess nutritional status. Three values that are particularly important in assessing nutritional status are serum albumin less than 3.5 g/dL,

TABLE 4–2 Body Mass Index (BMI Table)

BMI	19	20	21	22	23	24	25	26	27	28	29	30	31	32	33	34	35
Height								Weight (in pounds)									
4'10" (58")	91	96	100	105	110	115	119	124	129	134	138	143	148	153	158	162	167
4'11" (59")	94	99	104	109	114	119	124	128	133	138	143	148	153	158	163	168	173
5' (60")	97	102	107	112	118	123	128	133	138	143	148	153	158	163	168	174	179
5'1" (61")	100	106	111	116	122	127	132	137	143	148	153	158	164	169	174	180	185
5'2" (62")	104	109	115	120	126	131	136	142	147	153	158	164	169	175	180	186	191
5'3" (63")	107	113	118	124	130	135	141	146	152	158	163	169	175	180	186	191	197
5'4" (64")	110	116	122	128	134	140	145	151	157	163	169	174	180	186	192	197	204
5'5" (65")	114	120	126	132	138	144	150	156	162	168	174	180	186	192	198	204	210
5'6" (66")	118	124	130	136	142	148	155	161	167	173	179	186	192	198	204	210	216
5'7" (67")	121	127	134	140	146	153	159	166	172	178	185	191	198	204	211	217	223
5'8" (68")	125	131	138	144	151	158	164	171	177	184	190	197	203	210	216	223	230
5'9" (69")	128	135	142	149	155	162	169	176	182	189	196	203	209	216	223	230	236
5'10" (70")	132	139	146	153	160	167	174	181	188	195	202	209	216	222	229	236	243
5'11" (71")	136	143	150	157	165	172	179	186	193	200	208	215	222	229	236	243	250
6' (72")	140	147	154	162	169	177	184	191	199	206	213	221	228	235	242	250	258
6'1" (73")	144	151	159	166	174	182	189	197	204	212	219	227	235	242	250	257	265
6'2" (74")	148	155	163	171	179	186	194	202	210	218	225	233	241	249	256	264	272
6'3" (75")	152	160	168	176	184	192	200	208	216	224	232	240	248	256	264	272	279

(*Source:* Data from the *Evidence Report of Clinical Guidelines on the Identification, Evaluation, and Treatment of Overweight and Obesity in Adults,* 1998. NIH/National Heart Lung, and Blood Institute [NHLBI].)

TABLE 4–3 Body Mass Index (BMI Table) Classification Table

Classification	Men	Women
Normal	24–27	23–26
Moderately Obese	28–31	27–32
Severely Obese	>31	>32

(*Source*: Data from Department of Health and Human Services, *The Surgeon General's Report on Nutrition and Health*, DHHS [PHS] Publication 88-50210, Washington, DC: U.S. Government Printing Office, 1988.)

total lymphocyte count less than 1,800 mm, and an involuntary decrease in body weight greater than 15% (McVay-Smith, 2001). These three indicators have repeatedly been shown to correlate with nutritional status.

One of the most common and most useful measures to assess nutritional status is a dietary diary. Clients are instructed to keep a record of everything eaten for 3 days during the week prior to their clinic appointment or home visit. The record may be kept on a food intake record that allows listing of types of foods and amounts consumed during regular meals and snacks. When a record is kept accurately, daily food choices are compared with the *Food Guide Pyramid*, U.S. Department of Agriculture's Human Nutrition Information Service (see Chapter 7), or analyzed using published daily food guides or the many computerized dietary analysis packages available. Once the usual dietary patterns of the client have been identified, the nurse can provide needed nutritional assistance to the client (see Chapter 7). The nurse and nutritionists must work together to prepare materials that inform the client about the latest research on nutritional supplements, including vitamins and minerals (e.g., calcium, iron) as well as protein or complex carbohydrates. To review dietary assessment measures for use in primary care refer to *Practical Nutrition Assessment in Primary Care Settings: A Review* (Calfas, Zabinski, & Rupp, 2000).

Poor eating patterns, obesity, and malnutrition occur in all socioeconomic classes. In addition, dietary risk factors for chronic disease are widespread in the American population. Assessment of nutritional status and dietary habits is a critical part of a comprehensive health assessment for individuals, families, and specific target groups such as high-school students, pregnant women, and the elderly. For example, in a randomized, cross-sectional study of 266 nursing home residents using minimum data set variables, nurse researchers found that early identification and treatment of residents at risk for malnutrition improved their quality of life (Crogan & Corbett, 2002). Assessment determines which intervention is best to improve the nutritional status of the client.

Life Stress

Stress has been identified as a potential threat to mental health and physical well-being and has been associated with the occurrence of illnesses such as heart disease, cancer, and gastrointestinal disorders. Because of its apparent centrality to health, life stress should be

TABLE 4-4 Healthy and Unhealthy Weight Guidelines

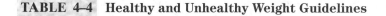

Are you at a healthy weight?

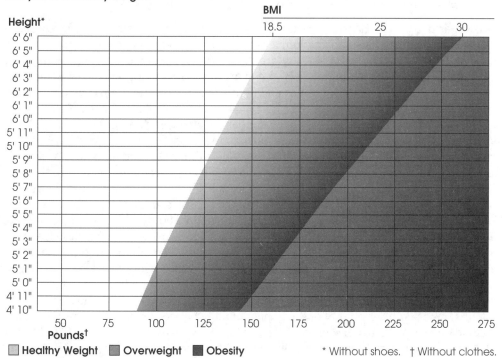

The BMI (weight-for-height) ranges shown above for adults. They are not exact ranges of healthy and unhealthy weights. However, they show that health risk increases at higher levels of overweight and obesity. Even within the healthy BMI range, weight gains can carry health risks for adults.

Directions: Find your weight on the bottom of the graph. Go straight up from that point until you come to the line that matches your height. Then look to find your weight group.

➤ BMI of 25 defines the upper boundary of healthy weight
➤ BMI of higher than 25 to 30 defines overweight
➤ BMI of higher than 30 defines obesity

(Source: *www.usda.gov/cnpp/Pubs/Dg2000*, p. 11)

evaluated as a part of comprehensive health assessment. Stress is typically evaluated with questionnaires that ask about difficulties or negative life experiences. Several of these instruments are described.

Stress Scales Assessing a person's vulnerability to stress and strengths to cope provides an essential measure of mental well-being. The Derogatis Stress Profile (DSP) is used to assess personal and professional stress in adolescents and adults (Derogatis & Fleming, 1997).

The 77-item instrument is designed to screen one's response to stress related to time pressure, driven behavior, attitude, relocation, work environment, family relationships, hostility, anxiety, depression, and health. The Perceived Stress Scale (Cohen, Kessler, & Gordon, 1997) measures moods and feelings about life stressors and is considered a measure of global stress. The 10-item scale is very easy to administer and score.

Hassles and Uplifts   Hassles are defined as the irritating, frustrating, distressing demands such as traffic jams, losing items, and arguments that may characterize everyday life. Uplifts, the counterpart of hassles, are defined as the positive experiences or joys of life, such as getting a good night's rest, receiving a letter from a friend, or spending time with a pet. Assessment of daily hassles and uplifts may be a better approach to the prediction of health or illness outcomes than the usual assessment of life events. If negative experiences such as hassles cause neuro-endocrine changes that predispose to illness, positive experiences such as uplifts may buffer stress disorders (Selye, 2000).

Kanner and Feldman (1991) explored the effects of hassles and uplifts, as well as perceived control of those events, among a group of 140 adolescents in relation to the experience of depression. Fewer hassles and more uplifts were related to less depression. Further, adolescents who felt they had control over hassles and uplifts in their lives were less depressed than those who reported less control. In a study of Navajo Indians, major life events and daily hassles were measured among adults presenting for either inpatient or outpatient care at a U.S. Indian Health Service facility. The number of outpatient visits and hospital admissions were monitored during the subsequent 2 years. Both major life events and daily hassles were associated with risk of hospital admission. Daily hassles were also associated with increased use of outpatient services. These findings support the potential cross-cultural validity of the impact of daily hassles on health status and related health care use (Williams, Zyzanski, & Wright, 1992). Mackey, Williams, and Tiller (2000), nurse researchers, studied stress in women with preterm labor (PTL) using the Daily Hassles Scale, a measure of day-to-day stressors or distressing experiences. They found that PTL women whose babies weighed 2,500 g or less had significantly higher scores on the Daily Hassles Scale.

Anxiety Inventory   Anxiety may also be assessed as part of the life-stress review. The State-Trait Anxiety Inventory consists of 20 items that assess the extent of anxiety a client feels at that moment (state anxiety), and 20 items to assess how the client generally feels (trait anxiety). Clients respond by rating themselves on a 4-point scale for each item (Spielberger, et al., 1983). A State-Trait Anxiety Inventory for Children, "How I Feel Questionnaire," has also been developed. Children respond by rating themselves on a 3-point scale. Both instruments and their administration manuals are available from Mind Garden, Palo Alto, California (Spielberger, et al., 1973). The State-Trait Anxiety Inventories provide an efficient yet reliable method to assess feelings of anxiety experienced by both child and adult clients.

Stress Warning Signals Inventory   In order to assist clients to understand how they respond to stress, they must be aware of the symptoms of an elevated stress level and how it affects them (Benson & Stuart, 1992). Once clients are aware of their own stress signals, they may use stress-management techniques (see Chapter 8) more effectively. Symptoms of stress may be physical, behavioral, emotional, or cognitive, as shown in Figure 4–4.

Stress Warning Signals

PHYSICAL SYMPTOMS

☐ Headaches
☐ Indigestion
☐ Stomachaches
☐ Sweaty palms
☐ Sleep difficulties
☐ Dizziness

☐ Back pain
☐ Tight neck, shoulders
☐ Racing heart
☐ Restlessness
☐ Tiredness
☐ Ringing in ears

BEHAVIORAL SYMPTOMS

☐ Excess smoking
☐ Bossiness
☐ Compulsive gum chewing
☐ Attitude critical of others

☐ Grinding of teeth at night
☐ Overuse of alcohol
☐ Compulsive eating
☐ Inability to get things done

EMOTIONAL SYMPTOMS

☐ Crying
☐ Nervousness, anxiety
☐ Boredom—no meaning to things
☐ Edginess—ready to explode
☐ Feeling powerless to change things

☐ Overwhelming sense of pressure
☐ Anger
☐ Loneliness
☐ Unhappiness for no reason
☐ Easily upset

COGNITIVE SYMPTOMS

☐ Trouble thinking clearly
☐ Forgetfulness
☐ Lack of creativity
☐ Memory loss

☐ Inability to make decisions
☐ Thoughts of running away
☐ Constant worry
☐ Loss of sense of humor

Do any seem familiar to you?

Check the ones you experience when under stress. These are your stress warning signs.

Are there any additional stress warning signals that you experience that are not listed? If so, add them here.

_____

_____

_____

_____

_____

FIGURE 4–4   **Stress Warning Signals**

(*Source*: From H. Benson and E. M. Stuart, 1993, *The Wellness Book: The Comprehensive Guide to Maintaining Health and Treating Stress-Related Illness*, New York: Scribner. Used with permission.)

Coping Measures   Coping is defined as an individual's ongoing efforts to manage specific internal and external demands that are appraised as exceeding personal resources (Folkman & Lazarus, 1988). Coping is a process that changes over time in relation to changing stressful events in one's life. The interaction of an individual with the environment determines how a stressful event is appraised and managed. Coping efforts in response to a stressful encounter are described as either problem focused or emotion focused.

Coping is most commonly measured with the Ways of Coping Questionnaire developed by Folkman and Lazarus (1988). The Likert-type measure consists of eight subscales that measure both emotion-focused and problem-focused coping strategies an individual uses when responding to a stress situation. Several other similar coping instruments are available that measure hardiness and sense of coherence, which are also considered personal resource constructs for responding to negative encounters.

The Schoolager's Coping Strategies Inventory is used to measure the type, frequency, and effectiveness of children's stress-coping strategies. Children between 8 and 12 years of age were asked in group discussions to identify the kinds of things that they do when they are experiencing stress. The resulting instrument and its psychometric evaluation are described by the developer (Ryan-Wenger, Sharrer, & Wynd, 2000). Younger (1993) reported on the development and testing of an instrument to measure mastery of stress in adults. Mastery is defined as a human response to difficult or stressful circumstances in which a person gains competence and control over the experience of stress. This 89-item instrument yields both a stress score and mastery score and is appropriate for administration to adults 19 years of age or older.

Spiritual Health

Spiritual health is defined as the ability to develop one's inner nature to its fullest potential. Spiritual health includes the ability to discover and articulate one's basic purpose in life; to learn how to experience love, joy, peace, and fulfillment; and how to help one's self and others achieve their fullest potential. The appraisal of spiritual health is critical in a holistic approach to health assessment because spiritual beliefs affect a client's interpretations of life events and health (Chuengsatiansup, 2003). Spirituality, religion, and health are clearly factors that need more research (Miller, & Thoresen, 2003), and standards to assess delivery and evaluation of spiritual care are needed as well (Cobb, Keeley, & Ahmedzai, 2003). However, "routinization of spiritual care" carries risks, and the supportive approach may be the best one for nurses to use (Johnson, 2001).

Daily spiritual experience is related to decreased use of alcohol, improved quality of life, and positive psychosocial status (Underwood & Teresi, 2002). McBride, Brooks, and Pilkington (1998) measured the relationship between a patient's spirituality and health experiences using the Index of Core Spiritual Experiences in 462 patients. Results showed a significant correlation between spirituality and health, supporting the importance of accessing spirituality. Another instrument developed and used by nurse researchers showed that practicing nurses perceive spirituality and spiritual care to be important (McSherry, Draper, & Kendrick, 2002). The Spiritual Involvement and Beliefs Scale (SIBS) is designed to be used across religious traditions to access actions as well as beliefs. The 26-item modified Likert instrument is easy to administer and score and avoids the use of cultural and religious bias (Hatch, Burg, Naberhaus, & Hellmich, 1998).

The Spiritual Perspective Scale (SPS) is a 10-item instrument that measures one's perceptions of the extent to which one's spiritual beliefs and one's daily interactions are consistent. Reed (1992), the author of the SPS, proposes that spirituality throughout one's life and especially during the later stages may help one manage life stresses more effectively. The SPS is easy to administer and score.

Areas of spirituality to be assessed include relationship with a higher being, relationship with self, and relationships with others (Greenstreet, 1999). Questions related to spiritual assessment are usually asked toward the end of the interview when the client and nurse are more at ease with each other. Clients need to be informed that assessing their spiritual well-being is integral to evaluating overall health.

Social Support Systems

It is important for both clients and health care providers to be aware of available sources of social support. Two approaches for reviewing the social support networks of clients are suggested. These approaches can be useful in giving both client and nurse increased insight into existing support resources. When assessing the adequacy of a client's support systems, it is important to be cognizant of factors that may cause the assessments to vary. Such things as the client's culture, stage of life-span development, social context (school, home, work), and role context (parent, student, professional) need to be considered for their influence on perceived and received support.

Support Systems Review   One straightforward, useful approach for assessment of support systems is to ask the client to list individuals who provide informational, emotional, appraisal, or instrumental support (Newcomb & Bentler, 1986). The client is then asked to indicate the relationship of the persons listed, such as family members, fellow workers, or social acquaintances. Next, persons who have been sources of support for 5 years or more are identified. This list enables the client to become aware of the stability of personal support systems. Last, the frequency and types of contact are identified. The type of contact may be face-to-face (visual) or nonvisual, which include telephone and e-mail communication. Examining the social network in this manner enables the client and the nurse to mutually assess the adequacy of support. If it is inadequate, strategies are generated about what can be done to enhance existing social networks. Figure 4–5 provides a sample support system review for a hypothetical client. After a review of the client's social support systems, the following questions can be explored:

- In what areas do you need more support: informational, emotional, instrumental, appraisal?
- Who within your present support system might provide the needed support?
- Who else do you think needs to become a part of your support system?
- What can you do to add the people you believe you need to your support system?

Answers to these questions suggest actions the client can take to expand sources of personal support.

Emotional Support Diagram   Sources of emotional support can also be diagrammed to assess the strength of support available. Figure 4–6 presents a sample emotional support diagram that is coded to indicate strong, moderate, and weak sources of support, as well as current conflicts with supportive individuals. The length of each line is used to indicate geographical proximity to the client. This approach is particularly appropriate for clients who need a visual presentation of their emotional support system in order to take action to sustain or enhance emotionally satisfying relationships.

List individuals who provide support to you. Next indicate the following relationships: Family member (FM); Fellow worker (FW); or Social Acquaintance (A). Frequency of Contact: Daily (D); Weekly (W); Monthly (M); or Rarely (R). Types of Contact: Face-to-Face (F); Telephone (T); E-mail (EM); or Smail (SM). If individual has been supportive for 5 years or more, place the number 5.

Individual	Relationship	Frequency	Type	Time
John	FM (husband)	D	F	5
Peter	FM (son)	D	F	5
Helen	FM (daughter)	D	F	5
Ted	FM (father)	W	T	5
Andrew	FW	D	F	-
Frances	FW	W	F	-
Rose	FW	W	T	5
Elsa	A	M	E	-
Jack	A	M	E	5

Ask the client to identify the type of support provided by individuals in the list. They may provide more than one type of support.

Sources of Emotional Support

FAMILY	WORK	SOCIAL GROUP
John	Frances	Elsa
Peter	Rose	Jack
Helen	Andrew	
Ted		

Sources of Instrumental Support

FAMILY	WORK	SOCIAL GROUP
John	Andrew	Jack
Ted		

Sources of Informational Support

FAMILY	WORK	SOCIAL GROUP
John	Andrew	Jack
Ted	Rose	

Sources of Appraisal Support

FAMILY	WORK	SOCIAL GROUP
John	Rose	Elsa

FIGURE 4-5 Support System Review: Social Network and Type of Support

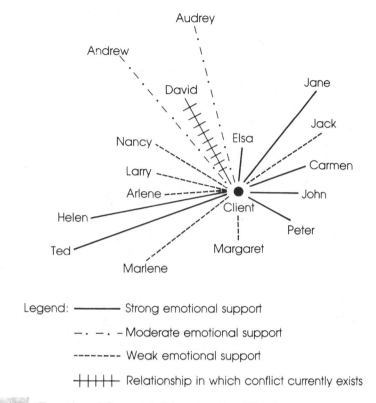

FIGURE 4–6 **Emotional Support Diagram for Client**

Review of sources of social support is an integral part of the assessment phase of health behavior. Through review, the client is able to recognize current sources of support and identify barriers in social relationships that may thwart desirable health actions. The nurse must always be alert to client situations where social support is minimal or nonexistent. Extensive review of support systems may cause anxiety and depression for the client. In this case, a more informal, nonthreatening approach should be used.

Several social support instruments are presented that represent the broad spectrum of measures used in clinical settings as well as research. The Medical Outcomes Study (MOS) Social Support Survey is a 19-item instrument that assesses emotional support, informational support, tangible support, positive social interaction, and affection (Sherbourne & Stewart, 1991). An instrument that determines the availability of and satisfaction with social support is the Social Support Questionnaire (SSQ). When the SSQ, a 27-item scale, was used with 295 students, those who reported more social support believed they could better manage life occurrences than those with less social support (McDowell & Newell, 1996). Perrin and McDermott (1997) and McDowell and Newell (1996) describe numerous other social support instruments used in social support research and practice.

Lifestyle

Increasing evidence indicates that individuals can maintain and enhance their well-being and prevent the early onset of disabling health problems by engaging in a health-promoting lifestyle. A thoughtful review of health habits with subsequent follow-up counseling and education may greatly increase the motivation and competence of clients to care for them in a responsible manner.

In the context of health, lifestyle is defined as discretionary activities that are a regular part of one's daily pattern of living and significantly influence health status. Health-promoting behavior is an expression of the human actualizing tendency that is directed toward optimal well-being, personal fulfillment, and productive living. The 52-item Health-Promoting Lifestyle Profile II (HPLP-II), a revision of the original instrument, consists of six subscales to measure major components of a health-promoting lifestyle: health responsibility, physical activity, nutrition, interpersonal relations, spiritual growth, and stress management. Scores are obtained for each subscale, or a total scale score is calculated to measure the overall health-promoting lifestyle (Sechrist, Walker, & Pender, 1987). Although the HPLP-II is frequently used in research, it can provide important information about a client's lifestyle when used in primary health care. Sample items for each of the subscales appear in Table 4–5.

An HPLP-II profile provides information to develop an individualized health-promotion plan that identifies lifestyle strengths and resources as well as areas for further growth. An adolescent version has been designed to identify health-enhancing behaviors, positive steps that enhance health, and well-being (Pender, 1997).

Stage-of-Change Assessment   Clients may be at one of several stages of readiness to change in relation to any given behavior change, based on various studies of behavioral changes from smoking cessation to exercise adoption. In the transtheoretical model

TABLE 4–5   Health-Promoting Lifestyle Profile II Subscales and Sample Items

Subscale	Sample Item
Health responsibility	Read or watch TV programs about improving my health.
	Question health professionals in order to understand their instructions.
Physical activity	Exercise vigorously for 20 or more minutes at least three times a week (brisk walking, bicycling, aerobic dancing, using a stair climber).
	Get exercise during usual day activities (such as walking during lunch, using stairs instead of elevators, parking car farther away from destination and walking).
Nutrition	Choose a diet low in fat, saturated fat, and cholesterol.
	Eat 2 to 4 servings of fruit each day.
Interpersonal relations	Spend time with close friends.
	Settle conflicts with others through discussion and compromise.
Spiritual growth	Feel connected with some force greater than myself.
	Am aware of what is important to me in life.
Stress management	Take some time for relaxation each day.
	Pace myself to prevent fatigue.

TABLE 4–6 Questions for Assessing Stages of Behavior Change

1. I currently do not (specify exact behavior, e.g., exercise 30 minutes three times a week, eat 2 to 4 servings of fruit daily) and do not intend to start in the next 6 months. (Precontemplation)

2. I currently do not (specify behavior), but I am thinking about starting to do so in the next 6 months. (Contemplation)

3. I have tried several times to (specify behavior) but am seriously thinking of trying again in the next month. (Planning)

4. I have (specify behavior) regularly for less than 6 months. (Action)

5. I have (specify behavior) regularly for more than 6 months. (Maintenance)

Prochaska and colleagues (2002) propose that stage-of-readiness will determine the intervention plan that is most effective. Stages of change for positive health behaviors may be assessed with the true-false questions presented in Table 4–6.

Following completion of lifestyle assessment, the interest of the client in making various changes may be assessed as well as the stage of the client in relation to each behavior. Prochaska and colleagues (2002) propose that "staging" a client in relation to various health behaviors allows for more precise tailoring of interventions.

Assessment of the Family

Family assessment, as well as individual assessment, is critical to successfully plan for health behavior change. The family is the primary social structure for health promotion within society. Health behaviors are learned within the context of the family, and the rudiments of health-enhancing or health-damaging lifestyles emerge. The family also acts as a powerful mediating factor in determining how its members cope with health concerns and challenges (Friedman, 1998). Thus, the family is a logical unit of assessment and intervention for health promotion, since it has the primary responsibility for (a) developing self-care and dependent-care competencies of the family, (b) fostering resilience of family members, (c) providing social and physical resources to the family group, and (d) promoting healthy individuals while maintaining family cohesion. Although women generally carry the major responsibility for health decision making and health education for the family, the task of fostering health and healthy behaviors should be "mainstreamed" as an integral part of family functioning.

The milieu for the promotion of health is likely to differ significantly across families, depending on their composition, structure, socioeconomic status, living environment, and cultural context. Healthy family traits may be expressed in many different ways. Family strengths may have many different modes of expression. One-parent families, blended families, not-married parents with children, and gay and lesbian families must all be taken into consideration. When conducting a family assessment the nurse must be attuned to this wide range of variation among families as well as variations produced by transitions in family life (Friedman, 1998). There is no one correct way to spend quality time together, promote physically active families, or express affection. Approaches to assessment that may be used in all types of families are described briefly.

Using a systems approach to family, Hanson and Kaakinen (2000) proposed the following assessment categories: (a) individual members, (b) subsystems (developmental, biological, psychological, and social characteristics), (c) interactional patterns (relationships, communication patterns, roles, and attachment patterns), (d) family processing, and (e) change or adaptive abilities. Clark (2003) described three categories of processes underlying a systems model of family assessment: those that regulate exchanges with the environment, processes designed to prevent an overload of the system, and internal processes that regulate the family's ability to adapt and change.

Friedman (1998) described a structural-functional approach to family assessment. Family is viewed as a system with communication patterns, power structure, role structure, family values, affective function, socialization function, health care function, and family stress, coping, and adaptation. Assessment based on systems theory provides insight concerning the internal processes of the family as well as the relationship of the family to the environment and larger social system. Family decision-making patterns in relation to health are identified in assessing power structure and the health care function.

Wright and Leahey (2000) adapted the Calgary Family Assessment Model (CFAM) for nurses to use to assess families. Their model consists of family structural assessment, family developmental assessment, and family functional assessment. In structural assessment, the family is analyzed in terms of both its internal and external structure. Aspects of the internal structure include family composition, rank order, subsystem, and boundary. Components of the external structure are culture, religion, social class status and mobility, environment, and extended family.

To assess family development the current stage of the family is appraised in relation to family developmental history. Family development focuses primarily on the traditional family developmental cycle, but it also includes assessment of alterations in the family developmental life cycle brought about by separation, divorce, single parenthood, and remarriage.

Family functional assessment is dichotomized as instrumental functioning and expressive functioning. *Instrumental functioning* refers to the routine activities of everyday living, while *expressive functioning* is elaborated as emotional communication, verbal communication, nonverbal communication, circular communication, problem solving, roles, control, beliefs, and alliances and coalitions. The reader is referred to Wright and Leahey's book (2000) for a detailed discussion.

A family health assessment scheme that focuses on assessment of tensions and stress created by situations in normal family life and on family health issues has been proposed by Mischke-Berkey, Warner, and Hanson (1996). The Neuman Health-Care Systems Model provides the blueprint for this assessment tool. Flexible and normal lines of defense as well as lines of resistance are important concepts in the model. Examples of family health assessment instruments are provided in works by Allender and Spradley (2001) and DeMarco, Ford-Gilboe, Friedemann, McCubbin, and McCubbin (2000).

An excellent compilation of approximately 20 measures of family functioning that is potentially useful in practice has been prepared by Sawin, Woog, and Harrigan (1995). Instruments include the Feetham Family Functioning Survey, Family Adaptability and Cohesion Scale, and the Family Hardiness Index. Any of these instruments may be used to assess families as a basis for developing a health promotion-prevention plan. The compilation includes a description of each instrument with sample items, psychometric properties, cross-cultural uses, gender sensitivity, applicability to variant family structures, list of selected studies using the instrument, critique, and source for accessing the instrument.

A major gap in family assessment is lack of an instrument that measures family dimensions of a health-related lifestyle. Nurse scientists need to develop valid and reliable measures to assess families' aggregate health behaviors. Areas suggested for assessment in such an instrument are shown in Table 4–7.

Family assessment complements individual assessment; thus, the two need to be considered as interrelated processes. To provide further guidance to nurses in working with families, a format for developing a family health promotion-prevention plan is presented in Chapter 5.

TABLE 4–7   Components of Family Assessment

Nutrition

1. Meals prepared in the home are generally consistent with the food guide pyramid.
2. Healthy snacks are consumed in the home.
3. Knowledge about healthy eating habits is shared among family members.
4. Mutual assistance occurs among family members for maintenance of recommended weights and avoidance of overweight and underweight.
5. Family members praise each other for healthy eating.
6. Family members encourage each other to drink 6 to 8 glasses of water per day.
7. Family members base purchase decisions on nutritional labels on food.

Physical Activity

1. Many family outings consist of vigorous or moderate physical activity.
2. Exercise equipment is available within the home.
3. Use of home exercise equipment is part of "family time."
4. Family members expect each other to be physically active.
5. A family membership is held in recreational facilities or programs.
6. Time together is seldom spent watching television or playing video games.
7. Family prefers to spend as much time out of doors as possible.

Stress Control and Management

1. Family manages time well to minimize stressful demands on members.
2. Family often relaxes, shares stories, and laughs together.
3. Emotional expression is encouraged within the family.
4. Family members share stressful experiences with each other.
5. Family members offer each other assistance with difficult tasks.
6. Family members seldom criticize each other.
7. Periods of relaxation and sleep are considered important by the family.

Health Responsibility

1. A schedule for preventive care visits is maintained by the family.
2. Family often discusses news and articles about health topics.
3. Family members are encouraged to seek health care early if a problem develops.

TABLE 4–7 Continued

Health Responsibility

4. Personal responsibility for health is encouraged by the family.
5. Family feels a sense of responsibility for the health of the family and each member.
6. Health professionals are consulted about health promotion as well as care in illness.
7. Appropriate protective behaviors are openly discussed and encouraged (abstinence, use of condoms, hearing protection, eye protection, sunscreen, helmets).

Family Resilience and Resources

1. Worship or spiritual experiences are a regular part of family activities.
2. Family members share a sense of "togetherness" despite difficult life events.
3. Family has a common sense of purpose in life.
4. Family members encourage each other to "keep going" when life is difficult.
5. Growth in positive directions is mutually encouraged within the family.
6. Health is nurtured as a positive family resource.
7. Personal strengths and capabilities are nurtured.

Family Support

1. Family has a number of friends or relatives that they see frequently.
2. Family is involved in community activities and groups.
3. Family members frequently praise each other.
4. In times of distress, the family can call on a number of other families or individuals for help.
5. Disagreements are settled through discussion rather than verbal abuse or physical violence.
6. Family members model healthy habits for each other.
7. Professional support services are sought when needed.

Assessment of the Community

A third essential component of health assessment is community analysis or appraisal. Community analysis is the process of assessing and defining needs, opportunities, and resources involved in initiating community health programs. It is critical to recognize that analysis is done with the community, not on or for the community. Local citizens and organizations must be involved in the assessment process in order to have "ownership" of the program and to build widespread commitment to community action (Haglund, Weisbrod, & Bracht, 1999). *Healthy People 2010* (2000) objectives are essentially community-oriented. The underlying premise of the 2010 initiative is that the health of individuals and their community is bound together. All sectors of the community must be activated to achieve the broad national goals set for the year 2010: increase quality and years of healthy life and eliminate health disparities. Objectives focused on injury and violence prevention; educational and community-based programs; occupational safety and health; environmental health; and maternal, infant, and child health all require community assessment and intervention.

Shuster and Colleagues (2000) identified five approaches to collecting data about communities: informant interviewing (directed conversation with community members); participant observation (sharing in community life activities); mobile survey (observation while driving about); secondary analyses (use of preexisting data); and community surveys (organized data collection efforts). Because community citizens constitute a critical primary data source, informant interviewing should always be used as one approach to data collection. An assessment methodology that combines at least three to four of the data collection methods is more likely to provide a holistic picture of the community than an assessment that relies on only one or two approaches.

One approach to community assessment is to collect information about the following community subsystems and their interrelationships: (a) values and culture, (b) politics, (c) education, (d) recreation, (e) transportation, (f) religion, (g) communications and media, (h) welfare, (i) economics, (j) utilities, (k) business and labor, (l) social life, (m) safety and protection, and (n) health. In assessing the health subsystem, population growth patterns, functional activity status, nutritional status, dominant lifestyle patterns, coping ability, community stressors, goal setting and achievement capabilities, and risk factors need to be assessed in addition to traditional indices of morbidity, mortality, and accessibility of health care resources.

The nature of the assessment is based on the time available and how the information will be used. Comprehensive assessment includes all relevant information about the community that is synthesized from existing documents and primary data collection. This approach is costly and time-consuming and is not recommended unless such a comprehensive study is absolutely essential before high-priority program goals are addressed. A familiarization assessment is more efficient and provides a broad rather than in-depth overview of the community at large. The windshield survey is an example. In a windshield survey, the nurse drives through the community and identifies multiple dimensions, including housing quality, recreation facilities, and the people residing in the area (Anderson & McFarlane, 2000).

Problem-oriented assessment begins with a single problem and assesses the community in terms of the problem, for instance, neighborhood violence. Aspects of the community relevant to the health issue are assessed to determine their contributory, ameliorative, or preventive effects. Subsystem assessment is focused on a particular sector of the community and permits an in-depth assessment of that sector. For example, the subsystem might be assessed to evaluate the impact of educational programs on the health and productivity of the community (Shuster & Goepinger, 2000).

Data collection methods are numerous and varied. Existing records can be examined to obtain as much information as possible before data collection is instituted. Key informants knowledgeable about the community provide another important data source. When primary data collection is necessary, focus group interviewing often is the method of choice because of the rich interactive data that can be obtained. Survey data can also be important as information from a large segment of the population is provided.

Screening is another method to collect data about the community. Screenings are conducted to detect a particular, unrecognized health problem in individuals who are members of a group at-risk for a certain disease or health problem. Information from screenings is an important component of the community assessment. The purpose of community screenings is to uncover health problems in an efficient and economically feasible manner. Screenings should be conducted only if the following factors are present: (a) the specific population has a high prevalence of the disease or health problem, (b) there is a successful treatment for the problem, (c) treatment is available if the condition is identified, and (d) screening instruments are valid and reliable (AMA Council on Scientific affairs, 1996). As with other components of the community assessment the cost of conducting screenings must be considered in the decision. For example, conducting a screening to detect osteoporosis requires special equipment, and the cost will be high due to the number of machines needed to screen in a time-efficient manner.

Community assessment provides information about a community's health status from which community diagnoses are derived. Thus, community assessment is a primary building block for planning, implementing, and evaluating community health promotion-prevention programs. The components of a community assessment have been identified (Clark, 2003) and have been organized and further expanded in Table 4–8. Examples of assessment instruments are available in most community health textbooks (Anderson & McFarlane, 2000; Clark, 2003; Shuster & Goepinger, 2000).

TABLE 4–8   Components of Community Assessment

Human Biology

1. Composition of population by age, gender, and race
2. Population patterns of longevity
3. Genetic inheritance patterns by gender and race
4. Disease incidence and prevalence compared to prior years, and to state and national statistics
5. Health status indicators (immunization levels, nutritional status, mobility)

Environment

1. Physical environment (urban/rural/suburban, housing, water supply, parks and recreation, climate, topography, size, population density, aesthetics, natural or manmade resources, goods and services, health risks)
2. Psychologic environment (productivity level, cohesion, mental health status, communication networks, intergroup harmony, future orientation, prevalence of stressors)
3. Social environment (income and education levels, employment, family composition, religious affiliations, cultural affiliations, language[s] spoken, social services, organization profile, leadership and decision-making structures)

Community Lifestyles

1. Consumption patterns (e.g., nutrition, alcohol)
2. Occupational groups
3. Leisure pursuits
4. Comunity health attitudes and beliefs
5. Patterns of health-related behaviors in aggregates
6. History of participation in community health action

TABLE 4–8 Continued

Health System

1. Health care services available (health promotion, prevention, primary care, secondary care, tertiary care, mental health)
2. Accessibility of promotive and preventive care (low income, homeless, varying racial and ethnic groups)
3. Financing plans for health care

(*Source*: Adapted from M. J. Clark, 2003, *Community Health Nursing*, Upper Saddle River, NJ: Prentice Hall. Used with permission.)

Assessment of communities is a complicated and time-consuming task. Collaboration is required among many individuals in the community as well as health professionals. However, such assessments are critical to identify community strengths and resources as well as diagnose community problems or deficits. Successful implementation of community health promotion-prevention programs depends in large part on accurate assessment of community characteristics.

Directions for Research in Health Assessment

Research that develops and tests instruments to assess health and health behaviors of individuals and aggregates from diverse racial, cultural, and socioeconomic backgrounds is a high priority. Reliable and valid instruments that are based on theory and research are needed in order to perform meaningful assessments. Accurate knowledge of the client, family, and/or community will facilitate the development and implementation of successful health-promotion interventions.

Directions for Practice in Health Assessment

Nurses must be able to use assessment measures to document areas for improvement to enhance the health status of individuals, families, and communities. Nurses who use nursing classification systems and collect data with valid and reliable assessment instruments contribute to evidenced-based practice. Assessment data about health status and behaviors provides the basis for clinical judgments and helps plan appropriate individual, family, and community interventions. Nurses must use their knowledge and influence to ensure that a portfolio of assessment instruments is available and used in the work setting. The nurse must know how to administer assessment instruments and explain the value of conducting systematic assessments to the client. The busy work environment may discourage the use of some assessment instruments since they require time to administer and follow-up. One way the nurse can manage the time issue is to seek innovative ways to communicate with clients through videotapes loaned to clients and brochures that explain assessment procedures. Information technology has made computerized assessment tools possible. Thus, clients may be able to complete self-assessments at home as time allows, with transmission of the information via computer prior to health care visits.

Practicing nurses must keep up-to-date and current about new assessment measures and strategies that may be quickly implemented and yet yield accurate data. Nurses influence the quality of the health-promotion plan of the individual, family, and community through a commitment to thorough assessment of health and health behaviors.

SUMMARY

Health assessment is carried out at the individual, family, or community level. Assessment is time-intensive for the nurse and the client, so measures must be carefully selected according to the client's characteristics and presenting health issues. The nurse and client need to mutually decide what assessments are needed to establish a relevant plan for health promotion.

LEARNING ACTIVITIES

1. Develop an assessment plan based on age-specific instruments for a child, young adult, and older adult.
2. Using Table 4–4, determine your own measure of body fat and outline a personal goal for improvement.
3. Investigate more fully one approach to assess a family and discuss its strengths and weaknesses for use in the clinical setting.
4. Identify the relationship between family and community assessments and how they affect the health outcomes of the family and community.
5. Discuss factors to consider in a community assessment, including factors to consider in the extent of assessment to be conducted.

SELECTED WEB SITES

American Public Health Association

http://www.apha.org/

Centers for Disease Control

http://www.cdc.gov

CLAS Guidelines:

http://www.omhrc.gov/Clas/index.htm

Healthfinder—Consumer Health and Human Services Information

http://www.healthfinder.gov/

Healthtouch—Prescription and Over-the-Counter Medications

http://www.healthtouch.com

National Cancer Institute

http://cancer.gov/cancerinformation

National Center for Health Statistics

http://www.cdc.gov/nchs

National Institutes of Health

http://www.nih.gov

Nursing Interventions Classification

http://www.nursing.uiowa.edu/centers/cncce/nic/index.htm

Nursing Outcomes Classification

http://www.nursing.uiowa.edu/noc/index.htm

PubMed—Corporate Sites

http://www.ncbi.nlm.nih.gov/PubMed/

Tufts University Nutrition Navigator

http://www.navigator.tufts.edu

REFERENCES

Allender, J. A., & Spradley, B. W. (2001). *Community health nursing: Concepts and practice* (5th ed.). Philadelphia: Lippincott.

AMA Council on Scientific Affairs. (1996). *Guide to clinical preventive services: Report of the U.S. preventive services task force* (2nd ed.). Baltimore, MA: American Medical Association.

American College of Sports Medicine. (1995). *Guidelines for testing and prescription* (5th ed.). Williams & Wilkins: A Waverly Company.

American College of Sports Medicine. (2001). *ACSM's resource manual for guidelines for exercise testing and prescription* (4th ed.). Williams & Wilkins: A Waverly Company.

Anderson, E. T., & McFarlane, J. M. (2000). *Community as partner: Theory and practice in nursing* (3rd ed.). Philadelphia: Lippincott.

Barnett-Damewood, M., & Carlson-Catalano, J. (2000). Physical activity deficit: A proposed nursing diagnosis. *Nursing Diagnosis: ND: The Official Journal of the North American Nursing Diagnosis Association, 11*(1), 24–31.

Beddoe, A. H. (1998). Body fat: Estimation or guesstimation? *Applied Radiation and Isotope, 49*(5–6), 461–463.

Bednarz, P. K. (1998). The Omaha System: A model for describing school nurse case management. *The Journal of School Nursing: The Official Publication of the National Association of School Nurses, 14*(3), 24–30.

Benson, H., & Stuart, E. M. (1992). *The wellness book.* New York: Birch Lane Press.

Calfas, K. J., Zabinski, M. F., & Rupp, J. (2000). Practical nutrition assessment in primary care settings: A review. *American Journal of Preventive Medicine, 18*(4), 289–299.

Carpenito, L. J. (2004). *Nursing diagnosis: Application to clinical practice.* Philadelphia: Lippincott.

Chuengsatiansup, K. (2003). Spirituality and health: An initial proposal to incorporate spiritual health in health impact assessment. *Environmental Impact Assessment Review, 23*, 3–15.

Clark, M. J. (2003). *Community health nursing: Caring for populations.* Upper Saddle River, NJ: Prentice Hall.

CLAS Guidelines. (2004). Accessed February 2004 at: *http://www.omhre.gov/CLAS.*

Cobb, H. J., Keeley, V. L., & Ahmedzai, S. H. (2003). The quality of spiritual care—developing a standard. *Int J Palliat Nurs, 9*(5), 208–215.

Cohen, S., Kessler, R. C., & Gordon, L. U. (1997). *Measuring stress.* New York: Oxford Press.

Cooper, K. H. (1999). *Fit kids! The complete shape-up program from birth through high school.* Nashville, TN: Broadman & Holman Publishers.

Crogan, N. L., & Corbett, C. F. (2002). Predicting malnutrition in nursing home residents using the minimum data set. *Geriatric Nursing, 23*(4), 224–226.

DeMarco, R., Ford-Gilboe, M., Friedemann, M., McCubbin, H. I., & McCubbin, M. A. (2000). Stress, coping, and family health. In V. H. Rice (Ed.), *Handbook of stress, coping, and health: Implications for nursing research, theory, and practice.* Thousand Oaks: Sage.

Derogatis, L. R., & Fleming, M. P. (1997). *Evaluating stress. The Derogatis stress profile (DSP): A theory driven approach to stress measurement.* Lanham, MD: Scarecrow Press.

Ervin, N. E. (2002). *Advanced community health nursing practice: Population-focused care.* Upper Saddle River, NJ: Prentice Hall.

Folkman, S., & Lazarus, R. S. (1988). Coping as a mediator of emotion. *Journal of Personality and Social Psychology, 54*(3), 466–475.

Freedson, P. S., Cureton, K. J., & Heath, G. W. (2000). Status of field-based fitness testing in children and youth. *Preventive Medicine, 31*, S77–S85.

Friedman, M. N. (1998). *Family nursing: Research theory and practice* (4th ed.). New York: Appleton Century-Crofts.

Gordon, M. (2002). *Manual of nursing diagnosis: Including all diagnostic categories approved by the North American Nursing Diagnosis Association* (10th ed.). St. Louis: Mosby.

Greenstreet, W. M. (1999). Teaching spirituality in nursing: A literature review. *Nurse Educ Today, 19*(8), 649–658.

Haglund, B., Weisbrod, R. R., & Bracht, N. (1999). Assessing the community: Its services, needs, leadership, and readiness. In N. Bracht (Ed.), *Health promotion at the community level.* Newberry Park, CA: Sage Publications Inc.

Hanson, S., & Kaakinen, J. (2000). Family development and family nursing assessment. In M. Stanhope & J. Lancaster (Eds.), *Community & public health nursing* (5th ed.). St. Louis: Mosby.

Hatch, R. L., Burg, M. A., Naberhaus, D. S., & Hellmich, L. K. (1998). The Spiritual Involvement and Beliefs Scale. Development and testing of a new instrument. *J Fam Pract, 46*(6), 476–486.

Healthy People 2010. 2nd edition (2000). Washington DC: U.S. Public Health and Human Services publications PHS 91-50212.

Houldin, A. D., Saltstein, S. W., & Ganley, K. M. (1987). *Nursing diagnosis for wellness: Supporting strengths.* Philadelphia, PA: J. B. Lippincott Co.

Johnson, C. P. (2001). Assessment tools: Are they an effective approach to implementing spiritual health care within the NHS? *Accident and Emergency Nursing, 9,* 177–186.

Kaiser, K. L., Hays, B. J., Cho, W., & Agrawal, S. (2002). Examining health problems and intensity of need for care in family-focused community and public health nursing. *Journal of Community Health Nursing, 19*(1), 17–32.

Kanner, A. D., & Feldman, S. S. (1991). Control over uplifts and hassles and its relationship to adaptational outcomes. *J Behav Med, 14,* 187–201.

Mackey, M. C., Williams, C. A., & Tiller, C. M. (2000). Stress, pre-term labor and birth outcomes. *Journal of Advanced Nursing, 32*(3), 666–674.

Marek, K. D. (1996). Nursing diagnoses and home care nursing utilization. *Public Health Nursing, 13*(3), 195–200.

Martin, K. S., & Norris, J. (1996). The Omaha System: A model for describing practice. *Holist Nurs Pract, 11*(1), 75–83.

McBride, J. L., Arthur, G., Brooks, R., & Pilkington, L. (1998). The relationship between a patient's spirituality and health experiences. *Fam Med, 30*(2), 122–126.

McDowell, I., & Newell, C. (1996). *Measuring health* (2nd ed.). New York: Oxford University Press.

McSherry, W., Draper, P., & Kendrick, D. (2002). The construct validity of a rating scale designed to assess spirituality and spiritual care. *Int J Nurs Stud, 39*(7), 723–734.

McVay-Smith, C. (2001). Nutrition assessment. *Nutrition, 17*(9), 785–786.

Miller, W. R., & Thoresen, C. E. (2003). Spirituality, religion, and health: An emerging research field. *American Psychologist, 58*(1), 24–35.

Mischke-Berkey, K., Warner, P., & Hanson, S. (1996). Family health assessment and intervention. In P. J. Bomar (Ed.), *Nurses and family health promotion: Concepts, assessments, and interventions.* Baltimore, MD: Williams & Wilkins.

Newcomb, M. D., & Bentler, P. M. (1986). Loneliness and social support: A confirmatory hierarchical analysis. *Personality and Social Psychology Bulletin, 12,* 520–535.

Pender, N. J. (1997). *The Adolescent Lifestyle Profile (ALP): Assessing health-related behaviors.* Unpublished Manuscript.

Perrin, K. M., & McDermott, R. J. (1997). Instruments to measure social support and related constructs in pregnant adolescents: A review. *Adolescence, 32*(127), 533–557.

Prochaska, J. O., Redding, C. A., & Covers, K. E. (2002) The transtheoretical model and stages of change. In K. Glang, B. K. Rimer, F. M. Lewis (Eds.), *Health behavior and health educations* (pp. 99–120). San Francisco: Jossey-Bass.

Reed, P. G. (1992). An emerging paradigm for the investigation of spirituality in nursing. *Research in Nursing and Health, 15,* 349–357.

Ryan-Wenger, N. M., Sharrer, V. W., & Wynd, C. A. (2000). *Handbook of stress, coping, and health: Implications for nursing research, theory, and practice.* Thousand Oaks, CA: Sage Publications, Inc.

Sawin, K. J., Harrington, M. P., & Wood, P. (1995). *Measures of family functioning for research and practice.* New York: Springer.

Sechrist, K. R., Walker, S. N., & Pender, N. J. (1987). Development and psychometric evaluation of the Exercise Benefits/Barrier Scale. *Res Nurs Health, 10,* 357–365.

Selye, B. L. (2000). Stress, coping, and health. *In* V. Rice (Ed.), *Handbook of stress, coping and health.* Sage Publications, Inc.

Sherbourne, C. D., & Stewart, A. L. (1991). The MOS Social Support Survey. *Social Science & Med.,* 32(6), 704–714.

Shuster, G. F., & Goepinger, J. (2003). Community as client: Using the nursing process to promote health. In M. Stanhope & J. Lancaster (Eds.), *Foundation of community and public health nursing practice.* St. Louis: Mosby.

Spielberger, C. D., Edwards, C. D., Lushene, R. E., et al. (1973). *State-Trait Anxiety Inventory for Children—Preliminary manual.* Palo Alto, CA: Mind Garden.

Spielberger, C. D., Gorsuch, R. L., Lushene, R., et al. (1983). *Manual for State-Trait Anxiety Inventory.* Palo Alto, CA: Consulting Psychologists Press Inc.

Underwood, L. G., & Teresi, J. A. (2002). The daily spiritual experience scale: Development, theoretical description, reliability, exploratory factor analysis, and preliminary construct validity using health-related data. *Ann Behav Med, 24*(1), 22–33.

Williams, R., Zyzanski, S. J., & Wright, A. L. (1992) Life events and daily hassles and uplifts as predictors of hospitalization and outpatient visitation. *Soc Sci Med, 34,* 763–768.

Wright, L. M., & Leahey, M. (2000). *Nurses and families: A guide to family assessment and intervention.* Philadelphia, PA: FA Davis Co.

Younger, J. B. (1993). Development and testing of the Mastery of Stress Instrument. *Nurs Res, 42,* 68–73.

5

Developing a Health Promotion-Prevention Plan

OBJECTIVES

1. Identify the nine steps in the health planning process.
2. Discuss the barriers the nurse must overcome in developing an individual and family health plan.
3. Describe strategies to increase the client's "ownership" of a health behavior-change plan.
4. Discuss strategies to implement to ensure that the health plan is an interdisciplinary process.
5. Discuss the barriers to effective individual and family behavior change.
6. Describe how community level plans and interventions influence individual and family health plans.

OUTLINE

- Guidelines for Preventive Services and Screenings
- The Health-Planning Process
  - A. Review and Summarize Data from Assessment
  - B. Reinforce Strengths and Competencies of the Client
  - C. Identify Health Goals and Related Behavior-Change Options
  - D. Identify Behavioral or Health Outcomes
  - E. Develop a Behavior-Change Plan
  - F. Reiterate Benefits of Change

    G. Address Environmental and Interpersonal Facilitators and Barriers to Change

    H. Determine a Time Frame for Implementation

    I. Formalize Commitment to Behavior-Change Plan

- Revisions of the Health Promotion-Prevention Plan
- Community-Level Health Promotion-Prevention Plan
- Directions for Research in Behavior Change
- Directions for Practice in Behavior Change
- Summary
- Learning Activities
- Selected Web Sites
- References

Clients must be active participants in interpreting assessment data and in planning. Client collaboration with the nurse for care promotes positive perceptions of worth. It also affirms the ability of individuals, families, or communities to self-regulate and to function on their own behalf in improving health and creating conditions supportive of healthy lifestyles. The role of the nurse is to *assist* clients with health planning rather than to *control* the process. During assessment, the nurse and client develop a mutual understanding of the client's (a) health status; (b) current health-behavior patterns; (c) attitudes and beliefs that affect health and health-related behaviors; (d) expectations of important referent groups; (e) potentially available behavioral options; (f) social-ethnic-cultural background; (g) potential or actual barriers to health-promoting self-care; and (h) existing support systems for health-promoting behaviors. Developing a systematic plan for behavior change provides an opportunity for the client to express stabilizing and actualizing tendencies in purposeful ways directed toward increasing wellness and enhancing life satisfaction.

Health planning is a dynamic process. Flexibility is critical to meet the changing needs of clients. The plan systematically lends direction but does not dictate goals that must be attained or behaviors that must be learned. The health promotion-prevention plan should be reasonable in terms of both demands on the client and the time frame allocated for accomplishment of desired health or health-related goals. Knowledge, skills, and strengths of the client should be used in the planning process. Capitalizing on positive health practices that are currently a part of personal or family lifestyle creates a sense of competence or efficacy as well as the behavioral control essential to successful behavior change. The nurse and the client should together assess the stage of change (precontemplation, contemplation, preparation, action, and maintenance) for behaviors the client wishes to modify. The client can then discuss with the nurse strategies for change that are likely to be most effective. The plan should be revised as needed to make behavior change a positive growth experience for clients. The ultimate goal of health planning and implementation is to make health promotion and prevention a way of life that individuals, families, and communities may manage and enjoy.

Innovative developments in information technology increasingly allow personalization of assessment and intervention protocols to the unique characteristics and needs of individual clients. Nurses should be actively involved in the design of health-assessment and health-planning software that is interactive and client friendly.

Guidelines for Preventive Services and Screenings

With increasing emphasis on the prevention of disease, varying sets of guidelines for the delivery of preventive services to individuals and families throughout the life span have been developed. These guidelines focus on clinical care directed toward prevention from specific diseases such as AIDS or behavioral morbidity such as substance abuse. The 1996 *Guide to Clinical Preventive Services*, 2nd edition (U.S. Preventive Services Task Force, 1996), recommended screenings as an important component of prevention. The value and benefits of age-specific periodic screenings based on gender and individual risk factors are available from the U.S. Office of Disease Prevention and Health Promotion. The U.S. Preventive Services Task Force identified counseling clients about their personal health habits as one of the most important components of the health visit. Nurses in all settings where primary care is delivered should become familiar with the following sets of guidelines to ensure that their clients benefit from "state-of-the-science" preventive services: *Guide to Clinical Preventive Services* (1996), *Clinician's Handbook of Preventive Services: Put Prevention into Practice* (1998), *AMA Guidelines for Adolescent Preventive Services: Recommendations and Rationale* (1994), and *Bright Futures: Guidelines for Health Supervision of Infants, Children, and Adolescents* (Green, 2002). These publications provide recommendations and rationale for a wide array of preventive measures.

The Health-Planning Process

The process for developing a health promotion-prevention plan is outlined below, with each step in the process discussed separately. These nine steps actively involve both the client and the nurse in the health-planning process:

1. Review and summarize data from assessment.
2. Reinforce strengths and competencies of the client.
3. Identify health goals and related behavioral-change options.
4. Identify behavioral or health outcomes that will indicate that the plan has been successful from the client's perspective.
5. Develop a behavior-change plan based on the client's preferences, on the stages of change, and on "state-of-the science" knowledge about effective interventions.
6. Reiterate benefits of change and identify incentives for change from the client's perspective.
7. Address environmental and interpersonal facilitators and barriers to behavior change.
8. Determine a time frame for implementation.
9. Commit to behavior-change goals and the support needed to accomplish them.

Review and Summarize Data from Assessment

During assessment, the nurse obtains a wealth of data from the client. The reduction of this data to useful and manageable information is accomplished by summarizing the client's results on the various assessment instruments and other data-gathering tools. From assessment activities, the nurse and client should have information available in the following domains as a basis for planning and action:

1. Physical health status
2. Status in relation to functional health patterns
3. Physical fitness
4. Nutritional status
5. Sources of life stress
6. Spirituality
7. Social support
8. Health-related lifestyle
9. Family health practices
10. Environmental and community supports or constraints for health behaviors

During one or more clinic appointments or home visits, the nurse should guide the client through the data summary process. The nurse and client should retain a copy of the assessment summary for continuing reference during the health-planning process.

Reinforce Strengths and Competencies of the Client

Each individual or family has in place a system of health care practices compatible with the client's cultural orientation. Thus, the nurse and client should achieve consensus on areas in which the client is already taking informed and responsible health action as well as on areas for further development of self-care competencies. Clients bring unique strengths to the health-planning task. These assets should be identified, acknowledged, and reinforced by the nurse. Because clients will carry out health behaviors in ways that fit their cultural beliefs, preferences, and current levels of knowledge and skill, existing cultural practices supportive of health should be integrated into the overall health plan. The client's sense of cultural or ethnic pride should be reinforced during the health-planning process.

Through teaching, guidance, and support, the nurse nurtures and enhances existing competencies to meet health needs. Self-care requirements and resources will vary according to the client's age, gender, developmental stage, and health status. The self-care needs of families will vary by family composition, developmental tasks being confronted, and role demands. Although clients will differ in their self-care and self-management competencies, it is important that the nurse emphasize to all clients their own importance as "primary self-care agent." Promoting client responsibility for health does not negate the importance of the nurse working to change the larger social infrastructure to make health-promoting options more available to groups and communities. Personal change and social change are both essential for effective health promotion and prevention.

A sample health promotion-prevention plan for an individual client is presented in Figure 5–1 and one for a family in Figure 5–2. In both planning tools, sections are provided in which client strengths can be identified.

Designed for: _James Moore_

Home Address: _714 George Street_

Home Telephone Number: _222-3333_

Occupation (if employed): _building services supervisor_

Work Telephone Number: _445-6666_

Cultural Identification: _African American_

Birth Date: _3/14/59_   Date of Initial Plan: _1/15/2005_

Client strengths:	Satisfactory peer relationships, spiritual strength, adequate sleep pattern
Major risk factors:	Elevated cholesterol, mild obesity, sedentary lifestyle, moderate life change, multiple daily hassles, few reported uplifts
Nursing diagnoses: (derived from assessment of functional health patterns)	Diversional activity deficit; altered nutrition: more than body requirements; caregiver role strain (elderly mother)
Medical diagnoses: (if any)	Mild hypertension
Age-specific screening recommendations: (derived from *Guide to Clinical Prev. Services*)	Blood pressure, cholesterol, fecal occult blood, malignant skin lesions, depression
Desired behavioral and health outcomes:	Become a regular exerciser (3x/week), lower my blood pressure, weigh 165 lb

FIGURE 5-1 **Example of an Individual Health Promotion-Prevention Plan**

Personal Health Goals (1 = highest priority)	Selected Behaviors to Accomplish Goals	Stage of Change	Strategies/ Interventions for Change
1. Achieve desired body weight	Begin a progressive walking program	Planning	Counter-conditioning Reinforcement management Patient contracting
	Decrease caloric intake while maintaining good nutrition	Action (eating 2 fruits and 2 vegetables daily; using low-fat dairy products for last 2 months)	Stimulus control Cognitive restructuring
2. Decrease risk for hypertension-related disorders	Change from high- to low-sodium snacks	Contemplation	Consciousness raising Learning facilitation
3. Learn to manage stress effectively	Attend relaxation classes and use home relaxation tapes	Contemplation	Consciousness raising Self-reevaluation Simple relaxation therapy
4. Increase leisure-time activities	Join a local bowling league	Contemplation	Support system enhancement

FIGURE 5–1 Continued

Identify Health Goals and Related Behavior-Change Options

The next step in the planning process is to identify personal or family health goals, prioritize them, and review related behavior-change options. Systematically reviewing the range of changes that are possible to achieve important health goals can assist clients in determining the behavioral changes on which they will focus in the initial health

---

Designed for (family name): ___The Marshalls___

Home Address: _1718 Green Street_

Home Telephone Number: ___777-4444___

Occupations of Employed
Members of Household: _Mother—Dental assistant_

Work Telephone Number: ___883-7777___

Family Form: __One-parent family__

Cultural Identification: __Asian American__

Family Members: Position in Family	Birth Date	Occupation/ Student/Retired
Joan (Mother)	9/65	Dental assistant
Dana (Daughter)	4/87	Student
Tiffany (Daughter)	7/91	Student
Eric (Son)	1/94	Student

Date of Initial Plan: ___1-15-2005___

Family strengths:	Open communication patterns, intrafamily cooperation, healthy snacks consumed at home
Major risk factors:	Mother recently divorced, oldest daughter has driver's license, high life change for family, minimal family physical activity
Nursing diagnoses:	Family coping: potential for growth
Medical diagnoses for family members:	None
Desired behavioral and health outcomes:	Active family outings, avoidance of early sexual activity and binge drinking among adolescent family members, injury prevention for children, adjustment to new family form

FIGURE 5–2   Example of a Family Health Promotion-Prevention Plan

promotion-prevention plan. Providing relevant information but letting the client deter-mine priorities for change constitutes educative–supportive care by the nurse. Clients should not be made to feel guilty or inadequate in regard to current health practices. During health counseling sessions, the nurse should create enthusiasm and excitement about growth in positive directions and the benefits of new health-related experiences.

Family Health Goals (1 = highest priority)	Selected Behaviors to Accomplish Goals	Stage of Change	Strategies/ Interventions for Change
1. Healthy adjustment to single-parent family status	Realign family responsibilities	Action (divorced 3 mo)	Social liberation Family process maintenance Caregiver support
	Increase spiritual resources (increase church attendance)	Contemplation	Spiritual support Helping relationships
	Discuss life purpose and goals among family members	Planning	Self-reevaluation Self-esteem enhancement Anticipatory guidance
2. Develop more active family lifestyles	Plan active family outings (biking, recreation center)	Planning	Exercise promotion Environmental reevaluation Modeling
3. Foster healthy sexuality among preadolescent and adolescents	Provide age-appropriate information	Action	Anticipatory guidance Parent education: adolescent stage
	Enhance self-esteem through praise, expression of affection, and assistance with skill development	Maintenance	Self-esteem enhancement Helping relationships

FIGURE 5–2 Continued

| 4. Encourage adolescents to avoid alcohol use | Hold family meetings to discuss binge drinking, drinking and driving, use of nonalcoholic alternatives | Contemplation | Parent education: adolescent stage Self-responsibility facilitation Substance use prevention |

FIGURE 5–2 **Continued**

Many clients will initially place high priority on areas of prevention in which the threat of illness is tangible and easily understood. Decreasing risk for specific chronic health problems fits the medical orientation to which most Americans have been socialized. A high level of client interest in reducing the risk of disease indicates to the nurse that prevention is likely the most meaningful area for emphasis in early health planning. Mastery of specific prevention measures will often motivate clients to consider making additional lifestyle changes directed toward health promotion in order to experience a higher level of health and well-being.

Clients often give important emotional cues concerning the behaviors they wish to change. Examples of such cues include:

"I hate myself when I gorge on fattening foods!"

"I get mad at myself for being so uptight!"

"I feel very sad when I think of how little time our family spends together."

"We need to improve our diet"

"We are very critical of each other"

"We don't participate in physical activities together."

The more open an individual or family is in discussing health concerns with the nurse, the higher the probability of developing a meaningful health promotion-prevention plan. The areas that the client is most reluctant to discuss, such as marital relationships, human sexuality, spirituality, and family cohesiveness, are often the most crucial areas for behavior change. A "safe" climate should be created in which the client can discuss personal health issues with assurance that communication will remain confidential.

Identify Behavioral or Health Outcomes

The nurse and client together should determine the desired health outcomes of the health promotion-prevention plan. Clear identification of outcomes both energizes and guides the client in changing or establishing new health behaviors. The client's perceptions concerning desired outcomes should determine the criteria used to evaluate whether the plan and its implementation have been successful. Have I reached my goal or made significant progress toward it is a critical question that must be asked periodically by the client to evaluate the viability of the health promotion-prevention plan.

Research literature supporting the link between particular interventions and desired outcomes should influence the process and the development of the plan. For example, the factors or strategies shown to affect the likelihood of maintaining a healthy diet should be integrated into the plan for persons wishing to address nutritional issues. The nurse should assist the client in setting realistic outcomes. For example, a behavioral goal of eating only at meals may be easier to attain than a goal of losing a certain number of pounds. Weight will most likely be reduced if the plan is followed, but tangible behaviors are more under the control of the client and thus easier to reinforce and manage. Long-term outcomes may be set but achieved through a progressive set of short-term goals that move the client toward the desired outcome.

Develop a Behavior-Change Plan

A constructive program of change is based on the client taking "ownership" of those behavior changes implemented everyday. The client should be assisted in examining major value–behavior inconsistencies that exist. Alternative actions that are both healthful and enjoyable to the client need to be substituted for the behaviors that are inconsistent with personal values. Many individuals and families have learned to prefer or value the American lifestyle that is frequently considered to be detrimental to health. Value clarification may be a useful tool in the development of an individual or family behavior-change plan (Chitty, 1997; Potter & Perry, 1997; Townsend, 1996).

Clients should select from the available options those behaviors that are appealing and that they are willing to try. The client's priorities for behavior change will reflect personal values, activity preferences, estimates of cognitive and psychomotor skills, affective responses to the various behavioral options, expectations for success in learning and carrying out the various behaviors, and ease with which the selected behaviors can be integrated into lifestyle. The client's stage of change in relation to each of the selected behaviors should be assessed.

Appropriate strategies and interventions to facilitate behavior change may be identified from the nursing intervention classification systems (Bowles & Naylor, 1996; Henry, Holzemer, Randell, Hsieh, & Miller, 1997; Johnson, Bulecheck, McCloskey, & Dochterman, 2003; Moorhead, McCloskey, & Bulecheck, 1993), transtheoretical model literature (Nigg et al., 1999), and from nursing and behavioral science literature on behavior change. The nurse should develop expertise in the activities that constitute the intervention and the appropriate sequencing of those activities. As the expert health care provider, the nurse can assist the client in gaining the behavior-change skills needed for the adoption and maintenance of positive health behaviors.

Reiterate Benefits of Change

Although clients are aware of the changes they want to make and the benefits of change, the positive benefits should be frequently reiterated by both the nurse and the client. The client should keep a list of benefits from the changes being made in a highly visible place so they may be reviewed frequently. This may be on the refrigerator, the bathroom mirror, the dashboard of the car, or the computer at work. Keeping health benefits "in front" of the client is a reminder that the behaviors in the health promotion-prevention plan are personally worthwhile and directed toward important life goals.

The benefits of change may include both health-related and non-health-related outcomes. Sensitivity to non-health-related benefits of change such as increased popularity or more time with friends is important, as these may be central to the client's motivation to engage in health promotion-prevention planning and implementation.

Address Environmental and Interpersonal Facilitators and Barriers to Change

Environmental features and interpersonal relationships supportive of positive change should be used to bolster the client's efforts to modify lifestyle. Social networks are important to help the client counter barriers to change. Encouragement from family and friends helps the client to persist when change efforts are difficult or competing demands or preferences vie for attention. All individuals and families experience barriers to changing behavior. Although some obstacles cannot be anticipated, others may be planned for and their potential negative impact considerably weakened. If the client is aware of possible barriers and has formulated plans for dealing with them if they arise, successful behavior change is more likely to occur.

Barriers to effective health behavior may arise from clients' internal conflicts, from significant others, or from the environment. Internal barriers to change may be lack of motivation, fatigue, boredom, giving up, lack of appropriate skills, or disbelief that behavior can be successfully changed. Family members may impose considerable barriers if they encourage continuation of health-damaging behaviors or if they actively discourage attempts at behavior change. Environmental barriers that may inhibit positive change include lack of space or appropriate setting in which to carry out the selected activity; dangers within the immediate environment, such as heavy traffic or high crime rate; or inclement weather. The nurse should assist the client in dealing with these environmental barriers or in locating other appropriate settings for health activities.

Determine a Time Frame for Implementation

Developing healthier behaviors should occur over time in order to allow new behaviors to be learned well, integrated into one's lifestyle, and stabilized. Attempting to change or initiate a number of new behaviors at one time may result in confusion, discouragement, and the client's abandonment of the health promotion-prevention plan. Whether the client is attempting to reduce the risk for chronic diseases or to enhance health status, gradual change is desirable. Just as health education for self-care must proceed at the pace of the learner rather than that of the nurse, changes in behavior must be sequenced in reasonable steps appropriate for the client.

Developing a time plan for implementation allows appropriate knowledge and skills to be mastered before a new behavior is implemented. For example, it is difficult to warm up before brisk walking or jogging if the client has no idea of what exercises are appropriate for warm-up. The time frame for developing a particular behavior may be several weeks or several months. If the client is rewarded for accomplishing short-term goals, this provides encouragement for continuing the pursuit of long-term goals and desired outcomes. A meaningful plan requires that deadlines be set for accomplishing specific goals. Adherence to deadlines should be encouraged, with changes made only when the time frame must be shortened or lengthened to make it more conducive to permanent behavior change.

Formalize Commitment to Behavior-Change Plan

Through identification of new behaviors that the client wishes to acquire, a verbal commitment is made to change. However, the client may be more motivated to follow through with selected actions if the personal commitment is formalized. A commitment to change may be formalized using one of the following options: (a) nurse–client contract agreements like those that appear in Figures 5–3 and 5–4, (b) self-contracts such as those shown in Figures 5–5 and 5–6, (c) public announcements to family members and friends of intentions to engage in new behaviors, (d) integration of new health behaviors into a daily or weekly calendar, and (e) purchase of necessary supplies (e.g., low-fat foods, exercise audiotapes) and equipment (e.g., exercise bike, walking shoes).

Behavioral contracts contain specific information about (a) the change to be made, (b) the way the change is to be accomplished, (c) the individual or family members who are to engage in the change, (d) the time frame for behavior change, and (e) the consequences of meeting or not meeting the terms of the agreement. A *nurse–client contract* provides direction through the identification of mutual objectives and the responsibilities of each party. Contracts allow clients to participate actively by choosing goals that can be realistically accomplished. Generally, the client is responsible for carrying out certain behaviors, whereas the nurse is responsible for providing information, training, counseling, or specific reinforcement rewards. The nurse bears the additional responsibility of providing helpful input and continuing feedback to the client concerning the adequacy of performance of activities identified in the contract. It is also critical that the nurse be consistent and conscientious in managing the reinforcement–reward contingencies of the contract. Failure in fulfilling this commitment will alter the trust and confidence placed in the nurse by the client.

In a nurse–client contract with a family, the agreement may be made to brisk walk, jog, or bicycle together two to three times each week or to modify their nutritional practices, such as increasing vegetables in their diet to three to four servings per day. Family members, because of their continuing contact and emotional bonding, serve as important sources of encouragement, reinforcement, and reward for one another.

The extent to which the contract has worked must be evaluated. Did the client accomplish the goal fully, partially, or not at all? If failure occurred, what were the reasons? How could the contract be reorganized so that the probability of successful completion is high? Does the contract need to be renegotiated? Should the contract be terminated? Careful analysis of the contracting process and evaluation of subsequent outcomes will permit the nurse and client to design contracts that successfully move clients toward desired health goals.

In a *self-contract* the client is responsible both for the behavioral commitment and for reinforcement of identified behaviors. Self-contracting is an effective approach for enhancing the client's control over behavior, thus creating a sense of independence, competence, and autonomy. The client does not become overly dependent on the nurse for reinforcement but instead serves as the source of rewards for positive health behaviors. Rewards may be extrinsic such as tangible objects (e.g., magazine, cosmetics) or experiences (e.g., warm bath, telephone call to a friend), or intrinsic (e.g., self-praise, feelings of pride). Rewards selected should be highly desirable to the client in order to have reinforcement value. A reward–reinforcement plan may be developed as illustrated in Figure 5–7.

Nurse–Client Contract and Agreement

Statement of Health Goal: _____ *Decreased feelings of stress and tension* _____

I _____ *Jim Johnson* _____ promise to _____ *use progressive relaxation* _____
        (client)

_____ *techniques upon arriving home from work each day* _____
                    (Client Responsibility)

for a period of _____ *one week* _____ , whereupon,

_____ *Kathy Turner* _____ will provide *(1) guest*
        (nurse)

coupon for 2 Spruill Coffees   *(2) Complimentary message*
                    (Nurse Responsibility)

on _____ *Saturday, March 7th* _____ to me.
                    (date)

If I do not fulfill the terms of this contract in total, I understand that the designated reward will be withheld.

Signed: _____
                                    (client)

         _____
                                    (date)

         _____
                                    (nurse)

         _____
                                    (date)

FIGURE 5–3 **Sample Nurse–Client Contract for an Individual Client**

Success in fulfilling the agreements in the contract enhances the client's self-esteem and problem-solving abilities. The client gains increased confidence in meeting future health needs. In reality, it is the client who must learn to manage a self-reward system that is supportive of new positive health practices.

Publicly announcing intentions to engage in a new behavior to family members and close friends is another way of solidifying commitment to a particular course of action. The expectations of other family members or friends that the client will be successful often enhance

---

Nurse–Client Contract and Agreement

Statement of Health Goal: _____ *Improve eating habits* _____

We _____ *The Nichols* _____ promise to _eat two servings of_
          (family)

_____ *vegetables and two servings of fruit daily* _____
                    (family responsibility)

for a period of _____ *one week* _____ whereupon,

_____ *Lana Buxton* _____ will provide _____ *guest passes* _____
          (nurse)

to Riverbanks Zoo _____
                    (nurse responsibility)

on _____ *Friday, April 10th* _____ to us.
                    (date)

If we do not fulfill the terms of this contract in total, We understand that the designated reward will be withheld.

Signed: _____
                              (family representative)

          _____
                              (date)

          _____
                              (nurse)

          _____
                              (date)

FIGURE 5–4   **Sample Nurse–Client Contract for a Family**

one's motivation for change behavior. Integrating new behaviors into one's calendar is an important way of building them into daily routines. For example, exercise time may be scheduled during the lunch hour and the appointment for exercise kept just as an appointment with one's friend or coworker. Lack of time is a frequent excuse for being unable to follow-through with newly adopted behaviors. When time is actually scheduled to accomplish health behaviors, the probability of their occurrence is significantly enhanced.

Self-Contract

Personal Health Goal: _____ *Change dietary habits* _____

I _____ *Doris Downs* _____ promise myself that I will _*follow*_

_____ *the sample menus for a 1,200 calorie diet for breakfast, lunch, and*

_____ *dinner* _____ for a period of _____ *four days* _____ ,

whereupon I will _____ *buy myself a new pair of earrings* _____

on _____ *Wednesday, June 8th* _____ .

Signed: _____

Date: _____

FIGURE 5–5 Sample Individual Self-Contract

Self-Contract

Family Health Goal: _____ *Get more exercise* _____

We _____ *The Stones* _____ promise each other that we will _____ *go* _____

_____ *swimming at the "Y" once a week* _____ for a period of _*three weeks*_

whereupon we will _____ *buy the newest version of Trivial Pursuit* _____

on _____ *Friday, February 10th* _____ .

Signed: _____

_____

_____

Date: _____

FIGURE 5–6 Sample Family Self-Contract

Behavior: Learn to Use Progressive Relaxation as One Approach to Handling Stress

Component of Behavior	Reward or Reinforcement
Attend first class session at 9 A.M. Saturday at the County Health Department	Watch the football game in the afternoon on TV
Use relaxation audiotape at home for 20 minutes of practice	
Sunday	Call John and visit for a while
Monday	Spend an hour at the driving range
Tuesday	Buy a new paperback novel
Wednesday	Praise myself for having practiced relaxation each day thus far
Thursday	Invite Harry and Jim over to play pool
Friday	Take my family to a movie
Attend second class session at 9 A.M. Saturday at the County Health Department	Take an orange juice break afterward with Bret, a class member
Practice relaxation techniques for 20 minutes providing my own cues rather than using the tape	
Sunday	Go for a short drive and enjoy the scenery
Monday	Spend 30 minutes reading my new novel
Tuesday	Buy myself a new bottle of aftershave lotion
Wednesday	Praise myself for persistence and successful practice
Thursday	Allow myself to linger in a warm shower longer than usual
Friday	Go biking with the family
Keep my weekly record of relaxation practice	The nurse will provide a copy of *Relaxation Response* by Herbert Benson

FIGURE 5–7 **Reward-Reinforcement Plan**

Purchasing necessary supplies and equipment is yet another way of making a commitment to behavior change. When equipment is purchased and a monetary investment is made, clients are much more likely to follow-through with the desired behavior. For example, people who have exercise equipment and exercise videos in their home are more likely to be active than persons who do not.

Revisions of the Health Promotion-Prevention Plan

A schedule for periodic review of the health promotion-prevention plan should be established. Revisions should be carried out during counseling sessions, with both the client and the nurse contributing to the process. Impetus for changes in the plan may result from mastery of target behaviors, changes in client's values and priorities, or awareness of new options available to the client. Outdated plans fail to provide impetus or direction for change and thus become uninteresting and meaningless to the client. Periodic revision and updating of the health plan provides a systematic approach for movement of the client toward more positive health behaviors and a higher level of health.

Community-Level Health Promotion-Prevention Plan

Community-level plans and interventions may be the most effective way to engage members in improving their health. Important health concerns such as youth and family violence, initiation of tobacco use, unintended pregnancy in adolescents, and unintentional injuries may require broad-based planning and intervention. School-based curricular (Institute of Medicine, 1997; U.S. Department of Health and Human Services, 2000) and community programs (Davidson, Durkin, Kuhn, et al., 1994; Rivara, Thompson, Thompson et al., 1994) may be the most effective way to address these health problems. The nurse must be aware of community-based initiatives and encourage client participation. The nurse may also serve as a consultant to communities implementing programs and be an advocate for developing community-based health plans and interventions (Murdaugh & Vanderboom, 1997; Tessaro, 1997).

Directions for Research in Behavior Change

Many nursing research questions relative to planning for health promotion and prevention have been identified. Nurses are in a pivotal position to address these questions and create new knowledge about the behavior-change process. Questions to be addressed include:

1. How can face-to-face and computerized feedback from health assessment be combined to optimize one's level of motivation for health promotion planning?
2. What interventions are most effective to reinforce clients' positive cultural health practices during health counseling?

3. During what stages of change for a given health behavior is intrinsic motivation likely to be more effective than extrinsic motivation?

4. What factors affect the rate of behavior change at different life stages?

5. What are the effects of successful behavior change on self-esteem, self-efficacy, and behavioral control?

6. What are the major barriers to implementing community intervention to improve the health of its members?

7. What types of community-based interventions are effective in improving the health of special populations?

Directions for Practice in Behavior Change

Developing a plan to counsel clients about their health behaviors is a major responsibility of nurses in practice. The nurse must possess the skills necessary to guide clients to participate in developing a realistic, positive plan. Nurses with a working knowledge of current guidelines will ensure that accurate, up-to-date information is incorporated into the plan. Understanding all information obtained from the assessment may mean that other disciplines are consulted to help interpret information or recommend appropriate goals. An interdisciplinary approach in which multiple experts are involved enables the client and nurse to set appropriate goals, develop interventions to meet the goals, and establish methods to evaluate the process. Support is critical during the change process, so the nurse also needs to learn to identify family and other support for the client, and to develop creative strategies to incorporate their support into the plan. The plan must be adapted to life-span issues and gender differences, as well as socioeconomic status.

Knowledge of cultural issues that may play a role is key to the design of a culturally sensitive, age- and gender-appropriate plan. Whenever possible, technology should be incorporated in developing the plan. Interactive software that provides feedback on achieving outcomes and formulates an ongoing review of the plan may motivate clients because they see immediate results of their input. Developing a health promotion-prevention plan is straightforward but complex, and the nurse will need to continually update skills to assist clients in this important process.

SUMMARY

The health promotion-prevention plans presented in this chapter provide individuals and families with a systematic approach to improving health practices and lifestyle. All clients should be provided with a health portfolio that contains a summary of their health assessment, their health promotion-prevention plan, and other relevant health records. It is imperative that clients have all the information and planning documents needed to follow through successfully with their desired behavior changes. Focusing on outcomes desired by the client will energize and direct implementation of the plan. Adjusting the plan as needed to ensure client success is vital to effective health-promoting care. Community-level plans that address broad-based health concerns are being developed. Increasing evidence supports the efficacy and effectiveness of developing health promotion-prevention plans at the community level.

LEARNING ACTIVITIES

1. Using the nine-step planning process, select a partner and develop an individual health plan for each other. Evaluate your experiences and outcomes.
2. Using the nine-step planning process, develop a health plan for a family with teenagers. Write a two-page summary of your experiences and outcomes.
3. Write a one-page summary of how the community influences the individual and family planning processes you developed in learning activities 1 and 2.

SELECTED WEB SITES

Agency for Health Research and Quality: Guide to Clinical Preventive Services

http://www.ahrq.gov/clinic/prevenix.htm

Biomedicine and Health in the News

http://library.uchc.edu/bhn/nyt.html

Centers for Disease Control and Prevention

http://www.cdc.gov

National Guideline Clearinghouse

http://www.guideline.gov

Occupational Safety and Health Administration

http://www.osha.gov

Office of Disease Prevention and Health Promotion

http://www.hhs.gov/diseases/index.shtml

Office of the Surgeon General, U.S. Public Health Service

http://www.surgeongeneral.gov

REFERENCES

American Medical Association. (1994). *AMA guidelines for adolescent preventive services: Recommendations and rationale.* Baltimore, MD: Williams & Wilkins.

Bowles, K. H., & Naylor, M. S. (1996, Winter). Nursing intervention classification systems. *Image J Nurs Sch, 28*(4), 303–308.

Chitty, K. (1997). *Professional nursing: Concepts and challenges.* Chattanooga, TN: University of Tennessee at Chattanooga.

Davidson, L. L., Durkin, M. S., Kuhn, L., et al. (1994). The impact of the Safe Kids/Healthy Neighborhoods Injury Prevention Program in Harlem, 1988 through 1991. *Am J Public Health, 84,* 580–586.

Green, M. (Ed.). (2002). *Bright futures: Guidelines for health supervision of infants, children, and adolescents.* Arlington, VA: National Center for Education in Maternal and Child Health.

Henry, S. B., Holzemer, W. L., Randell, C., Hsieh, S. F., & Miller, T. J. (1997). Comparison of nursing interventions classification and current procedural terminology codes for categorizing nursing activities. *Image J Nurs Sch, 29*(2), 133–138.

Institute of Medicine. (1997). *Schools and health: Our nation's investment.* Washington, DC: National Academy Press.

Johnson, M., Bulecheck, G., McCloskey Dochterman, J. (2003). *Nursing outcomes classification 3e, Interventions classification and nursing diagnoses: NANDA, NOC, and NIC* linkages. St. Louis: Cumasky Co.

Moorhead, S. A., McCloskey, J. C., & Bulecheck, G. M. (1993). Nursing interventions classification. A comparison with the Omaha System and the home healthcare classification. *J Nurs Adm, 23*(10), 23–29.

Murdaugh, C. L., & Vanderboom, C. (1997). Individual and community models for promotion wellness. *J Cardiovasc Nurs, 11*(3), 1–14.

Nigg, C. R., Burbank, P. M., Padula, C., Dufresne, R., Rossie, J. S., Velicer, W. F., Laforge, R. G., & Prochaska, J. O. (1999). Stages of change across ten health risk behaviors for older adults. *Gerontologist, 39*(4), 473–482.

Potter, P. A., & Perry, A. G. (1997). *Fundamentals of nursing: Concepts, process and practice.* St. Louis: Mosby.

Rivara, F. P., Thompson, D. C., Thompson, R. S., et al. (1994). The Seattle Children's Bicycle Helmet Campaign: Changes in helmet use and head injury admissions. *Pediatrics, 93,* 567–569.

Tessaro, I. (1997). The natural helping role of nurses in promoting healthy behaviors in communities. *Adv Pract Nurs Q, 2*(4), 73–78.

Townsend, M. C. (1996). *Psychiatric mental health nursing: Concepts of care* (3rd ed.). Oklahoma City: 1996.

U.S. Department of Health and Human Services. (2000). *Healthy People 2010* (conference edition, Educational and Community–Based Programs). Washington, DC: U.S. Government Printing Office.

U.S. Department of Health and Human Services (1998). *Clinician's handbook of preventive services: Put prevention into practice,* 2nd edition, Washington D.C.: U.S. Government Printing Office.

U.S. Preventive Services Task Force. (1996). *Guide to clinical preventive services* (2nd ed.). Baltimore, MD: Williams & Wilkins.

Part 3

Interventions for Health Promotion and Prevention

6

Physical Activity and Health Promotion

Regular physical activity is essential for healthy, energetic, and productive living. Modern life with its automobiles, televisions, computers, video games, and low levels of physical activity in school and work environments necessitates the commitment of significant leisure time to physical activity in order to gain resultant health benefits. *Physical activity* is defined as any bodily movement produced by skeletal muscles that results in expenditure of energy (expressed as kilocalories) and includes a broad range of occupational, leisure-time, and routine daily activities. These activities may require either light, moderate, or vigorous effort (U.S. Department of Health and Human Services, 1998). *Leisure physical activity* is physical activity undertaken during discretionary time. *Lifestyle physical activity* is characterized as integration of numerous short bouts of moderate activity into daily living. *Exercise* is leisure-time physical activity conducted with the intention of developing physical fitness (U.S. Department of Health and Human Services, 1999). *Physical fitness* is a measure of a person's ability to perform physical activities that require endurance, strength, or flexibility and is determined by a combination of level of physical activity and genetically inherited physical characteristics (U.S. Department of Health and Human Services, 1999). The term *physical activity* is used in this chapter to encompass a broad range of activities that, if performed regularly, will improve health. Because of the centrality of physical activity to health, this chapter focuses on the benefits of physical activity, guidelines for activity, the determinants of physical activity for children and adults, primary care and community interventions to promote physical activity, and the importance of health providers routinely incorporating physical activity counseling into the care of clients of all ages.

Maintenance of regular physical activity is largely dependent on sources of personal and social motivation within a person's day-to-day environment. Family and peers play a powerful role in encouraging active lifestyles. Many individuals begin physical activity on their own; some are able to continue this important health behavior. Others rely on the school or work environments to create programs that help them achieve their physical activity goals. Many others cycle through periods of activity and inactivity, never establishing regular physical activity patterns. Within the last decade, there has been an alarming increase in the prevalence of overweight and obesity among both adults and adolescents.

Among adults who are overweight, it is important for them to know that elevated body weight is potentially a preobese state. One goal of *Healthy People 2010* is to increase the number of healthy-weight adults (defined as a body mass index equal to or greater than 18.5 and less than 25) ages 20 years and older from a baseline of 42% to 60%. Another goal is to reduce the percentage of obese adults ages 20 and older from 23% to 15% (U.S. Department of Health and Human Services, 2000). The cost of obesity to U.S. businesses in 1998 was estimated at over $75 billion ($92.6 billion in 2002 dollars) (health expenditures, sick leave, life insurance, and disability insurance) (Finkelstein, Fiebelkorn, & Wang, 2003). The 1996 National Longitudinal Study of Adolescent Health (Popkin & Udry, 1998) found 24% of white adolescents, 31% of black and Hispanic adolescents, and 42% of Native American adolescents to be overweight (≥ 85th percentile).

Healthy People 2010, the 10-year health plan for the American people, identified the important goals of improving health, fitness, and quality and years of healthy life of Americans through daily physical activity. The report notes the disparity in level of physical activity among population groups. The percent of the population reporting no leisure time activity is higher among women than men, among African Americans and Hispanics than whites, among older than younger adults, and among the less affluent than the more affluent. Participation in all types of physical activity declines strikingly during the adolescent years. A total of 15 physical activity objectives to be achieved by the end of the decade have been identified. Selected objectives include (U.S. Department of Health and Human Services, 2000):

- Increase from 15% (baseline) to 30% the proportion of adults who engage regularly, preferably daily, in moderate activity for at least 30 minutes per day.
- Increase from 20% (baseline) to 30% the proportion of adolescents who engage in moderate physical activity for at least 30 minutes on 5 or more days per week.
- Increase from 64% (baseline) to 85% the proportion of adolescents who engage in vigorous physical activity that promotes cardio-respiratory fitness 3 or more days per week for 20 or more minutes per occasion.
- Increase from 32% (baseline) to 50% the proportion of adolescents who spend at least half of school physical education class time being physically active.
- Increase from 60% (baseline) to 75% the proportion of children and adolescents who view television 2 or fewer hours per day.
- Increase the proportion of work sites offering employer-sponsored physical activity and fitness programs.

Achieving these goals will increase the level of health and well-being of persons of all ages and increase the prevalence of healthy lifestyles in the population.

Health Benefits of Physical Activity

Regular physical activity contributes to physiologic stability and high-level functioning and assists individuals in actualizing their physical performance potential. Regular activity also decreases the risk for obesity, heart disease, diabetes, hypertension, and stroke, and is associated with a decreased risk for colon cancer. Being physically active enhances psychological well-being, reduces the risk of depression, and improves mood as well as self-concept and self-esteem. Research studies provide evidence of the causal link between inactivity and cardiovascular disease. Indeed, millions of Americans are at risk for a wide range of chronic diseases and mental health problems that might well be prevented by active lifestyles. Among children and adolescents, weight-bearing exercise is needed for normal skeletal development and attainment of peak bone mass. Regular physical activity increases strength, agility, and prevents falls among older adults and increases their independence in activities of daily living. It improves the functional capacity of individuals with disabilities (U.S. Department of Health and Human Services 1998, 2000). Research to increase knowledge concerning the actual mechanisms connecting physical activity and health is needed but many studies clearly indicate a variety of beneficial effects from regular patterns of activity (U.S. Department of Health and Human Services, 1998).

To achieve health benefits, regular physical activity of moderate to vigorous intensity is essential. Moderate-intensity activity refers to a level of effort that burns 3.5 to 7 kilocalories per minute (kcal/min) or 3 to 6 metabolic equivalents (METS). Activities at this level include walking briskly, bicycling on level terrain, swimming, or dancing. Vigorous-intensity activity is at a level of effort that burns more than 7 kcal/min or greater than 6 METS. Such activities include jogging, swimming continuous laps, or bicycling uphill. The minimum amount of activity required for health benefits burns approximately 150 kcal of energy per day or approximately 1,000 kcal per week. The exercise prescription for middle-age men is about 2,000 kcal per week, or the equivalent of walking 3 miles a day. The time needed each day to achieve this goal depends on the intensity level of the activity and the number of days of activity each week (U.S. Department of Health and Human Services, 2000). Research is lacking for a precise exercise prescription for women and other subgroups, but a recent study suggests that a goal of 10,000 steps per day or 5 miles would classify a person as "active" (Tudor-Locke, 2003).

It is difficult to sort out the health benefits solely from physical activity, because being active may trigger other health behaviors such as changes in dietary and smoking habits and adoption of more effective methods of coping with stress. Positive effects of regular physical activity are summarized in Table 6–1. For a detailed discussion, see Bouchard, Shephard, and Stevens (1994).

Genetic and Environmental Effects on Activity Level

The interaction between genetic and environmental influences on level of physical activity is receiving increased attention from researchers. Rapid advances in the field of genetics will offer new and vital information for nurses concerning the effects of the genotype–environment interaction both on predisposition to physical activity and on health-related fitness responses from physical activity. Scientific breakthroughs in understanding genetic individuality will become increasingly important in assessing differences in risk for diseases associated with inactivity.

TABLE 6–1 **Positive Effects of Physical Exercise**

Cardiopulmonary and Blood Chemistry Effects

Reduce systolic and diastolic blood pressure
Increase blood oxygen content
Decrease total cholesterol
Increase high-density lipoproteins
Reduce serum triglycerides
Increase peripheral blood circulation and return
Reduce resting heart rate by increasing stroke volume
Increase blood supply to heart and myocardial efficiency
Increase heart rate recovery after exercise

Immunologic–Oncologic Effects

Reduce incidence of selected types of cancer
Improve prognosis posttreatment for cancer
Increase circulating leukocytes

Endocrine and Metabolic Effects

Improve glucose tolerance
Decrease reactivity to psychosocial stressors
Decrease body fat
Increase endogenous opioid peptides, particularly beta-endorphins
Enhance oxidation of fatty acids
Enhance elimination
Increase metabolism rate

Musculoskeletal Effects

Increase lean muscle mass
Maintain bone mass
Prevent or ameliorate chronic back and joint pain
Increase muscle strength and endurance

Psychosocial Effects

Improve self-concept
Improve body image
Decrease anxiety and depression
Improve mental alertness
Enhance general mood and psychological well-being
Enhance sexual satisfaction
Increase stress resistance

According to Baranowski and associates (2000) genetic research is likely to identify foods that do not increase fat deposits, ages when the body is more receptive to change, and people with certain genes that are more receptive to specific behavior changes. These findings would allow for tailoring of specific behavior models to the relevant genotypic mechanism.

The association of genetics and childhood environments to lifelong exercise participation is receiving more study. Simonen, Videman, Kaprio, Levalahti, and Battie (2003) found that 43% of the variation in exercise in adulthood was attributed to familial factors. Participation in exercise in adolescence was associated with continued exercise in adulthood. Early childhood environmental factors were strong influences for exercise throughout adulthood.

Obesity and regional fat distribution, factors that may contribute to activity or inactivity, have definite inherited components. The estimated variance due to genotype is 5% for body mass index and 25% for percent body fat and truncated abdominal fat (Bouchard & Perusse, 1994).

Life-Span Patterns of Physical Activity

Interest in life-span patterns of physical activity has been fueled by the realization that a number of risk factors for cardiovascular disease including obesity, high blood pressure, and elevated cholesterol are often evident early in childhood. Further, of the four major modifiable risk factors for coronary heart disease, elevated cholesterol, smoking, hypertension, and inactivity, the latter—lack of regular physical activity—is the most prevalent in the population. A survey conducted by the Centers for Disease Control and Prevention (CDC) indicated that only 40% of the population is active enough to gain physical and mental health benefits (Karch, 2000).

Habits of physical activity begun early in life are likely to persist over time. It is much easier to focus on developing positive physical activity patterns initially than on changing unhealthy behaviors once they are stabilized as habits. Although vigorous activity is likely to result in the most health benefits, the accumulation of 30 minutes or more of moderate physical activity on most days of the week may be more acceptable to currently sedentary individuals. Lifestyle activity provides flexibility for increasing energy expenditure through altering patterns of daily activities such as walking to work or school, taking the stairs, and being active during lunchtime or after school or work. Activities other than participation in organized sports are attractive to a broader range of the population (Marcus & Forsyth, 1999). Gender and type of physical activity influences the amount of exercise one does and should be considered in planning programs to reverse the decline during the adolescent years, with females becoming increasingly more sedentary than males (van Beurden et al., 2003).

Understanding the determinants of physical activity in various age groups is essential to effective interventions and counseling by health care providers to promote active lifestyles. More research is needed that examines developmental transitions in physical activity attitudes and beliefs from childhood through adulthood to explain variability in physical activity behavior for individuals across the life span (Sallis et al., 2000).

Determinants of Physical Activity in Children and Adolescents

A commonly held misperception is that children and adolescents are perpetually active and physically fit. Nothing could be further from the truth. Various studies indicate that greater than one-third of youths have adopted sedentary lifestyles by 10 years of age (Baranowski et al., 2000). The long-term goal of physical activity research among youths is to identify factors influencing level of activity as a basis for designing culturally appropriate interventions to increase activity and improve related short- and long-term health outcomes. Of particular interest are the ways in which developmental and social transitions, which occur with great rapidity during late childhood and early adolescence, affect participatory patterns. Pubertal changes (onset of menarche, changing patterns of body fat distribution) and social transitions (moving from elementary school to junior high school and on to senior high school) undoubtedly exert important influences on sports participation and patterns of physical activity. To date, most studies have been cross-sectional, identifying only correlates or potential influences on physical activity. Longitudinal studies are needed to identify changing activity patterns and probable influences on physical activity across childhood and adolescence. Prediction of physical activity behavior is difficult as influences may fluctuate in their predictive importance for different gender, race, or socioeconomic groups and at different developmental time points. Thus, it is important to specify clearly the group(s) being studied and their stage of development.

Physical Activity Related to Gender

Physical activity patterns and related influences vary by gender across many studies. Among 732 fourth and fifth graders, significant declines in physical activity occurred over 20 months. Gender-specific factors appeared to influence this decline. For boys, changes in attitude toward physical education, perceived competence or self-efficacy, parental transport to activities, and level of activity of the parent were related to the decline. For girls, changes in activity preferences and parental transport to activities were related to the decline (Trost, Pate, Ward, Saunders, & Riner, 1999). Sallis, Alcaraz, McKenzie, and Hovell (1999) studied 198 sixth graders and found that for boys, physical activity self-efficacy, social norms regarding physical activity, and involvement in community sports organizations predicted level of physical activity. For girls, only physical activity self-efficacy predicted activity level (Sallis et al., 1999).

In a longitudinal study, 111 families with fifth- and sixth-grade children were followed for 3 years to determine influences on physical activity over time. In the first phase of the study, enjoyment of exercise was the only variable related to activity for girls. Three years later, exercise knowledge, mother's physical activity, and friend–family modeling and support were related to activity among girls. Enjoyment of exercise and friend–family modeling and support were related to level of activity for boys. Three years later, physical activity self-efficacy, exercise knowledge, and interest in sports media correlated with physical activity. Trends in the data appear to indicate that social support became more important for girls over time whereas personal interest and self-efficacy became more important for boys. Determinants of physical activity differed for boys and girls and changed over the period of development that was studied (DiLorenzo, Stucky-Ropp, Vanderwal, & Gotham,

1998). Continuing assessment of factors influencing physical activity as the children transitioned to middle school and high school would provide valuable information about gender-specific developmental changes in the determinates of physical activity.

Garcia and colleagues (1995), in applying the Health Promotion Model to physical activity behavior in a racially diverse population, found definite gender differences between physical activity beliefs and behaviors of fifth, sixth, and eighth graders. Compared to boys, girls reported less representation of self as athletic and lower levels of past and current physical activity. The benefits to barriers differential (benefits-of-physical activity score minus barriers-to-physical activity score), access to recreational facilities and programs, and gender were significant predictors of physical activity measured several weeks later. Grade, health status, physical activity self-efficacy, social support, and social norms appeared to exert indirect effects on physical activity by modifying the balance between perceived benefits and barriers to being active. Race influenced physical activity through differential access to recreational facilities.

Family influences during childhood have a positive effect on the physical activity patterns that children develop. More active parents have been shown to have more active children of both genders. Trost and colleagues (2003) found that parental support is an important influence on physical activity in young people in grades 7 through 12.

Physical Activity Related to Ethnicity and Socioeconomic Status

A study of 2,285 children in fourth to sixth grades in a multiethnic, low-income urban neighborhood revealed that 20% of the girls and 25% of the boys were inactive. Children of Asian origin were less active than children in other ethnic groups. Socioeconomic status particularly influenced participation in organized sports outside of school where cost of participation and transportation may have posed major problems to parents. Correlates of low levels of activity included no participation in organized sports at or outside of school, lower physical activity self-efficacy, and lack of parental support for engaging in physical activity. Physical activity programs should promote high levels of perceived competence (self-efficacy) among youths and involve parents in family-oriented activities. Further, interventions should be developed to encourage parents to be positive role models of physically active lifestyles (O'Loughlin, Paradis, Kishchuk, Barnett, & Renaud, 1999). In another study of 1,871 multiethnic high school students, boys reported a level of physical activity 41% higher than girls. The most common activities for boys were weight lifting, baseball, basketball, jogging, and bicycling. The most common activities for girls were dancing, walking, calisthenics, and baseball. African Americans reported twice as much dancing as did other groups and Asian Americans reported more tennis than did other groups. Boys reported more modeling and support from friends to be active than did girls. Girls reported more barriers to being active and disliked physical education more than did boys. In terms of ethnic differences, Asian Americans and Latinos reported the lowest level of neighborhood safety for physical activity, and African Americans and Latinos reported the fewest convenient facilities for physical activity. African Americans reported the highest level of television viewing per week (Sallis, Zakarian, Hoveil, & Hofstetter, 1996). Caution should be exercised in interpreting the findings of many multiethnic studies because ethnicity–race is often confounded with social class so differences may be due to class rather than cultural background. Studies of physical activity determinants among youth that clearly separate these social and economic influences are needed. A multiethnic, developmental approach to the promotion of physical activity takes into consideration the level of maturity of youth, their decision-making ability, and culture-specific sources of motivation.

Factors Related to Increased Physical Activity

According to a recent comprehensive review of 108 studies of correlates of physical activity (Sallis, Prochaska, & Taylor, 2000), factors that increase the likelihood of children (4 to 12 years) being active include *history of being active, preference for physical activity over sedentary pursuits, goals or intentions to be active, lack of barriers to physical activity, access to recreational facilities and programs,* and *time spent outdoors.* Among adolescents (13 to 18 years), *history of being active, achievement orientation, intention to be active, perceived physical competence, opportunities to be active such as involvement in community sports, sensation seeking,* and *not being sedentary after school and on weekends* is associated with a more active lifestyle. *Active parental support such as transport or payment of activity fees, encouragement from significant others,* and *level of activity of siblings* were important social influences on adolescents. More studies are needed of the determinants of activity in diverse groups of children and adolescents to better understand how to tailor effective programs. Nurses should address important correlates of physical activity in their counseling with children and adolescents as these influences, when addressed, have the potential for increasing the development of an active lifestyle.

Role of Schools in Promoting Physical Activity

Schools play a major role in promoting the involvement of children in recreational activities that they can enjoy for a lifetime. By involving children on a daily basis in physical activity, teaching the personal value of regular activity, and encouraging continuing involvement in moderate or vigorous activities both at school and at home, schools contribute to the goal of an "active" generation. The level of structured activity in physical education classes has declined with just over one-third of elementary and secondary schools offering classes.

Role of Community in Promoting Physical Activity

Family-based activities, community-based recreational programs, and physical activity counseling by nurses and physicians in primary care should supplement school-based programs. Family-based programs encourage parents to be active with their children in relationship-building experiences. For example, weekend family bike outings and parent–child aerobic or recreational activities create opportunities for parents to be role models for active lifestyles (Ganley & Sherman, 2000). Community-based programs such as community runs, community all-sports days, and neighborhood walking groups will establish norms of physical activity participation for youths. Childhood and adolescence are ideal periods in the life span to cultivate regular physical activity that can reap positive health benefits throughout life.

Determinants of Physical Activity in Adults

Most of the theories and models used in adult physical activity studies to date have their origins in social psychology: social cognitive theory, theory of reasoned action, theory of planned behavior, Health Belief Model, protection-motivation theory, and the Health Promotion Model. In a classic article, Godin and Shephard (1990) reviewed the use of attitude–behavior models in promotion of physical activity. They identified *past behavior, self-efficacy, barriers to physical activity, outcome expectancies (positive and negative)*, and *intentions* as useful in predicting level of physical activity among adults. However, they concluded their review by pointing out that attitude–behavior models seldom explain more than 35% of the variance in physical activity behavior. Models that sometimes explain more variance do so inconsistently. The authors suggest that this may be due to the fact that the models used to study physical activity have focused on predisposing factors or those factors that result in the initiation of physical activity. Other factors that need to be studied include facilitating factors, such as accessibility and availability of facilities, and reinforcing factors, such as rewards and incentives that accompany or follow moderate or vigorous physical activity and contribute to its persistence. De Bourdeaudhuij and Sallis (2002) studied the contribution of four major psychosocial variables including social variables, self-efficacy, perceived benefits, and barriers to explain the variance in moderate to vigorous exercise. Their findings, supporting the findings of Godin and Shephard (1990), indicated that the relative contribution of their study variables did not contribute significantly to the explanation of physical activity and was of unequal importance in different age groups and gender. With advances in the field of genetics, the interaction of genetic makeup, psychological factors, and environmental factors in the determination of level of physical activity in adults requires further investigation. For example, it is likely that one's genetic makeup explains one's receptivity to physical activity and why some people are more successful in changing their exercise patterns. King, Stokols, Talen, Brassington, and Killingsworth (2002) discuss the limitations of the personal-level literature and propose approaches to studying physical activity behavior that include concepts and beliefs from social-ecology and urban-planning theories. These theories propose that environmental stress, neighborhood disorder, urban planning and design (automobile-oriented or pedestrian-oriented environments), and other macroenvironmental factors are also important mediators of physical activity.

In a study of 2,020 adults, the determinants of exercise behavior were studied using the Health Promotion Model (HPM) as the framework. The sample consisted of subgroups of working adults, community-dwelling older adults, cardiac rehabilitation patients, and ambulatory cancer patients. Perceiving many benefits from exercise, few barriers to exercise, and good perceived health status predicted greater involvement in exercise behavior. In the two populations (working adults, older adults) in which exercise efficacy was tested, higher perceived efficacy predicted greater involvement in exercise behavior. Among working adults, level of prior exercise program participation was highly predictive of continuing participation. Among older adults, preference for a moderate-to-high level of physical exertion and being high in self-motivation also contributed to the explanation of exercise frequency. The variance in exercise predicted across the four subgroups ranged from 23% to 59% (Pender et al., 1990).

Whereas in the past most studies of physical activity focused on males, there is increasing interest in the determinants of physical activity among women. Interest in the health benefits of moderate physical activity, that is, accumulation of at least 30 minutes most days of the week, has particular importance for women who are more likely to adopt moderate compared to vigorous physical activity. It is estimated that only 40% of women participate in regular physical activity (Seefeldt, Malina & Clark, 2002). Women's roles such as multiple family obligations and work pressures decrease their time for physical activity. Zaravar and Nies (1997) found that as women experienced increased daily hassles related to household activity, family, friends, and personal life, there was a decrease in physical activity. Unmarried women generally profile as more active than do married women with children at home (Brown & Trost, 2003). However, less is known about how physical activity is affected by role changes in women's lives such as parenthood, employment, children leaving home, or retirement (Pinto, Marcus, & Clark, 1996).

O'Brien Cousins and Gillis (2004) found that middle-age women differed from middle-age men in that they valued and understood the need for physical activity while the men were more concerned about the competitiveness of activities. Lack of social support to be physically active from a spouse or close friends may reinforce sedentary lifestyles. Low physical activity self-efficacy is characteristic of many females throughout the life span and may undermine efforts to increase level of activity. In some neighborhoods, safety issues and lack of facilities tailored to women's needs further impede adoption of active lifestyles. Home-based programs compared to structured health club programs are more accessible and affordable, particularly for women with limited economic resources. Home-based programs should be fun and allow inclusion of other family members in physical activities. The occupational dimension of physical activity is important for women. Wilbur, Naftger-Kang, Miller, Chandler, and Montgomery (1999) found that women with higher occupational energy expenditure had higher HDL cholesterol and lower total cholesterol than did women with lower occupational energy expenditure. Because over 65% of women work outside the home, work sites provide a critical environment for promoting increased physical activity during work hours.

A consistent finding is that after adoption of regular exercise, adults have difficulty maintaining regular exercise patterns, which results in a usual rate of dropout from organized programs of about 50% in the first 3 to 6 months. Further, those who might benefit most, such as overweight persons, are most susceptible to dropping out due to a low level of tolerance for physical activity. Influences on physical activity for middle-age adults include *past program participation, self-efficacy, benefits, barriers, spouse support, peer support, perceived available time*, and *access to facilities* (King et al., 2002; O'Brien Cousins, & Gillis, 2004).

Older adults merit special consideration in discussions of determinants of physical activity. Feeling better physically and improving fitness (endurance, muscle strength, balance) are frequent reasons given for participating in physical activity. Barriers to physical activity, an important consideration for the elderly, need further exploration because although work and family demands may lessen with age, convenience of facilities, cost, opportunities for physical activity with others, fear of resultant illness or injury, disability, and sensory impairment become more salient with age. Concern about existing medical conditions may be a further deterrent to an active lifestyle. Perceived barriers, self-efficacy expectations, and age were found to be important predictors of participation in physical activity among older adults (Conn, 1997, 1998). A study of women over 70 years of age found that they needed to feel socially supported by family, friends, and caregivers and they had to feel confident in their ability to participate in physical activity (O'Brien

Cousins, 1996). A 2001 study examined motivations between young people and older adults and found that older adults valued physical activity more for mental alertness while younger people valued the fun aspect of physical activity (Campbell, MacAuley, McCrum, & Evans, 2001).

Shephard (1994) suggests that focusing on personal beliefs rather than subjective norms (expectations of Others) may be more effective in motivating older adults to be active. However, O'Brien Cousins and Gillis (2004) studied "self talk," a concept explained by Thompson and Hoekenga (1998), in this manner: "All of us have a sort of ongoing internal dialogue within our minds. Sometimes when we concentrate especially hard, we may even 'talk through' our thought processes out loud. The statements that we make to ourselves silently (and occasionally out loud) are referred to as 'self talk' " (p. 49). O'Brien Cousins and Gillis (2004) found that "self talk" was not a useful tool for many active exercisers and actually was a negative force for some. Providing transportation, facilitating companionship for physical activity, building on prior activity habits, and tapping existing skills that have developed over a lifetime are other variables that may facilitate regular physical activity.

Older adults consist of the young old (65 to 74 years), middle old (75 to 84 years), and very old (over 85 years). Ability to be physically active as well as relevant determinants undoubtedly varies over this age spectrum. Almost all studies of determinants of physical activity in older adults have focused on the young old. In order to optimize physical activity potential for those 75 years of age or older, further studies of exercise capabilities and determinants are needed that investigate physical activity in the middle old and very old (Conn, Valentine, & Cooper, 2002).

The Process of Physical Activity Behavior Change

The use of process models to specify the mechanisms underlying the adoption and maintenance of physical activity behavior is advocated by a number of investigators (Bock, Marcus, Rossi, & Redding, 1998; Prochaska & Marcus, 1994). The transtheoretical model or stages-of-change model has been applied by Marcus and colleagues (2000) to physical activity behavior. This model proposes that individuals engaging in a new behavior move through a series of changes: precontemplation (not intending to make changes), contemplation (considering changes), planning or preparation (making minor changes), action (actively engaged in major behavior change), and maintenance (sustaining the behavior over time). The processes and strategies used to promote change are linked specifically to the stage of change of the client. In testing the model on 1,172 participants in a work site health-promotion project, Marcus and colleagues concluded that the constructs of the theory can be applied to physical activity. Experiential processes suggested as useful interventions in the precontemplation and contemplation stages include consciousness raising and self-reevaluation. Behavioral processes proposed as useful interventions in the preparation, adoption, and maintenance stages include helping relationships, counterconditioning, reinforcement management, and stimulus control. The study revealed that women were more likely than men to be in the contemplation or action stages and less likely to be in the maintenance stage. Working women with young children in the home were more likely to be in the lower stages of exercise adoption than were women without young children

(Brown & Trost, 2003). In a study of 286 women age 50 to 64, precontemplators were significantly older, had lower exercise knowledge, perceived lower psychological benefits from exercise, had lower family support for exercise, and did not perceive exercise as important compared to the action group. Both the precontemplation and the contemplation groups perceived more barriers to exercise than did the action group. Persons in maintenance also scored the highest on the pro scale (benefits of exercise) and lowest on the con scale (costs of exercising) as predicted by the theory (Marcus et al., 1994). These findings support predictions based on the transtheoretical model.

Cardinal (1999) proposed an extension of the transtheoretical model of physical activity behavior to include a sixth stage identified as the transformed stage. He defines the transformed stage as having participated regularly in physical activity for 5 or more years and being 100% confident in personal ability to remain physically active for life. In a study of 551 members of a physical education and recreation professional organization, those in the transformed stage had a higher reported level of physical activity and a more positive attitude toward role modeling an active lifestyle than did those in the maintenance group. Understanding the stages of physical activity behavior will provide important information for appropriately tailoring interventions to groups at differing points in the change process.

While much of the literature continues to focus on strategies for changing individual behavior, it is important to recognize the interest in broader, multilevel, ecological approaches (models) to promote changes in behavior. As discussed earlier, at best, current models and theories explain only 20% to 40% of the variance in physical activity. New models such as the comprehensive model of physical activity posited by Spence and Lee (2003) would incorporate both intra- and extra-individual influences that contribute to change in the individual and test the interplay among environmental settings and biological and psychological factors.

Interventions in Primary Care to Promote Physical Activity

Nurses and physicians in primary care have multiple opportunities to engage in physical activity counseling. The American Nurses' Association's *Clinician's Handbook of Preventive Services: Put Prevention into Practice* (1998) recommends that every primary care visit be seen as an opportunity to promote an active lifestyle. In a 2000 national survey, 58% of the adult nurse practitioners surveyed indicated that they routinely advised clients to engage in moderate-intensity physical activity for a total of 30 minutes on most days of the week, which is the latest recommendation for sedentary adults from the American College of Sports Medicine and the Centers for Disease Control and Prevention (Burns, Camaione, & Chatterton, 2000). Nursing diagnoses from the North American Nursing Diagnosis Association (NANDA) in the category of Activity-Exercise Pattern include diversion activity deficit and high risk for activity intolerance. The reader is referred to the NANDA taxonomy (2003) for further diagnostic information about definitions, defining characteristics, and etiologic or related factors. Nursing interventions to address these diagnoses include behavior modification and exercise promotion (McCloskey & Bulechek,

2003). Nursing outcomes or goals of client care achieved through these nursing interventions include improvements in circulatory status, endurance, muscle function, leisure participation, and physical fitness (Johnson, Maas, & Moorhead, 2000).

Counseling in primary care should assist children and adolescents to select activities they enjoy and not focus solely on competitive sports. Children should be encouraged to engage in activities that can be carried into adulthood and are easily incorporated into their daily life year-round. Appropriate safety equipment should be used in order to prevent injuries and youth should be counseled to avoid use of any anabolic steroids. By offering simple recommendations to children and parents the health care provider will play a key role in promoting lifelong physical activity (Ganley & Sherman, 2000).

Adult clients in primary care should be asked about their physical activity habits at work, at home, and during leisure to determine if these activities are of sufficient frequency, intensity, and duration to confer health benefits. Adults should be assisted in planning a program of physical activity that is medically safe, enjoyable, convenient, realistic, and structured to achieve self-selected goals. Routine monitoring, follow-up, and booster sessions are essential to assist clients in maintaining their exercise programs. Home exercise programs may work for some adults, whereas for others structured programs may need to be offered at work sites or convenient community locations. Group activities may be particularly appealing to adults who prefer the social support and comradeship of group programs.

Few studies have been conducted of physical activity counseling interventions in primary care. Calfas and colleagues (1996) evaluated the Patient-Centered Assessment and Counseling on Exercise (PACE) Program (1999) developed to promote adoption of physical activity in adults. The intervention protocol is based on social cognitive theory and the transtheoretical model. PACE incorporates proven behavioral change techniques, tailors physical activity counseling to the individual client, and incorporates both moderate and vigorous activity guidelines. The intervention is designed to alter factors known to influence physical activity such as self-efficacy, social support, perceived benefits, and perceived barriers. The protocol includes physical activity assessment forms and stage-specific counseling protocols. For example, the "Getting Out of Your Chair" protocol is geared to working with clients in the precontemplation and contemplation stages, the "Planning the First Step" protocol to those in the preparation or planning stage, and the "Keeping the Pace" protocol to those in the adoption or maintenance stages. The physical activity assessment is completed by the client in the waiting room and scored by office personnel. The client is then given the appropriate counseling protocol for stage of exercise, and the primary care provider places the assessment and protocol on the client's chart for use during the visit. The provider counsels the client and arranges for appropriate follow-up by phone, mail, or office visit.

The effectiveness of the protocol for the contemplation stage was tested with 98 intervention clients and 114 control primary care clients who were sedentary at the beginning of the study. Intervention clients received the office-based intervention and a 10-minute booster phone call to answer questions and discuss progress. The control group received the regular office visit. A significant number of clients moved from the contemplation to action stage in the intervention compared with the control group. Intervention subjects increased 40 minutes per week in self-reported walking compared to a 10-minute-per-week increase in the control group. These results were supported by accelerometer readings. The study demonstrated that brief activity counseling in primary care followed by a booster phone call—both matched to the client's stage of physical activity—produced meaningful increases in activity among sedentary adults. By identifying the client's stage of physical activity prior to the visit, the primary care provider may efficiently tailor counseling to the client's specific needs (Calfas et al., 1996). Calfas, Sallis, Oldenburg, and French (1997) examined the possible mechanisms fostering physical activity change as a result of the intervention. They found that the intervention increased reported use of cognitive and behavioral processes to facilitate adoption of physical activity, but they did not find any increase in physical activity self-efficacy or social support for being active. The brevity of the intervention may have precluded these psychological and social effects. Studies are needed of other physical activity interventions structured to impact more directly an array of factors known to affect levels of physical activity.

The PACE + Program included the same exercise protocol used in the PACE project, and added a nutrition protocol and an assessment of strategies such as mail and phone-based follow-up, to maintain behavior changes over time. Four primary care sites were selected for the intervention conducted by physicians and nurse practitioners. Both providers and patients reported satisfaction with computer and provider counseling. The patients rated the phone follow-up more satisfactory than the mailings. Both patients and providers recommended that the program be added to other primary care offices as a regular offering (Calfas et al., 2002).

The Activity Counseling Trial (ACT) was another major study of a primary care–based physical activity counseling intervention sponsored by the National Heart, Lung, and Blood Institute. This was a 5-year, multicenter, randomized controlled trial with 874 adults in primary care between the ages of 35 and 75 years assigned to one of three educational interventions: standard care control, staff-assisted intervention, or staff–counseling intervention. Standard care consisted of advice to exercise by a physician or health educator. The staff-assisted intervention included advice but added in-clinic counseling by a health educator and interactive mail follow-up. The staff–counseling intervention further added telephone counseling and classes to the intervention components in the other two groups. Study findings showed that men and women in all three groups—"advise only," "assistance," and the "counseling" group—improved their cardiovascular fitness and physical activity (Blair et al., 1998; King et al., 1998; NIH, 2001).

Barriers to physical activity counseling sometimes cited by health professionals include lack of time, lack of reimbursement, absence of theoretically sound protocols to guide counseling with diverse groups, lack of perceived effectiveness as a counselor, and lack of proper training to fulfill this role. If nurses are to provide quality counseling to clients regarding their physical activity, they must work to overcome these barriers. Providers who model active lifestyles themselves are likely to be much more effective counselors than their sedentary counterparts. According to social learning theory, observation of others is a powerful mode for transmitting attitudes, beliefs, patterns of thought, and behaviors. Clients are quick to recognize the extent to which their provider has actually experienced the challenges and the "ups and downs" of adopting and maintaining a regular program of physical activity. The physical appearance of health care providers also provides powerful cues to clients as to whether they actually "practice what they preach" (Pender et al., 1994).

Tailoring Physical Activity Interventions

Interventions that tailor physical activity counseling and behavioral interventions to individuals based on motivational readiness and other psychological influences proven to affect physical activity are now being developed and tested. Information technology will revolutionize physical activity interventions in the next decade, providing interactive, personalized, and web-based formats for counseling. A review of 28 studies of media-based interventions indicated that mass-media campaigns had little impact on physical activity behavior. Interventions using printed self-help media and telephone contacts were effective in the short term in changing level of activity. Interventions with more intensive contacts and tailored to the target audience were most effective (Marcus, Owen, Forsyth, Cavill, & Fridinger, 1998). A review of tailored print communications found them to be superior to nontailored interventions in 75% of the studies reviewed (Skinner, Campbell, Rimer, Curry, & Prochaska, 1999).

In a randomized, controlled study of 194 sedentary adults recruited from the community, Marcus and colleagues (1998) tested the efficacy of an individually tailored intervention matched to stage of readiness to change. This intervention consisted of individually tailored reports generated by a computer expert system and stage-matched self-help manuals. The initial assessment and interventions were mailed to participants. The control group was mailed a standard self-help intervention. At 6 months the group receiving the tailored intervention outperformed the control group on minutes of physical activity per week, reaching 30 or more minutes of moderate activity on most days of the week, and on reaching the action stage of physical activity. Surprisingly, there were no group differences in the psychological constructs associated with physical activity in other studies, for example, self-efficacy, decisional balance, or processes of change. In another controlled trial of 763 sedentary patients, brief advice and a pamphlet tailored to stage of change were given to the intervention group. The control group received brief advice and a standard pamphlet. There were no group differences in physical activity or movement across the stages of change (Bull, Jamrozik, & Blanksby, 1999).

The effective content and processes in tailored interventions, the conditions under which they positively impact behavior, and the extent to which these interventions are effective with differing population groups are areas needing further exploration. The cost effectiveness of various tailoring methods for physical activity counseling also needs to be determined to optimize efficient use of time by health care providers.

Intensity of Physical Activity

Vigorous physical activity has been widely advocated with at least 20 minutes spent three times per week at 60% or more of maximum heart rate. Recently, moderate physical activity (less than 60% maximum heart rate) has been proposed as having some of the same health-protective benefits as vigorous activity. The national recommendation for *moderate physical activity* is accumulating 30 minutes daily on most days of the week through a combination of activities. Because some people dislike strenuous physical activity, moderate activities may have fewer barriers to participation and therefore may be incorporated more easily into an individual's daily routine (U.S. Department of Health and Human

TABLE 6–2 **Sedentary and Active Approaches to Daily Living**

Sedentary	Active
Take the elevator or escalator	Climb the stairs
Call on the telephone	Walk down the hall or walk next door
Drive to lunch	Walk to lunch
Sit in a chair throughout a meeting	Get up quietly and walk about the room
Park right next to your destination	Park some distance away from your destination
Remain sedentary at your desk	Take several minutes to do arm and leg exercises
Use the remote control for the TV	Get up and walk to the TV when you want to change the channel
Visit with your colleagues in the "break room"	Take a walking break and visit

Services, 1998). Blair, Kohl, and Gordon (1992) suggest that lifestyle exercise in which a person engages in numerous short bouts of physical activity throughout the day (stair climbing, walking to and from a distant parking place) resembles the physical activity measured in epidemiological studies that have found cumulative energy expenditure to be inversely related to cardiac risk. Some combination of lifestyle physical activity and moderate or vigorous leisure-time physical activity is probably closer to the ideal for most individuals. Sedentary and active approaches to daily living are presented in Table 6–2.

Special considerations in optimizing tolerance of physical activity are warming up and cooling down properly. *Warming up* is important to increase blood flow to the heart and skeletal muscles, enhance oxygenation of tissues, and increase flexibility of muscles before physical activity. The warming-up period allows the heart rate and body temperature to increase gradually and the joints to become more flexible prior to physical activity. A gradual increase in heart rate reduces chances of arrhythmias. Warming up can include activities such as walking briskly, arm circles, jumping jacks, leg exercises, or wall push-ups. The warming-up period need take no longer than 7 to 10 minutes and should be followed immediately by moderate or vigorous physical activity. Following physical activity, a *cool-down* period is essential. Taking time to cool down for a period of 5 to 10 minutes following physical activity is important because activity raises heart rate, blood pressure, body temperature, and lactic acid within the muscles. Cooling down allows the heart rate to decrease gradually, preventing pooling of blood in muscles and resultant lightheadedness. It helps eliminate lactic acid within muscles and maintains blood flow to and from the muscle. During the cooling-down period, it is important to keep the lower extremities moving in activities such as slow walking, jogging, or cycling. At the end of the cooling-down period, the client's heart rate should be below 100 (American College of Sports Medicine, 2000).

Risks of Physical Activity

An overly aggressive approach to physical activity may exaggerate existing clinical conditions and put patients, particularly older adults, at risk for untoward effects. If an individual has an undiagnosed heart condition, strenuous physical activity could create arrhythmias. Persons with cardiovascular disease or other chronic conditions should be cautioned to avoid activity at levels that are physiologically untenable or result in untoward symptoms. Overstressing muscles and joints may result in muscle soreness and joint pain. Individuals over 50 years of age or with an existing chronic illness should be evaluated medically before starting regular physical activity. A program of gradually increasing physical activity is recommended, with much more emphasis on moderate rather than vigorous activity for older adults. Appropriate physical activity should optimize the benefits while minimizing the risks.

Interventions in the Community to Promote Physical Activity

Interventions to promote physical activity may occur in schools, work sites, community organizations, and families. These interventions generally reach a larger group than one-on-one primary care interventions. The numerous community physical activity intervention studies preclude an exhaustive review. Thus, in this section several examples of community interventions are presented.

A school-based intervention, the Cardiovascular Health in Children Study, was conducted in 18 elementary schools in North Carolina. The schools were randomized and a sample of 2,109 third- and fourth-grade children were placed in one of three groups: a public health classroom-based intervention; a risk-based intervention for those with one or more cardiovascular risk factors; or a control group. All children in the classroom-based intervention received a physical activity intervention three times per week that included warm-up, 20 minutes of physical activity, and a cool-down period. In the risk-based intervention group, only at-risk children received the physical activity intervention. Posttest data were collected 2 weeks after the 8-week intervention. Both intervention groups improved their cardiovascular risk profiles. However, the classroom-based intervention was easier to implement and reached a wider group of children (Harrell, McMurray, Gansky, Bangdiwala, & Bradley, 1999).

The Child and Adolescent Trial for Cardiovascular Health (CATCH) compared 56 intervention schools given a multicomponent behavioral intervention over three grades with 40 control schools. Enhancement of physical education classes, home curricula, and family fun nights were part of the 3-year physical activity program for the intervention group. The intensity of physical activity in physical education classes increased significantly more in the intervention group than in the control group. Although total minutes of activity did not differ between youths in intervention and control schools, reported vigorous activity was significantly higher in students at the intervention schools. These increases were maintained at follow-up testing 3 years later. The results of this study suggest that changes in physical activity initiated in elementary school can persist into early adolescence (Luepker et al., 1996; Nader et al., 1999).

Project Active is another example of a community-based intervention. This study focused on 235 sedentary men and women between the ages of 35 and 60 years of age. Volunteers were randomly assigned to a structured exercise program or a lifestyle physical activity program. Social cognitive theory and the transtheoretical model provided the theoretical basis for study interventions. Participants randomized to the structured program group received a traditional exercise program at 50% to 85% of maximal aerobic power for 20 to 60 minutes for 3 to 5 days per week. Individual supervised sessions were offered to this group at a state-of-the-art fitness center 5 days a week for 6 months. Participants in the lifestyle group were advised to accumulate at least 30 minutes of moderate-intensity physical activity on most days of the week. This group met and learned cognitive and behavioral strategies matched to their stage of change or level of motivational readiness. After 6 months of intervention, both groups were significantly more fit than at baseline. Of the structured group, 85% were meeting physical activity criterion for their group. Of the lifestyle group, 78% were meeting the physical activity criterion for their group. For both groups, those who increased their use of cognitive and behavioral strategies increased in self-efficacy, perceived more benefits than barriers, and were more likely to achieve the physical activity criterion. Both groups experienced reduction in cardiovascular risk. The importance of this study is the finding that a lifestyle approach compared to a structured approach to physical activity achieved comparable results. Sedentary adults can make significant progress in becoming more fit and lowering cardiovascular disease risk without attending a traditional exercise program (Dunn, Garcia, Marcus, Kampert, & Kohl, 1998; Dunn et al., 1997; Kohl, Dunn, Marcus, & Blair, 1998).

Community interventions are an effective approach to increasing physical activity in population groups. If large numbers of communities implement these interventions, it would contribute significantly to attaining the physical activity goals of *Healthy People 2010* by the end of the decade.

Directions in Physical Activity Research

This chapter has provided a discussion of the benefits of physical activity, factors influencing physical activity among youth and adults, and physical activity interventions in primary care and in the community. Research continues to be needed to better understand how to tailor exercise programs to the needs of different populations. Particular focus should be placed on developing and testing interventions that assist very young children to adopt physical activity as enjoyable and rewarding. How to sustain physical activity in adolescence also needs further study. Focusing on behavior development rather than behavior change is critical as behaviors once developed during youth are highly resistant to change.

Suggestions for future research include:

1. Investigate the influences in infancy and early childhood that promote the development of physically active lifestyles.

2. Explore how important developmental milestones or life transitions (e.g., school transition, marriage, pregnancy) influence readiness and opportunities to be physically active.

3. Describe the mechanisms that explain transition across stages of physical activity from precontemplation to transformation.

4. Investigate the influence of multiple roles and daily hassles on the adoption and maintenance of physical activity among women.

5. Investigate the interaction of genetic makeup, environment, and behavior on the adoption and maintenance of physical activity.

6. Test the effectiveness of computer-assisted physical activity interventions tailored to motivational readiness, age, gender, race–ethnicity, and socioeconomic status.

7. Test the effectiveness of family, school, work site, and community interventions to increase physical activity.

8. Test the effectiveness of changing both policies (environmental, educational, and health policies) and community environments to increase physical activity in populations.

Directions for Practice to Promote Physical Activity

Throughout this chapter, benefits of physical activity, determinants of physical activity, and approaches for increasing physical activity have been emphasized. This information can guide evidence-based nursing practice in counseling persons of all ages about the adoption of regular physical activity. Within any given age, gender, or cultural group, nurses should start by assessing the client's level of physical activity and the influences known to predict physical activity. For example, when working with children, the nurse should assess patterns of physical activity; preferred activities; perceptions of barriers to being active; perceptions of self-efficacy; intentions to be active; availability of active parents, siblings, and peers; access to safe recreational facilities; and time spent outdoors. For older adults, current health status, existing medical conditions, disabilities, fear of injury, preference for activities requiring exertion, as well as perceived benefits and self-efficacy for being active, need to be assessed. Physical activity counseling and behavioral intervention programs may then be developed for the individual that focus on the most relevant sources of motivation as well as their personal concerns.

Tailoring the behavioral intervention program to the individual is likely to enhance its effectiveness. Nurses should consider developing or using existing computer-based tailoring programs to optimize their physical activity counseling skills. It is also important to follow-up assessment and counseling in the office with mail or phone follow-ups at periodic intervals. These contacts should focus on assessing the stage of physical activity of the client, providing advice regarding appropriate strategies to increase or maintain activity, and helping them deal with any barriers to being active that they have encountered. Generally, in-office or phone follow-up is considered more effective than mail follow-up. Nurses should access web sites that provide additional information concerning recommendations and considerations related to physical activity for different populations.

The nurse should work with the health care team to set up office systems that will facilitate regular physical activity counseling for all clients. Physical activity components of health-promotion and prevention systems should consist of screening systems for assessing patterns of physical activity, clear agency guidelines for physical activity counseling, chart reminders for counseling at client visits, relevant client education materials, and follow-up protocols to "bolster" interventions. When health care agencies systematize counseling protocols, physical activity counseling is much more likely to be carried out as an integral part of care by all health professionals.

SUMMARY

Nurses, as key health professionals, need to assume responsibility for using current and emerging knowledge to assist clients to develop lifelong habits of physical activity. Physical activity must be an integral part of personal lifestyle if it is to have optimum effects on health. Maintaining physical fitness can be enjoyable and rewarding for persons of all ages and contribute significantly to extending longevity and improving the quality of life.

LEARNING ACTIVITIES

1. Review the positive effects of physical exercise. Develop an exercise plan for a healthy young adult to improve two selected outcomes. Tailor the plan based on the young adults age and socioeconomic status.
2. Review the proposed suggestions for research in physical activity and suggest two additional areas that need further investigation.
3. Find percentage and estimated cost of obesity for your region on the Centers for Disease Control and Prevention web site listed below.

SELECTED WEB SITES

A Guide from the National Institute on Aging and National Aeronautics and Space Administration

http://weboflife.nasa.gov/exerciseandaging/cover.html

American College of Sports Medicine

http://www.acsm.org

American Heart Association

http://www.americanheart.org/catalog/Health_catpage9.html

Centers for Disease Control and Prevention, Division of Nutrition and Physical Activity

http://www.cdc.gov/nccdphp/dnpa/obesity/index.htm

Mayo Clinic Rochester Aerobic Exercise and Fitness Guidelines

http://www.mayo.edu:80/ cv/wwwpg_cv/cv-whc/mc1952/mc1952.htm

Office of the Surgeon General

http://www.surgeongeneral.gov/ophs/pcpfs.htm

Statistics Related to Overweight and Obesity

http://www.niddk.nih.gov/health/nutrit/pubs/statobes

The Cooper Institute

http://www.cooperinst.org/7.html

The President's Council on Physical Fitness

http://www.fitness.gov

REFERENCES

American College of Sports Medicine. (2000). *ACSM's guidelines for exercise testing and prescription* (6th ed.). Philadelphia: Lippincott, Williams, & Wilkins.

American Nurses' Association. (1998). *Clinician's handbook of preventive services: Put prevention into practice* (2nd ed.). Waldorf, MD: American Nurses Publishing.

Baranowski, T., Mendlein, J., Resnicow, K., Frank, E., Cullen, K. W., & Baranowski, J. (2000). Physical activity and nutrition in children and youth: An overview of obesity prevention. *Preventive Medicine, 31,* S1–S10.

Blair, S. N., Applegate, W. B., Dunn, A. L., Ettinger, W. H., Haskell, W. L., et al. (1998). Activity counseling trial (ACT): Rationale, design, and methods. *Medicine and Science in Sports and Exercise, 30*(7), 1097–1106.

Blair, S. N., Kohl, H. W., III, & Gordon, N. F. (1992). Physical activity and health: A lifestyle approach. *Med Exerc Nutr Health, 1,* 54–57.

Bock, B. C., Marcus, B. H., Rossi, J. S., & Redding, C. A. (1998). Motivational readiness for change: Diet, exercise, and smoking. *Am J Health Behavior, 22*(4), 248–258.

Bouchard, C., & Perusse, L. (1994). Heredity, activity level, fitness and health. In C. Bouchard, R. J. Shephard, & T. Stephens (Eds.), *Physical activity, fitness and health: International proceedings and consensus statement* (pp. 106–118). Champaign, IL: Human Kinetics.

Bouchard, C., Shephard, R. J., & Stephens, T. (Eds.). (1994). *Physical activity, fitness and health: International proceedings and consensus statement.* Champaign, IL: Human Kinetics.

Brown, W. J., & Trost, S. G. (2003). Life transitions and changing physical activity patterns in young women. *Am J Prev Med, 25*(2), 140–143.

Bull, F. C., Jamrozik, K., & Blanksby, B. A. (1999). Tailored advice on exercise—Does it make a difference? *Am J Prev Med, 16*(3), 230–239.

Burns, K. J., Camaione, D. N., & Chatterton, C. T. (2000). Prescription of physical activity by adult nurse practitioners: A national survey. *Nurs Outlook, 48,* 28–33.

Calfas, K. J., Long, B. J., Sallis, J. F., Wooten, W. J., Pratt, M., & Patrick, K. (1996). A controlled trial of physician counseling to promote adoption of physical activity. *Prev Med, 25,* 225–233.

Calfas, K. J., Sallis, J. F., Oldenburg, B., & French, M. (1997). Mediators of change in physical activity following an intervention in primary care: PACE. *Prev Med, 26,* 297–304.

Calfas, K. J., Sallis, J. F., Zabinski, M. F., Wilfley, D. E., Rupp, J., Prochaska, J. J., Thompson, S., Pratt, M., & Patrick, K. (2002). Preliminary evaluation of a multicomponent program for nutrition and physical activity change in primary care: PACE+ for adults. *Preventive Medicine, 34,* 153–161.

Campbell, P. G., MacAuley, D., McCrum, E., & Evans, A. (2001). Age differences in the motivating factors for exercise. *Journal of Sport and Exercise Psychology, 23,* 191–199.

Cardinal, B. J. (1999). Extended stage model of physical activity behavior. *Journal of Human Movement Studies, 37,* 37–54.

Conn, V. S. (1997). Older women: Social cognitive theory correlates of health behavior. *Women and Health, 26*(3), 71–85.

Conn, V. S. (1998). Older adults and exercise: Path analysis of self-efficacy related constructs. *Nurs Res, 47*(3), 180–189.

Conn, V. S., Valentine, J. C., & Cooper, H. M. (2002). Interventions to increase physical activity among aging adults: A meta-analysis. *Ann Behav Med, 24,* 190–200.

De Bourdeaudhuij, I., & Sallis, J. (2002). Relative contribution of psychosocial variables to the explanation of physical activity in three population-based adult samples. *Preventive Medicine, 34,* 279–288.

DiLorenzo, T. M., Stucky-Ropp, R. C., Vanderwal, J. S., & Gotham, H. J. (1998). Determinants of exercise among children. II. A longitudinal analysis. *Prev Med, 27,* 470–477.

Dunn, A. L., Garcia, M. E., Marcus, B. H., Kampert, J. B., & Kohl, H. W. III. (1998). Six-month physical activity and fitness changes in Project Active, a randomized trial. *Medicine and Science in Sports and Exercise, 30*(7), 1076–1083.

Dunn, A. L., Marcus, B. H., Kampert, J. B., Garcia, M. E., Kohl, H. W., et al. (1997). Reduction in cardiovascular disease risk factors: Six-month results from Project Active. *Prev Med, 26,* 883–892.

Finkelstein, E. A., Fiebelkorn, I. C., & Wang, G. (2003). National medical spending attributable to overweight and obesity: How much, and who's paying? *Health Affairs, W3,* 219–226.

Ganley, T., & Sherman, C. (2000). Exercise and children's health: A little counseling can pay lasting dividends. *The Physician and Sports Medicine, 28*(2), 1–8.

Garcia, A. W., Norton, M. A., Frenn, M., et al. (1995). Gender and developmental differences in exercise beliefs among youth and prediction of their exercise behavior. *J School Health, 65*(6), 213–219.

Godin, G., & Shephard, R. J. (1990). Use of attitude-behavior models in exercise promotion. *Sports Med, 10*(2), 103–121.

Harrell, J. S., McMurray, R. G., Gansky, S. A., Bangdiwala, S. I., & Bradley, C. B. (1999). A public health vs. a risk-based intervention to improve cardiovascular health in elementary school children: The Cardiovascular Health in Children Study. *Am J Public Health, 89*(10), 1529–1535.

Johnson, M., Maas, M., & Moorhead, S. (Eds.). (2000). *Nursing Outcomes Classification (NOC)* (2nd ed.). St. Louis: Mosby.

Karch, B. (2000). A case for physical activity in health promotion. *Health promotion: Global perspectives, 2*(6), 1.

King, A. C., Sallis, J. F., Dunn, A. L., Simons-Morton, D. G., Albright, C. A., et al. (1998). Overview of the Activity Counseling Trial (ACT) intervention for promoting physical activity in primary care settings. *Medicine and Science in Sports and Exercise, 30*(7), 1086–1096.

King, A. C., Stokols, D., Talen, E., Brassington, G. S., & Killingsworth, R. (2002). Theoretical approaches to the promotion of physical activity: Forging a transdisciplinary paradigm. *Am J Prev Med, 23*(2S), 15–25.

Kohl, H. W., Dunn, A. L., Marcus, B. H., & Blair, S. N. (1998). A randomized trial of physical activity interventions: Design and baseline data from Project Active. *Medicine and Science in Sports and Exercise, 30*(2), 275–283.

Luepker, R. V., Perry, C. L., McKinlay, S. M., Nader, P. R., Parcel, G. S., et al. (1996). Outcomes of a field trial to improve children's dietary patterns and physical activity: The Child and Adolescent Trial for Cardiovascular Health (CATCH). *JAMA, 275,* 768–776.

Marcus, B. H., Bock, B. C., Pinto, B. M., Forsyth, L. H., Roberts, M. B., et al. (1998). Effects of an individualized, motivationally tailored physical activity intervention. *Annals of Behavioral Medicine, 20*(3), 174–180.

Marcus, B. H., Dubbert, P. M., Forsyth, L. H., McKenzie, T. L., Stone, E. J., Dunn, A. L., & Blair, S. N. (2000). Physical activity behavior change: Issues in adoption and maintenance. *Health Psychol, 19*(1, suppl), 32–41.

Marcus, B. H., & Forsyth, L. H. (1999). How are we doing with physical activity? *Am J Health Prom, 14*(2), 118–124.

Marcus, B. H., Owen, N., Forsyth, L. H., Cavill, N. A., & Fridinger, F. (1998). Physical activity interventions using mass media, print media, and information technology. *Am J Prev Med, 15*(4), 362–378.

Marcus, B. H., Pinto, B. M., Simkin, L. R., et al. (1994). Application of theoretical models to exercise behavior among employed women. *Am J Health Prom, 9*(1), 49–55.

McCloskey, J. C., & Bulechek, G. M. (Eds.). (2003). *Nursing Interventions Classification (NIC)* (4th ed.). St. Louis: Mosby.

Nader, P. R., Stone, E. J., Lytle, L. A., Perry, C. L., Osganian, S. K., et al. (1999). Three-year maintenance of improved diet and physical activity: The CATCH cohort. *Archives of Pediatric and Adolescent Medicine, 153,* 695–704.

NIH. (2001). NHLBI study finds brief counseling by health professionals boosts patients' physical fitness. Accessed at *http://www.nhlbi.nih.gov/new/press/01-08-07.htm.*

North American Nursing Diagnosis Association. (2003). *Nursing diagnoses: Definitions and classification.* Philadelphia: NANDA.

O'Brien Cousins, S. (1996). Exercise cognition among elderly women. *Journal of Applied Sport Psychology, 8,* 131–145.

O'Brien Cousins, S, & Gillis, M. M. (2004). "Just do it . . . before you talk yourself out of it": The self-talk of adults thinking about physical activity. *Psychology of Sport and Exercise,* in press.

O'Loughlin, J., Paradis, G., Kishchuk, N., Barnett, T., & Renaud, L. (1999). Prevalence and correlates of physical activity behaviors among elementary schoolchildren in multiethnic, low income, inner-city neighborhoods in Montreal, Canada. *Annals of Epidemiology, 9,* 397–407.

PACE manual: Patient-centered assessment and counseling for exercise and nutrition. (1999). San Diego, CA: San Diego State University Foundation.

Pender, N. J., Sallis, J. F., Long, B. J., et al. (1994). Health-care provider counseling to promote physical activity. In R. K. Dishman (Ed.), *Advances in exercise adherence* (pp. 213–235). Champaign, IL: Human Kinetics.

Pender, N. J., Walker, S. N., Sechrist, K. R., et al. (1990). *The Health Promotion Model: Refinement and validation.* Final Report to the National Center for Nursing Research, National Institutes of Health (Grant no. NR 01121). DeKalb, IL: Northern Illinois University Press.

Pinto, B. M., Marcus, B. H., & Clark, M. M. (1996). Promoting physical activity in women: The new challenges. *Am J Prev Med, 12,* 395–400.

Popkin, B. M., & Udry, J. R. (1998). Adolescent obesity increases significantly in second and third generation U.S. immigrants: The National Longitudinal Study of Adolescent Health. *J Nutri, 128,* 701–706.

Prochaska, J. O., & Marcus, B. H. (1994). The transtheoretical model: Applications to exercise. In R. Dishman (Ed.), *Advances in exercise adherence* (pp. 161–180). Champaign, IL: Human Kinetics.

Sallis, J. F., Alcaraz, J. E., McKenzie, T. L., & Hovell, M. F. (1999). Predictors of change in children's physical activity over 20 months: Variations by gender and adiposity. *Am J Prev Med, 16*(3), 222–229.

Sallis, J. F., Patrick, K., Frank, E., Pratt, M., Wechsler, H., & Galuska, D. A. (2000). Interventions in health care settings to promote healthful eating and physical activity in children and adolescents. *Preventive Medicine, 31*, S112–S120.

Sallis, J. F., Prochaska, J. J., & Taylor, W. C. (2000). A review of correlates of physical activity of children and adolescents. *Medicine and Science in Sports and Exercise, 32*(2), 963–975.

Sallis, J. F., Zakarian, J. M., Hovell, M. F., & Hofstetter, C. R.. (1996). Ethnic, socioeconomic, and sex differences in physical activity among adolescents. *Journal of Clinical Epidemiology, 49*(2), 125–134.

Seefeldt, V., Malina, R. M., & Clark, M. A. (2002). Factors affecting levels of physical activity in adults. *Sports Medicine, 32*(3), 143–168.

Shephard, R. J. (1994). Determinants of exercise in people aged 65 years and older. In R. Dishman (Ed.), *Advances in exercise adherence* (pp. 343–360). Champaign, IL: Human Kinetics.

Simonen, R. L., Videman, T., Kaprio, J., Levalahti, E., & Battie, M. C. (2003). Factors associated with exercise lifestyle—a study of monozygotic twins. *Int J Sports Med, 24*(7), 499–505.

Skinner, C. S., Campbell, M. K., Rimer, B. K., Curry, S., & Prochaska, J. O. (1999). How effective is tailored print communication? *Annals of Behavioral Medicine, 21*(4), 290–298.

Spence, J. C., & Lee, R. E. (2003). Toward a comprehensive model of physical activity. *Psychology of Sport and Exercise, 4*, 7–24.

Thompson, S., & Hoekenga, S. J. (1998). Understanding and motivating older adults. In R. T. Cotton (Ed.), *Exercise for older adults.* San Diego, CA: American Council on Exercise.

Trost, S. G., Pate, R. R., Ward, D. S., Saunders, R., & Riner, W. (1999). Correlates of objectively measured physical activity in preadolescent youth. *Am J Prev Med, 17*(2), 120–126.

Trost, S. G., Sallis, J. F., Pate, R. R., Freedson, P. S., Taylor, W. C., & Dowda, M. (2003). Evaluating a model of parental influence on youth physical activity. *Am J Prev Med, 25*(4), 277–282.

Tudor-Locke, C. (2003). *Manpo-Kei: The art and science of step counting: How to be naturally active and lose weight!* New Bern, NC: Trafford.

U.S. Department of Health and Human Services. (2000, January). *Healthy People 2010* (conference edition, in two volumes). Washington, DC: U.S. Government Printing Office.

U.S. Department of Health and Human Services, Center for Disease Control and Prevention, National Center for Chronic Disease Prevention and Health Promotion. (1998). *Physical activity and health: A report of the surgeon general.* Boston: Jones & Bartlett.

U.S. Department of Health and Human Services. Public Health Service, Centers for Disease Control and Prevention, National Center for Chronic Disease Prevention and Health Promotion, Division of Nutrition and Physical Activity. (1999). *Promoting physical activity: A guide for community action.* Champaign, IL: Human Kinetics.

Van Beurden, E., Barnett, L. M., Soc, B., Zask, A., Dietrich, U. C., Brooks, L. O., & Beard, J. (2003). Can we skill and activate children through primary school physical education lessons? "Move it Groove it"—a collaborative health promotion intervention. *Preventive Medicine, 36*, 493–501.

Wilbur, J., Naftger-Kang, L., Miller, A. M., Chandler, P., & Montgomery, A. (1999). Women's occupations, energy expenditure, and cardiovascular risk factors. *J Women's Health, 8*(3), 377–387.

Zaravar, P. W., & Nies, M. A. (1997). Daily hassles and exercise frequency in women. *Home Health Care Management and Practice, 10*(1), 54–58.

7

Diet, Nutrition, Prevention, and Health Promotion

OBJECTIVES

1. Discuss the nutrition goals of *Healthy People 2000,* success in meeting these goals, and the nutrition goals of *Healthy People 2010.*
2. Describe the Food Guide Pyramid and its role in setting guidelines for healthy eating.
3. Examine factors that influence eating behaviors and the research supporting each factor's role in determining eating behaviors.
4. Contrast the differences in nutritional needs of infants and children, adolescents, and older adults.
5. Examine the causes of overweight/obesity and the primary goal of intervention in weight loss.

OUTLINE

- The Role of Diet and Nutrition in Prevention and Health Promotion
- Factors Influencing Eating Behavior
  A. Genetic–Biologic Factors
  B. Psychologic Factors
  C. Sociocultural Factors
  D. Environmental Factors
- Nutritional Needs of Special Populations
  A. Infants and Children
  B. Adolescents
  C. Older Adults

Good nutrition is important to the nurturance of health. Accumulating evidence indicates that eating patterns play a major role in preventing disease and in creating the capacity for energetic and productive living. Although much is yet to be learned through nutritional research about mechanisms underlying the relationship between nutrition and health, community-based health education programs and national dietary and food production policies are focused on promoting optimum nutrition among persons of all ages. One of the goals of *Healthy People 2010* (U.S. Department of Health and Human Services, 2000) is to promote health and reduce chronic disease with diet and weight management. A significant number of the nutrition objectives relate to reducing the proportion of children, adolescents, and adults who are overweight or obese. The objectives that address nutrition and overweight measure in some way the implementation of the Dietary Guidelines for Americans (U.S. Department of Agriculture and U.S. Department of Health and Human Services, 2000). Other nutrition objectives relate to increasing the quality of food choices made by children and adolescents at school and increasing the proportion of work sites that offer nutrition or weight management classes or counseling.

Of the 27 nutrition objectives in the *Healthy People 2000* initiative, targets for only five were met. These included two related to the availability of reduced-fat foods and the prevalence of growth retardation. A majority of the remaining objectives showed progress, including those related to the intake of fruits, vegetables, grain products, total fat, saturated fat, availability of nutrition labeling, breast-feeding, nutrition education in schools, and work site nutrition and weight management programs. The objective to reduce salt intake in the elderly was not met. Of particular concern was the result that objectives to increase intake of calcium and reduce the number of overweight and obese persons moved away from the targets (Glanz, 1999; U.S. Department of Health and Human Services, 2000). The number of children and adults who are overweight or obese increased substantially (U.S. Department of Health and Human Services, 2000).

Because nurses are the health professionals most often in extended contact with clients, they are a valuable resource to individuals, families, and communities in providing information and assistance in regard to healthy nutrition. The professional nurse must be able to deal not only with therapeutic aspects of nutrition but also with nutrition as a critical element in prevention and health promotion. Nutritionists and psychologists are valuable colleagues of the nurse in planning sound nutrition education programs for individuals, families, or entire populations.

The Role of Diet and Nutrition in Prevention and Health Promotion

Poor eating habits are often established during childhood. More than 60% of young people eat too much fat, and less than 20% eat the recommended amount of fruits and vegetables each day (U.S. Department of Agriculture and U.S. Department of Health and Human Services, 2000). A study of the prevalence and trends, 1999 to 2000, among U.S. children and preadolescents showed that approximately 10.4% of children 2 to 5 years of age and approximately 15.3% of preadolescents age 6 to 11 years are overweight (Ogden, Flegal, Carroll, & Johnson, 2002). The prevalence of overweight children does not differ based on race–ethnicity, income, or education (Goran, 1998). For children and adolescents (2 to 20 years of age) the National Center for Chronic Disease Prevention and Health Promotion (CDC) has developed gender-specific body mass index (BMI—index of the relationship between an individual's height and weight) charts to respond to the changes in body fat as children mature. Nurses and other health care professionals use the following percentile points to identify underweight and overweight children: underweight—BMI for age < 5th percentile; at risk of overweight—BMI for age 85th to < 95th percentile; and overweight—BMI for age > 95th percentile. For example, if a child is in the 60th percentile, it means that 60% of children of the same gender and age have a lower BMI than the child (for growth charts and additional information visit the CDC National Center for Health Statistics web site noted at the end of the chapter). BMI decreases during preschool years and increases into adulthood. There is evidence that among boys, there is a prepubertal increase in subcutaneous fat that is lost during adolescence, whereas prepubertal fat in girls continues through puberty and into adulthood (U.S. Department of Health and Human Services, 2000). The American Dietetic Association (2004) position statement on dietary guidance for healthy U.S. children 2 to 11 years of age identified inadequate intakes of calcium and fiber-rich foods as critical nutritional concerns. Stewart, Seemans, McFarland, Weinhufer, and Brown (1999) compared the dietary fat and cholesterol intake in young children to the National Cholesterol Education Program guidelines. The subjects were 468 children, second to fifth graders. The mean percentages of intake from total fat, saturated fat, monounsaturated fat, and polyunsaturated fat were higher than the recommended levels. A study of 200 obese children revealed that 35% of the parents did not believe their child to be obese and 53% reported they could control what their child ate. Parents expressed concern about heart disease as a consequence of childhood obesity but did not perceive their own child to be at risk (Myers & Vargas, 2000). Hernandez, Uphold, Graham, and Singer (1998) documented obesity in preschool children. They collected data from 309 charts of children enrolled in a Head Start program and found 99 (32%) to be obese. A study of trends and prevalence over 23 years among adolescents up to 17 years of age documented the same increase in weight gain as younger children, 11% were overweight and 14% were obese (Goran, 1998).

Overweight and obesity affect 55% to 66% of the adults in the United States. Percentages vary due to the use of different measurement tools such as the BMI, which is an index of the relationship between an individual's height and weight or use of a height and weight chart for determining weight. Over the last two decades, the percentage of obese adults has increased from 14.5% to 22.5% of the population. Approximately 25% of adult women and 20% of adult men are obese (BMI 30 or greater, which equates to 30 pounds or more; Freedman, Khan, Serdula, Galuska, & Dietz, 2002). Refer to Chapter 4, Table 4–1, for the BMI chart and standards for adults. African American and Hispanic women are more likely to be obese compared to white women, and the proportion of African American women who are obese is 80% higher than the proportion of African American men who are obese (U.S. Department of Health and Human Services, 2000). The National Health and Nutrition Examination Survey data found that 50% of African American women ages 20 years and older were obese (Freedman et al., 2002). These percentages were found across socioeconomic strata (Flegal, Carroll, Ogden, & Johnson, 2002). Because weight management is difficult for most people, the *Healthy People 2010* goal of 15% or less of adults having a BMI of 30 or more is very challenging (U.S. Department of Health and Human Services, 2000).

The overconsumption of saturated fats, cholesterol, sugar, and salt has been linked to four of the leading causes of death: coronary heart disease, some types of cancer, stroke, and Type II diabetes. These diseases cost the U.S. economy over $200 billion in health care expenses and lost productivity (U.S. Department of Health and Human Services, 2000). Evidence documents a *strong* link between diet and atherosclerotic cardiovascular diseases and hypertension and is *highly suggestive* for certain forms of cancer, especially those of the esophagus, stomach, large intestine, breast, lung, and prostate. Certain dietary patterns also appeared to predispose individuals to obesity, the risk of noninsulin-dependent diabetes mellitus, chronic liver disease, and possibly osteoporosis. Although these chronic diseases are complex, involving genetic and environmental determinants, modifications in diet may play a significant role in reducing the risk of occurrence (U.S. Department of Health and Human Services, 2001).

For example, about 1.5 million Americans suffer myocardial infarctions, nearly 500,000 die each year, and many more have angina pectoris (U.S. Preventive Services Task Force, 1996). Coronary heart disease (CHD) costs the U.S. economy approximately $100 billion annually. A number of factors influence the development of cardiovascular disease. Factors that offer little possibility for control are genetic predisposition, gender, and advancing age. Factors over which individuals can have control include high blood cholesterol, cigarette smoking, high blood pressure, excessive body weight, and long-term physical inactivity. Addressing controllable risk factors can decrease deposits of cholesterol and other lipids, resultant cellular reactions, and the thickening of coronary artery walls and subsequent risk of myocardial infarction and sudden death (U.S. Department of Health and Human Services, 2001).

A considerable amount of observational evidence from case-control and cohort studies provides evidence that dietary factors may be associated with both the occurrence of cancer and protection against cancer (Bergmann & Boeing, 2002; Chen & Holick, 2003; Martinez, 2004). Dietary constituents suspect in the occurrence of cancer include excessive intake of fat, kilocalories, nitrites, mutagens (contained in smoked, charbroiled, fried, or pickled meats), meats, and alcohol. Milk; fruits; vegetables; dietary fiber; vitamins A, C, and E; carotenoids; folate; and calcium have been suggested as protectants against cancer.

Bingham and associates (2003) prospectively studied the association between incidence of colorectal cancer and dietary fiber in over 500,000 participants ages 25 to 70 years old that were taking part in a larger European study. Participants completed dietary questionnaires over 6 years between 1992 and 1998 and were followed up for cancer incidence. The greater amount of fiber that one consumed, the less incidence of colorectal cancer was found in this population. For populations with low fiber dietary intake it was interpreted that with an approximate doubling of total fiber intake from food the risk of colon cancer could be reduced by 40%.

The *Dietary Guidelines for Americans, 2000* (U.S. Department of Agriculture and U.S. Department of Health and Human Services, 2000) form the basis for a federal nutrition policy. In general these guidelines answer the question concerning how Americans over 2 years of age should eat for good health. Too many Americans eat too many calories; too much fat, cholesterol, and sodium; too few complex carbohydrates; and not enough fiber, which contributes to the high rates of chronic disease in the United States. The dietary guidelines for the prevention of chronic diseases appear in Table 7–1. The *Food Guide Pyramid*, consistent with these guidelines and published by the U.S. Department of Agriculture (1996), appears in Figure 7–1. The pyramid has replaced the "Basic Four Food Groups" model and is useful for simple dietary screening and as a foundation for general nutrition education. Of calories consumed daily, 30% or less should be from fat (less than 10% saturated fatty acids, 10% polyunsaturated fatty acids, and 10% monounsaturated fatty acids). No more than 300 mg of dietary cholesterol should be consumed daily. The amount of saturated fat in some commonly eaten foods is shown in Table 7–2 and the upper limit on fat based on calorie intake is presented in Table 7–3. Significant controversies exist (Gifford, 2002) about the meaning and implications of the 2000 Dietary Guidelines and the Food Guide Pyramid. One of the issues that contributes to this controversy is the need to separate the amount of recommended animal fat from that of plant oils clearly in the guidelines and in the pyramid. The public must comprehend the message that within a limitation on overall intake of fat, the type of dietary fat consumed is critical to healthy diets. Another issue is the treatment of daily servings from separate food groups. The U.S. Department of Agriculture projected unrealistically small serving sizes, making the pyramid user "unfriendly" and confusing to the public. The most confusing issue is that the pyramid uses ounces to describe size and the Nutrition Facts Label uses grams to determine serving size. While work to address these issues continues, it is accepted that implementation of these

---

TABLE 7–1 Nutrition and Your Health: Dietary Guidelines for Americans

1. Aim for a healthy weight.
2. Choose a variety of grains daily, especially whole grains.
3. Choose a variety of fruits and vegetables daily.
4. Choose a diet that is low in saturated fat and cholesterol and moderate in total fat.
5. Choose beverages and foods to moderate your intake of sugars.
6. Choose and prepare foods with less salt.
7. If you drink alcoholic beverages, do so in moderation.

(*Source:* From *U.S. Dietary Guidelines, 2000*, U.S. Department of Agriculture/U.S. Department of Health and Human Services, 2000.)

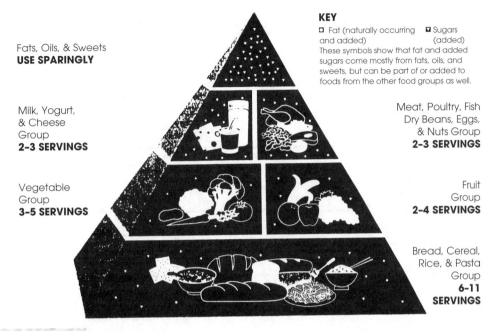

KEY

◻ Fat (naturally occurring   ◼ Sugars
and added)   (added)
These symbols show that fat and added
sugars come mostly from fats, oils, and
sweets, but can be part of or added to
foods from the other food groups as well.

Fats, Oils, & Sweets
USE SPARINGLY

Milk, Yogurt,
& Cheese
Group
2–3 SERVINGS

Meat, Poultry, Fish
Dry Beans, Eggs,
& Nuts Group
2–3 SERVINGS

Vegetable
Group
3–5 SERVINGS

Fruit
Group
2–4 SERVINGS

Bread, Cereal,
Rice, & Pasta
Group
**6–11
SERVINGS**

FIGURE 7–1   **Food Guide Pyramid: A Guide to Daily Food Choices**

(From U.S. Department of Agriculture and U.S. Department of Health and Human Services, 1996, *The Food Guide Pyramid*, Washington, DC: U.S. Department of Agriculture and U.S. Department of Health and Human Services.)

recommendations would result in an approximate reduction of 10% or more in the average blood cholesterol level of the U.S. population and lead to an approximate reduction of 20% or more in coronary heart disease, significantly improving the health and quality of life of the population. Concerns about an overconsumption of carbohydrates have been raised in relationship to reduced fat intake. The current incidence of overweight and obesity and resulting chronic diseases supports a diet that consists of fewer calories, low percentage of animal fat, and moderate serving sizes. The 2005 revised guidelines are projected to address many of the concerns about the 2000 guidelines, but the important goal is to increase the number of Americans who use the guidelines and eat a balanced, nutritional diet.

The high-fat, low-carbohydrate diet made popular by Adkins is currently being studied and some findings indicate that weight loss is greater over time than the loss experienced on other diets. Caution is recommended as the long-term effects of a high-saturated fat, low-carbohydrate diet have not been studied sufficiently. Weight loss is the result of lower intake of calories than expended calories regardless of type of diet. Weight loss is also influenced by the types of food consumed such as whole grains, dairy, and non-animal fat.

Most studies on diet and health focus on a single nutrient, food, or food group. For example, studies have looked at vitamin E intake and its relationship to heart disease. Researchers at Queen's Colleges, New York City, studied dietary patterns using diet data from 42,000 women who participated in a 2-year breast-cancer study. Those who ate more variety of foods from several of the recommended food categories were found to have a

TABLE 7–2 **A Comparison of Saturated Fat in Some Foods**

Food Category	Portion	Saturated Fat Content in Grams
Cheese		
Regular Cheddar cheese	1 oz.	6.0
Low-fat Cheddar cheese*	1 oz.	1.2
Ground Beef		
Regular ground beef	3 oz., cooked	7.2
Extra lean ground beef*	3 oz., cooked	5.3
Milk		
Whole milk	1 cup	5.1
Low-fat (1%) milk	1 cup	1.6
Breads		
Croissant	1 medium	6.6
Bagel*	1 medium	0.1
Frozen Desserts		
Regular ice cream	1/2 cup	4.5
Frozen yogurt*	1/2 cup	2.5
Table Spreads		
Butter	1 tsp.	2.4
Soft margarine*	1 tsp.	0.7

*The food categories listed are among the major food sources of saturated fat for the United States.
(*Source:* From U.S. Department of Agriculture, U.S. Department of Health and Human Services)

TABLE 7–3 **What Is Your Upper Limit on Fat for the Calories You Consume?**

Total Calories Per Day	Saturated Fat in Grams	Total Fat in Grams
1,600	18 or less	53
2,000*	20 or less	65
2,200	24 or less	73
2,500*	25 or less	80
2,800	31 or less	93

*Percent Daily Values on Nutrition Facts Labels are based on a 2,000 calorie diet. Values for 2,000 and 2,500 calories are rounded to the nearest 5 grams to be consistent with the Nutrition Facts Label.
(*Source:* From U.S. Department of Agriculture, U.S. Department of Health and Human Services)

30% lower death rate during 6 years of follow-up. It is possible that complex interaction among foods and nutrients in the overall diet produces some protective mechanism (Rosenberg, 2000).

Undernutrition is also a problem in many segments of the population, resulting in retardation in linear growth of preschool children. It is estimated that 11% of U.S. households did not have sufficient food sometime during 2001. That represents 11.5 million households (Nord, Andrews, & Carlson, 2002). Chronic iron deficiency in childhood may have adverse effects on growth and development. The prevalence of iron deficiency is higher in African American children compared to white children and higher in children of families below the poverty level than in children of more affluent families. Inadequate calcium intake in youth may be related to failure to attain peak bone mass during the years of bone mineralization (up to age 20 years), possibly resulting in later predisposition to osteoporosis. Eating disorders such as anorexia nervosa and bulimia are nutritional threats to the health of youth, particularly young women, which are not well understood. Anorexia nervosa affects 1 in 100 adolescents between 12 and 18 years of age (National Center for Health Statistics, 1997). In the nursing home settings, the elderly may experience weight loss due to undernutrition because they are not adequately fed (Kayser-Jones & Schell, 1997). In a nonrandomized study of undernourished nursing home patients (defined by BMI, weight loss, and anthropometrics), those who gained at least 10 pounds due to increased nutritional supplements had fewer recurring infections and were less likely to die (Keller, 1995). Further research is needed to explore mechanisms underlying nutritional problems as a basis for effective interventions.

Factors Influencing Eating Behavior

A wide variety of factors influence *overt* eating behavior. These factors are classified as genetic–biologic, psychologic, sociocultural, and environmental. The multicausal nature of eating behavior makes it highly complex and resistant to change. Eating behaviors are an integral part of individual, family, and community lifestyles. Effective modification requires consideration of the factors that determine eating behavior and the use of appropriate behavior-change techniques.

Genetic–Biologic Factors

Some advances have been made in identifying the relationship between appetite and metabolic factors as they relate to fat and protein intake. Several new peptides have been identified that play a role in regulating energy expenditure, appetite, and metabolic factors (Bessesen, 2000). Fuel metabolism generates signals that control food intake, and evidence exists that the interaction of carbohydrate and fat fuel may play a role in overeating (Friedman, 1998). Also, the recent discovery of the "obese" ("ob") gene offers the potential of understanding what stimulates and inhibits the processes of eating behaviors in humans. With this discovery, new drugs will be developed that will regulate appetite and calorie expenditure (Ravussin & Bouchard, 2000). Genetics influence taste and account for some of the variation in the desire for certain foods by some people and not others (Duffy & Bartoshuk, 2000) and appear to confer specific dispositions to the development of obesity (Blundell & Cooling, 1999). Although one study found evidence that genetic factors influenced the frequency of food intake, no relationship was found to exist between genetic effects on weight gain and actual increase in weight (Heitmann, Harris, Lissner, & Pedersen, 1999).

The biologic changes of aging have a marked effect on eating behavior. A progressive loss of taste buds on the anterior tongue occurs with age, resulting in decreased sensitivity to sweet and salty tastes. In contrast, taste buds sensitive to bitter and sour increase with age. This taste distortion may result in decreased enjoyment of food and decreased intake of nutrients. Decreased gastric secretions may result in limited absorption of iron, calcium, and vitamin B_{12}. Decreased gastric motility augments the need for foods high in fiber (fresh fruits, raw vegetables, whole-grain breads, and cereals) and increases the importance of water consumption to promote regularity in bowel evacuation. A decrease in basal metabolic rate with aging has also been associated with a decrease in caloric intake. Many elderly people suffer from isolation and depression. Altered hypothalamic-pituitary-adrenal–axis regulatory mechanisms have been noted in depression, including excessive cortisol secretion and an elevation in corticotropin-releasing factor, a potent inhibitor of food intake (MacIntosh et al., 1999).

In regard to other physiologic influences, energy requirements also appear to be highly salient biologic determinants of eating behavior. Individuals exhibit awareness and sensitivity to low energy levels (Martinez, 2000). Fatigue, listlessness, and apathy may indicate a caloric intake that is inadequate to meet energy needs. More studies are needed to document how various biologic factors affect eating behavior.

Psychologic Factors

Increasing knowledge of proper nutrition by itself does not necessarily improve eating habits. Adolescents report that saturated fat and foods high in sugar should not be eaten in excess, but this knowledge has only a slight influence on the consumption of foods high in these constituents (Richter et al., 2000). Motivation and other psychologic factors must be addressed among persons of all ages if healthy nutritional practices are to become a reality for a larger portion of the population. Psychologic factors have positive or negative effects on eating behaviors. Perceiving many benefits from good dietary practices encourages individuals to select foods that are high in nutrients, low in animal fat and refined carbohydrates, high in fiber, and low in sodium and food additives. Health-conscious decisions about nutrition may be taught as early as preschool with systems such as "green" foods such as fruits and vegetables (foods high in nutrition), "red" foods such as candy and soft drinks (foods low in nutrition), and "yellow" foods such as ice cream and red meats (foods with limited but some nutritional value that are to be eaten sparingly). A positive self-concept also creates a psychologic climate that encourages persons of all ages to take care of themselves and control what they eat because they place a high value on their own health and well-being.

Emotions, such as depression, low self-esteem, and lack of personal control over one's life, particularly overeating behavior, markedly impair nutritional practices. Negative emotions, such as anger, frustration, and insecurity, lead to disturbances in eating behavior that lead to undernutrition (e.g., anorexia nervosa, bulimia) or overnutrition (obesity). These problems frequently are indicative of a personal search for comfort, security, and nurturance. Focusing on enhancing or modifying self-concept and reducing depression may well be necessary before nutritional behaviors are changed. Provision of nutritional guidance without attention to coexisting psychologic states may exaggerate rather than ameliorate nutritional problems.

Habits constitute another important determinant of eating behavior. A habit is defined as a behavior that occurs often and is performed automatically or with little conscious awareness. Habits are performed so frequently that many cues within the environment serve as signals for the behavior. They often result in a psychologic addiction to certain behaviors because they become a pervasive part of lifestyle. Such behaviors are known as consummatory because the response itself (eating) provides the reinforcement. People may also become psychologically addicted to the consequences of habitual behaviors such as the "energy spurt" experienced after the ingestion of highly refined sugars (doughnuts, sweet rolls, snack foods) or caffeine (sodas, coffee, chocolate). Habits often result in poor dietary practices because little or no conscious thought is given to eating behavior. Habits also depend on the availability of foods that are readily consumed without preparation. Fast foods that are high in animal fats and refined carbohydrates and low in protein, minerals, and vitamins often meet this requirement. To change lifestyle behavior, most notably, modification of eating behavior, self-management skills are necessary. Habits can be changed and new attitudes and behavior can be adopted to replace old habits (Brownell, 1999; Fredericks, 1999; O'Neil, 2001).

Sociocultural Factors

Social determinants of food choice include moral or health concerns (whether one chooses to eat genetically modified foods), optimistic bias (whether one believes others are at a greater risk for negative health outcomes), and ambivalent attitudes about healthy eating habits (Shepherd, 1999). The dietary habits of young children are profoundly impacted by family food preparation and eating behaviors. Numerous organizations have recommended that total fats and cholesterol be restricted in the diets of children over 2 years of age (saturated fats to 10% of calories, total fats to 30% of calories, and dietary cholesterol to less than 300 mg/d). African American children and children from low-income families have diets least consistent with recommendations (Purcell, O'Brien, & Parks, 1996). Parental beliefs about good nutrition for children may not match these recommendations and thus may actually contribute to an unhealthy diet. For example, in a study of 547 children between the ages of 2 and 5, the major food source of saturated fat for the total group was whole milk, which contributed 16.1% for white children, 18.5% for African American children, and 26.9% for Hispanic children of saturated fat consumed. Many parents who drink reduced-fat or skim milk themselves will give their children over 2 years whole milk in the belief that it is better for them. When the diets of African American children were examined separately, their major sources of total dietary fat were franks, sausages, luncheon meats, and bacon, with whole milk as a close second. This finding suggests cultural differences that may need to be considered in dietary counseling. Almost a third of total cholesterol consumed by children comes from eggs or egg products, with additional cholesterol added by whole milk, sweets, and beef. Children's diets may be considerably improved by changing the beliefs and practices of their care providers, including parents, other relatives, and child care or preschool personnel. Substituting 1% milk for all the whole milk consumed, skim milk cheese for whole milk cheese, and skim milk for all the low-fat milks consumed would markedly decrease total fat intake. Not all children find the substitutes acceptable and not all would use them all the time. However, moderate changes in food consumption patterns results in favorable changes in dietary intake for most children (U.S. Department of Agriculture and U.S. Department of Health and Human Services, 2000).

Mass media is another aspect of an individual's sociocultural environment that exerts considerable influence over health behaviors. Television and print media provide models of various behaviors that result in vicarious learning about the social desirability of eating behaviors and their positive and negative consequences. For example, in examining nutrition, dieting, and fitness messages in a magazine widely read by adolescent women from 1970 to 1990, Guillen and Barr (1994) reported that both nutrition-related and fitness-related coverage emphasized weight loss and physical appearance. Less emphasis was placed on the role of good nutrition in improving health and well-being. The volume of content on nutrition and weight loss did not change over time but the hip:waist ratio of models decreased, becoming less curvaceous and more linear. This is a clear indication that the cultural norm expected of women, "thinness," is becoming *more* evident in media despite national concern about unhealthy nutrition practices among adolescent women that may lead to eating disorders. The peak onset of eating disorders occurs during adolescence (Boschi et al., 2003). Ironically, in the same magazine, candy and snacks were the most frequently advertised food products. Rapid changes in body shape may make adolescents particularly vulnerable to these confusing messages (Guillen & Barr, 1994). This is cause for concern, because early adolescence is a time of high nutritional demands due to high growth rates, energy demands, and calcium and iron requirements related to the onset of puberty and menstruation. Likewise, mass media may be used effectively to promote positive change. In one West Virginia town, paid advertising and public relations were successful in increasing the number of low-fat or skim-milk drinkers. Following the campaign and at a 6-month follow-up, 34% of those who switched from whole milk continued to report using low-fat or skim milk. The sale of low-fat and skim milk increased significantly (Reger, Wootan, & Booth-Butterfield, 1999).

Ethnic and cultural backgrounds serve as important influences on eating behavior. Ethnic foods are a source of pride and identity for many groups and may have deep emotional meaning for individuals because of their association with their country of origin or because of fond childhood memories of holidays on which particular foods were served. Food-consumption patterns of some ethnic groups provide good role models for other cultural groups within American society and often the opposite as well. For example, Watanabe and colleagues (2003) studied the impact of Westernization of the lifestyle on two groups of Japanese people. Two hundred and seventy-one nondiabetic Japanese living in Hiroshima and 222 nondiabetic Japanese Americans living in Hawaii were studied. Risk factors for atherosclerosis such as serum lipids, blood pressure, BMI, insulin resistance, and smoking habits showed that Japanese Americans had a more rapid progression of atherosclerotic disease risk much earlier when compared with native Japanese. The link of cardiovascular disease to diet has been clearly established. Soy food consumption was studied in 75,000 Chinese women ages 40 to 70 years old (Zhang et al., 2003). Soy intake was recorded during interviews and the cohort was followed biennially. Based on incident cases of coronary heart disease it was concluded that an increased soy food intake resulted in a decrease in coronary heart disease. The nurse should be alert to cultural groups that can serve as positive role models for healthy eating behaviors to Americans. Sharing health-promoting cultural practices with the larger society is an important asset of the increasing cultural diversity in North America.

Recognition of and respect for individual food preferences is important for professional nurses in dealing with adults from a wide variety of cultural backgrounds. Suggestions for health promotion in diverse cultural communities that can be extrapolated to the promotion of good nutrition in various ethnic groups include (Gutierrez, 1994; Zephier et al., 1997):

- Understand cultural beliefs about the interrelationships between food and health.
- Recognize how food consumption practices contribute to cultural identity.
- Assess the extent to which acculturation to dominant-group nutritional behaviors has taken place.
- Consult with nutritionists or nurses of similar ethnic backgrounds to clients.
- Form a group of lay consultants on nutritional practices from the target ethnic community.
- Recognize nutritional attributes of ethnic foods.
- Reinforce ethnic nutritional practices that are positive.
- Make recommendations, when necessary, for changing ingredients to lower saturated fats, cholesterol, and sodium or increase fiber while still retaining taste.
- Provide information on nutrient values of ethnic foods to clients.
- Work with ethnic restaurants to offer healthy choices that are acceptable to target populations.
- Promote increased consumption of nutritious ethnic foods among the general population.
- Incorporate healthy ethnic food choices into work site and school site cafeterias and vending machines.

The nurse should also be sensitive to the difficulties that ethnic groups may have in identifying the contents of foods packaged in the United States and in understanding nutrition labeling. Inability to obtain foods familiar to them and trying to eat foods that are unfamiliar may be a source of considerable frustration and distress. Lack of money, language barriers, day-to-day stresses of an unfamiliar environment, and confusing messages on mass media about nutritious foods often serve as barriers to good nutrition among members of varying ethnic groups (Wellman, 1994).

As part of their clients' sociocultural milieu, health professionals serve as important role models in terms of healthy eating patterns. Thus, nurses and other health professionals should not only advocate healthy diets for others but also put the dietary guidelines into practice as a part of their own lifestyles. Modeling recommended eating behaviors as well as struggling with the issues that surround maintenance of positive nutritional practices will indicate sincerity and commitment to good health practices that speaks louder than words to the clients that they serve.

Environmental Factors

The American food environment is slowly changing to support healthier eating behavior on the part of all Americans. For example, new mandatory labels on all packaged foods contain more complete, useful, and accurate nutrition information than ever before. Improved labeling may assist individuals and families in making healthier food choices. Parents should include children and adolescents in grocery shopping and make them a part of the search for healthy, appealing foods. Learning by active decision making about food selections is one way to increase the nutrition awareness of youth. In 1994, nutrient content claims (e.g., reduced fat) and health claims (e.g., decreases cholesterol) on food-product labels became regulated to eliminate misleading statements. A section called Nutrition Facts on each packaged food product now provides per-serving values of nutrient information. Daily value percentages of nutrients are derived from recommended daily allowances (RDAs) and are based on a 2,000 calorie diet (Morbidity and Mortality Weekly Report, 1998). Legislation and regulation to achieve truth in advertising and open disclosure of information on food constituents is an important step toward facilitating consumers' awareness and use of knowledge to make nutritious point-of-choice decisions about food purchases.

Many environmental barriers to healthful eating still remain. The complexities of modern life make it difficult for many individuals to consistently maintain access to foods rich in important nutrients. For example, Americans spend nearly half of their food budget on takeout, restaurant, and convenience foods with one-third of the total food dollars on fast food (American Dietetic Association, 2004). Foods prepared away from home are higher in fat, cholesterol, and sodium, and lower in calcium and fiber (U.S. Department of Heath and Human Services, 2000). The major environmental factors influencing eating patterns appear to be accessibility, convenience, and cost. These factors can present barriers to positive nutritional practices during the action phase of health behavior. Seasonal variation in availability of foods such as raw vegetables and fresh fruits determines both accessibility and costs. Seasonal patterns in the types of fruits and vegetables used by clients need to be followed to maximize nutrient quality and minimize cost. Use of frozen fruits and vegetables in their natural juices rather than those canned during off-season is recommended to decrease the intake of sugar and salt. Home-frozen products are an important source of nutrients at reasonable cost.

Ease of preparation also plays an important role in food selection. Quick and effortless preparation techniques appeal to many families because of busy work schedules. In addition, attractiveness of prepared foods is an important consideration. Assisting the client in selecting nutritious foods that are quickly prepared and aesthetically appealing increases the likelihood of sustaining positive eating behavior. Cost of food is also a critical consideration for many families, given the increasing numbers of families living at or below the poverty level. Sources of complex carbohydrates (fruits, vegetables, and grains) may exceed the cost of highly refined sugar products. Proteins also vary greatly in per-unit cost. Assisting families in identifying low-cost, high-nutrition options within their "choice" environments is an important responsibility of the nurse providing nutritional guidance to diverse populations.

In modern society, food additives are used to retard spoilage and prevent deterioration of quality, improve nutritional value, enhance consumer acceptability, and facilitate preparation.

Types of additives include preservatives, coloring agents, flavorings, bleaching and maturing agents, and nutrition supplements. By law, labels of many products must list the manufacturer, packer, and distributor, and the amount of each ingredient. Even when ingredients are listed, information on the products is often by itself insufficient to guide knowledgeable food selection. Not only are potentially carcinogenic additives used in the preparation of foods (e.g., nitrosamines in bacon and saccharin in low-caloric carbonated beverages), but unintentional food additives such as pesticides and other agricultural chemicals may appear in foods. A great deal of research must be done on the safety of large numbers of food additives. Unfortunately, some of the synergistic, cumulative, and long-term effects of many additives will be determined only after years of use and exposure within human populations.

Nutritional Needs of Special Populations

Infants and Children

The caloric and nutrient intakes of children are critical for supporting growth and development. Infants whose diet is primarily mother's milk or infant formula consume 40% or more of their calories from fat, which is appropriate during infancy. When children reach 2 years of age, however, they should be encouraged to consume a diet lower in total fat, saturated fat, and cholesterol than the usual American diet (36% to 40%) as a basis for lowering the risk for chronic diseases in later years.

Iron deficiency is also a problem for 21% of low-income children 1 to 2 years of age and for 10% of low-income children 3 to 4 years of age. Chronic iron deficiency may have adverse effects on both early and later growth and development. Anemia, an index of iron deficiency, can result in decreased physical ability, impaired body temperature regulation, lowered resistance to infection, and alterations in intellectual performance. A healthy start for infants means encouraging mothers to breast-feed or use iron-rich formulas for formula-fed infants. It is important that during pregnancy and lactation mothers maintain sufficient iron intake through iron-rich foods or supplements, as this increases the likelihood that their children will not be iron deficient during the early years of life (Morbidity and Mortality Weekly Report, 1998; U.S. Congress, Office of Technology, Assessment, 1991).

Research suggests that parents influence the dietary choices made by preschoolers. Parents have less influence on food choices made by school-age children (American Dietetic Association, 2004; U.S. Department of Health and Human Services, 2000). Infants and children in child-care facilities should be provided with adequate nutrition. Cost consciousness on the part of caretakers should not interfere with the provision of good nutrition. It is important that parents monitor the food provided to their children in care facilities until they are assured that healthy nutrition guidelines are followed.

Adolescents

Adolescence is a period of biologic and social change. Body size, composition, functions, and physical abilities are changing rapidly. Undernutrition slows height and weight growth and may delay puberty. Among adolescents, minimal dietary requirements are those that maintain an optimal rate of pubertal development and growth. Adolescents who are vigorously active also have increased energy needs. Thus, adolescents should consume diets providing more total nutrients than they consumed as young children. Moderation is a good rule, as adolescents whose caloric intake is too high will gain weight, potentially leading to obesity. Those whose caloric intake is too low will experience loss of energy, weight loss, and, in the extreme, eating disorders that can lead to health problems and even premature death (Boschi et al., 2003). Adolescents with chronic diseases such as diabetes have special nutrition needs, because absorption, metabolism, or excretion of particular nutrients may change both as a result of adolescent biologic changes and as a result of their disease (Morbidity and Mortality Weekly Report, 1996).

In terms of fat intake, adolescents should be given dietary counseling on how to reduce total fat to less than 30% of calories per day with less animal fat, and cholesterol to less than 300 milligrams per day to lower risk factors for chronic disease. Because adolescents consume many fast foods at lunchtime or during the evening hours, selecting low-animal-fat fast foods is a real challenge. As an example of high-fat, fast food meals, a meal of a double burger with sauce, milkshake, and French fries contains 46% of its total calories from fat. Because the goal should be less than 30% calories from fats, it is easy to see why consumption of such meals day after day can create conditions of high risk for cardiovascular disease as early as adolescence. There is accumulating evidence that this "risk" carries over into adulthood (U.S. Preventive Services Task Force, 1996).

Adolescent girls in the United States typically begin menstruating at 12 1/2 years of age. Menstrual losses increase the need for iron, as does physical activity. Thus, particular attention should be given to adequate intake of this mineral in the diet for women in general and, in particular, for female athletes. The mineral calcium helps to build strong bones. It is also thought that adequate intake of calcium throughout childhood to age 25 will reduce the risk of osteoporosis in later life. Thus, girls should receive counseling on selecting diets that ensure adequate calcium and iron intake (U.S. Preventive Services Task Force, 1996).

Adolescents have special nutritional needs that require the attention of adolescents themselves as well as that of their families and primary care health professionals. Nurses have the opportunity to play a critical role in heightening awareness of the importance of good nutrition to overall adolescent health and performance. The challenge is to make nutritious food options appealing to adolescents who may eat primarily for taste rather than for nutritional or health reasons. Peer support for healthy eating practices is also critical, as the desire to be accepted by peers is extremely high during the adolescent years. Meal skipping contributes to poor nutrition and should be discouraged. Eating fast food but selecting lower-fat options creates opportunities for adolescents to be with their peers and yet limit fat intake. Pressure on fast food establishments to offer healthier options is also essential to creating a supportive environment for healthy nutritional practices among adolescents. Health professionals have increasingly used schools in the last few years as a vehicle for early health promotion and prevention activities. School lunch programs are more carefully monitored than in the past, and since at risk children are often eligible for reduced or free breakfast and/or lunch, these children's nutritional statuses are improved. The Child and Adolescent Trial for Cardiovascular Health (CATCH) Eat Smart program attempted to reduce the amount of saturated fat and total fat of school lunch in the 56 intervention schools. The 5-year follow-up post intervention showed that the intervention schools had further lowered the mean percentage of total calories from saturated and all fats to 10.4% and 31%, respectively. Sodium intake levels increased in both the intervention and control schools (Osganian et al., 2003). In addition, efforts on the part of major national health organizations and health professionals should be directed toward ensuring that nutritional education is a part of all kindergarten through grade 12 education programs. Efforts should also be made to integrate nutrition concepts throughout the entire curriculum including courses where it is not traditionally taught, such as math, chemistry, and history (Morbidity and Mortality Weekly Report, 1996).

Older Adults

Research on the nutritional needs of the elderly is expanding rapidly as the American population ages. Aging is thought to alter nutrient requirements for calories, protein, and other nutrients as a result of changes in lean body mass, physical activity, and intestinal absorption. Although many older Americans maintain healthy eating patterns, for some, changing nutritional needs may be accompanied by deterioration in diet quality and quantity, jeopardizing nutritional status, quality of life, and functional independence. Many elderly people skip meals and exclude whole categories of food from their diet because of reduced appetites, infrequent grocery shopping, lack of energy to cook, and difficulties in chewing and swallowing. For these individuals, supplementation may be required but should be initiated in consultation with health professionals. Too much self-medication may result in toxic levels of some vitamin and mineral supplements. In many communities Meals on Wheels, a senior nutrition program, provides meal(s) for the elderly in their homes. The Meals on Wheels program is an excellent use of public funds.

The interaction of foods and drugs must be considered. With polypharmacy common in older adults, some may take medications that interact with foods, decreasing nutrient absorption. Foods and drugs may interact, increasing the absorption of some foods and drugs and decreasing the absorption of others. The rate of absorption or the total level of absorption of drugs or nutrients may be affected. For example, crackers, dates, jelly, and other carbohydrates may slow down the rate of absorption of analgesics and limit their effectiveness in reducing pain. Milk, eggs, cereals, and dairy products may inhibit the absorption of iron. Antibiotics such as tetracycline are less readily absorbed when milk, dairy products, or iron supplements are taken. Prune juice, bran cereal, and high-fiber foods may increase intestinal emptying time to the point where some drugs cannot be adequately absorbed. There is a need for further exploration of food–drug interactions that commonly occur among the elderly (Blandford, 1998).

For individuals over 65 years of age, recommended eating patterns lower in saturated fatty acids, total fat and saturated fats, and cholesterol help maintain desired body weight and lower the risk of cardiovascular heart disease (CHD). High-fat diets contribute to the overall risk of CHD. Risk factors are as follows: being male or a postmenopausal female, having a family history of premature CHD, cigarette smoking, hypertension, high LDL cholesterol level, low HDL cholesterol concentration, diabetes mellitus, history of cerebrovascular or occlusive peripheral vascular disease, and obesity. All of these factors except cigarette smoking are influenced by diet in some way. Thus, there is international consensus among scientists that CHD is linked to nutritional patterns throughout life, with the damage manifest most frequently in middle-age and older adults. Daily activity along with an adequate diet can prevent premature mortality from heart disease and maintain vigor into old age (Food and Drug Administration and National Institutes of Health, 2000; Morbidity and Mortality Weekly Report, 1998).

The diets of older Americans generally would be healthier if they contained more complex carbohydrates and fiber. Many elderly people have chewing and swallowing disorders that make eating fruits and vegetables difficult. Average daily fiber intake among the elderly is less than half the recommended 20 to 35 grams. Health benefits attributed to fiber include proper bowel function, reduced risk of colon cancer, reduction of serum cholesterol, and improved glucose response. Six servings of whole grains are the recommended minimum for the elderly.

Energy requirements decline with reductions in body size, lean body mass, basal metabolism rate, and decreased physical activity. Because physical activity maintains muscle mass, it is highly desirable to keep physically active in later years. Diets of the elderly may also be deficient in protein along with calories as the result of an inability to chew meat or afford the cost of protein-rich foods. Infections, trauma, and other metabolic stresses may increase protein needs. Protein–calorie malnutrition may lower resistance to disease and delay recovery from illness (Morbidity and Mortality Weekly Report, 1998). Refer to Chapter 4 for suitable methods to assess an elderly client's nutritional status.

Older adults of limited economic means should be assisted in selecting low-cost foods that meet recommended nutritional requirements. They may need guidance on using label information to select foods and on how to prepare foods so that they are easier to chew and swallow. Nutrition is integral to quality of life for the elderly. Thus, it is a primary area for focus by nurses providing care to the elderly in primary care and long-term care settings.

Interventions to Change Eating Behaviors

The functional health pattern inclusive of eating behaviors is the Nutritional-Metabolic Pattern. Gordon (2002) describes this area of functional assessment as patterns of food and fluid consumption relative to metabolic need. Nursing diagnoses relevant to health promotion include *altered nutrition:* high risk for more than body requirements, *altered nutrition:* more than body requirements, and *altered nutrition:* less than body requirements. Diagnoses focus on the categories of obesity and undernutrition. An overview of definitions, defining characteristics, and etiologic or related factors are found in Gordon's (2002) *Manual of Nursing Diagnosis.*

Improving eating patterns involves changing knowledge, attitudes, and skills as well as the food consumption environment. The following strategies are recommended:

- Improving accessibility of nutrition information, nutrition education, nutrition counseling and related services, and healthful foods in a variety of settings and for all subpopulations.

- Focusing on preventing chronic disease associated with diet and weight, beginning in youth.

- Strengthening the link between nutrition and physical activity in health promotion.

- Maintaining a strong national program for basic and applied nutrition research to provide a sound science base for dietary recommendations and effective interventions.

- Maintaining a strong national nutrition-monitoring program to provide accurate, reliable, timely, and comparable data to assess status and progress and to be responsive to unmet data needs and emerging issues.

- Strengthening state and community data systems to be responsive to the data users at these levels.

- Building and sustaining broad-based initiatives and commitment to these objectives by public and private sector partners at the national, state, and local levels (U.S. Department of Health and Human Services, 2000).

Altering nutrition education, the food acquisition environment, and food consumption patterns will contribute to health. To alter nutrition education, there must be wide exposure of the general population at all ages to nutrition education through mass media, education at schools and work sites, do-it-yourself nutrition education packages, and nutrition counseling in primary health care services. New information technology must be used while at the same time making sure that nutrition education approaches are user friendly. Interactive computer nutrition programs, nutrition videos, and integration of healthy nutrition messages into packaging are all important in broad-based nutrition education. The dietary advice offered needs to evolve as scientific discoveries about the contribution of diet to health take place (Kumanyika et al., 2000; McCann & Bovbjerg, 1998; Wing, 2000). Research studies are needed to present evidence for the efficacy of the interventions for low-income or ethnic minorities (Ammerman, Lindquist, Lohr, & Hersey, 2002) and focus on policy and environmental interventions (Kumanyika, 2001).

The food acquisition environment still must undergo considerable change. It is affected by legislation and regulation regarding production of food and by availability of food options (Kumanyika, 2001). Populations at schools and work sites are captive and rely primarily on others to provide and prepare their food for a considerable part of the day. The availability of healthy options within the environment, such as from cafeterias and vending machines, greatly affect nutrition behaviors. Furthermore, healthy food choices must have appeal in terms of taste and texture. Widespread research in the food production industry is creating more food options that are both consistent with dietary recommendations and acceptable to the public.

Food consumption patterns are affected not only by knowledge and availability but also by the decision-making patterns of the individual or family. Kiosks at grocery stores and shopping malls to query about nutrients in specific foods as well as simple coding systems for fat, sodium, and fiber content all provide cues and easy assistance to consumers in making food selections.

Meta-Analysis of Clinical Studies and Randomized Clinical Trials

In a review of dietary fat reduction research, Barnard, Akhtar, and Nicholson (1995) found that studies that had the strictest fat intake reduction resulted in the greatest success. Some studies set less stringent fat restrictions to make the diet more acceptable to the study participants, and it appeared to minimize the degree of change needed and discouraged people from making the commitment to reduce their fat intake. Other study characteristics that predicted success were focused on participants who had cardiac problems, participants who initiated the program while in a hospital, family involvement, frequent monitoring, prepackaged meals, and meatless or vegetarian meals. Support groups were not found to contribute to the reduction of fat intake. Barnard looked at a total of 18 studies that were 1 year or longer and found that the mean fat intake was 29%. This compared with a mean intake of 28% fat reported in 21 shorter studies showing that the length of the intervention did not make a difference in the reduction of the participants' fat intake. Brunner and colleagues (1997) found similar outcomes in their review of several randomized, controlled intervention studies and 10 other studies. However, in all of the studies the greater the number of intervention contacts, the greater the positive change.

The development of randomized clinical trials to study long-term success of strategies for changing eating behavior is an increasingly important goal for scientists in the fields of nutrition and behavior. Although it is not always possible to generalize the findings of clinical trials to the general population due to the stringent criteria for inclusion of participants, the findings do make an important contribution to the knowledge about changing eating behaviors (Barnard et al., 1995; Kumanyika, 2001).

The Eating Patterns Study

The Eating Patterns Study (Beresford et al., 1997) is a randomized controlled study of 2,111 patients in six primary care practices. The study participants were 90% white and had at least some college education. The primary care offices were randomized to have intervention or no-intervention conditions. The low-intensity intervention included a self-help book, *Help Yourself*, introduced by a physician and a 2-week follow-up letter. A food frequency questionnaire and a foods habit questionnaire were administered over the telephone at 3-month and 1-year intervals after the baseline data were collected. The control group offices received no intervention. Intake of fat was reduced in the intervention and control groups, with the amount of reduction of fat significantly more in the intervention group controlling for age, gender, and baseline value.

Participants in the intervention group had greater success than did others in the intervention group if they had the responsibility for food shopping and preparation, were motivated to change, and indicated they used the self-help book. The summary of research findings to date indicates that in large, intensive, community-based studies, fat intake can be modified in participants who are well-screened and motivated to change. In smaller studies with less intense interventions, smaller changes are found to occur (Kumanyika et al., 2000).

Work Site Intervention Study

Sorenson and colleagues (1999) studied the dietary fat, fiber, and fruit and vegetable intake in a 2-year multi-work site intervention. The intervention included joint planning and implementation of work site programs by workers and management, increased healthy foods available at the work site, and programs offered to support individual change. Questionnaires were used to collect data over time. The intervention resulted in an increased fruit and vegetable intake (0.23 servings per day) compared to the control sites (0.10 servings per day). Managers and professional staff increased their intake of fruits and vegetables more than did other workers, but they did not improve their fiber intake to the extent that other workers did. The number of community-based studies conducted to study fruit and vegetable intake is limited. The results of the few studies available show that small increases in fruit and vegetable consumption are achievable (Kumanyika et al., 2000).

The Waianae Diet Program

The Waianae Diet Program (Shintani, Beckham, Kanawaliwali, et al., 1994) is an excellent example of a culturally sensitive program to change eating behaviors of the native Hawaiian population, who have a disproportionately high rate of obesity. In 1993, the program received the Distinguished Community Health Promotion Program Award from the U.S. Secretary for Health and Human Services. The primary intervention was a 3-week program of adhering to a strict, traditional Hawaiian diet with medical monitoring. Historical evidence suggests that prior to the adoption of Western diets, Native Hawaiians had little cardiovascular disease or obesity.

The intervention included a number of components. In the evenings, community participants ate traditional foods such as taro (a starchy root similar to potato), poi (a mashed form of taro), sweet potatoes, yams, breadfruit, greens, fruit, seaweed, fish, and chicken. This diet approximates that of ancient Hawaiians, which was estimated to contain less than 10% fat, 12% to 15% protein, and 75% to 78% carbohydrates. Participants also attended educational sessions, which include cultural teachings, nutrition education, and motivational sessions. They were taught techniques for using the diet as a template for making food choices. A whole-person approach, with emphasis on spiritual aspects of living and group *ohana* (family-like) support, had additional features. Participants were particularly encouraged to act as role models for the modified eating behaviors they learned. The program is viewed as a strategy for community empowerment, bringing community members together to address a problem they want to solve.

The results show that the Waianae Diet Program was successful. Weight, cholesterol, low-density lipoproteins (LDL), triglycerides, glucose, and systolic and diastolic blood pressures were decreased significantly in participants. A long-term evaluation was conducted over 7 1/2 years on 82 participants in the original study (Shintani, Beckham, Tang, O'Connor, & Hughes, 1999). The evaluation showed that an average weight loss of 15.1 pounds was maintained over 7 1/2 years. The unique aspects of the program offered particular insight into how changes in dietary behavior may be integrated into the cultural, spiritual, recreational, and social aspects of participants' life perspective. This whole-person approach, espoused by nursing, may decrease the problems with compliance to new dietary behaviors evident in so many prior studies.

The Partners in Prevention Nutrition Program

This intervention (McCann & Bovbjerg, 1998) used a stage-of-change approach based on the transtheoretical model developed by Prochaska and colleagues (2002) to match tailored communications about dietary behavior to the needs of participants at different points in the change process. The 558 adult participants were recruited from four family practices in central North Carolina. The study sample was 73% female, 62.3% married, 19%

minority (predominantly African American) with a mean education level of 13.6 years, average age of 40.8 years, and median income level of $30,000 to $39,000. A randomized trial was used with pretest and posttest measures to determine the impact of tailored versus nontailored nutrition education materials on the consumption of fat, fruit, and vegetables. Current dietary intake, stage of change in regard to dietary behavior, self-efficacy for dietary change, beliefs concerning perceived susceptibility to diet-related diseases, perceived benefits of dietary change to avoid health problems, and other psychosocial and physical variables were assessed at baseline. Participants were categorized at baseline as being in one of the following stages: precontemplation (not seriously thinking about change), contemplation (seriously thinking about change within the next 6 months), preparation (planning to change within the next 30 days), or action or maintenance (currently trying to change). Participants were randomly assigned to one of three groups: tailored nutrition messages, nontailored nutrition messages, or a control group that received no nutrition messages. Messages were mailed to participants 3 weeks after the collection of baseline data. The tailored intervention consisted of a one-time, mailed nutrition information packet customized to the participant's stage of change, dietary intake, and psychosocial information. For example, contemplators received information designed to decrease barriers to change and increase self-efficacy. Those individuals already trying to change received tailored recipes and messages aimed at preventing relapse. The nontailored messages provided standard risk information about the relation of diet to disease and gave dietary recommendations based on the 1990 *Dietary Guidelines for Americans* (Crane, Hubbard, & Lewis, 1998). The control group completed pretest and posttest surveys but received no nutrition information. Members of the tailored message group, when surveyed approximately 6 months later, had significantly decreased total fat by 23% compared to 9% in the nontailored group and 3% in the control group. The tailored group reported decreased saturated fat by 26%, compared to 11% in the nontailored group and 3% in the control group. The tailored message did not affect reported intake of fruits and vegetables. Also, more individuals in the tailored message group, compared to the other groups, could remember receiving and reading the nutrition information packet. Thus, the stage-of-change approach to dietary modification looks promising. Further research is needed to determine whether interventions based on the transtheoretical model may be used to promote maintenance of dietary changes (McCann & Bovbjerg, 1998).

Maintaining Recommended Weight

Obesity in adults is generally defined as a BMI of greater than or equal to 30 kg/m (U.S. Department of Health and Human Services, 2000). Whereas the physical basis for excessive weight gain is relatively simple and straightforward (i.e., the ingestion of more calories than needed for energy expenditure), the actual causes of being overweight are complex. They include:

1. Heredity
2. Cognitive factors (e.g., unrealistic personal standards and expectations)
3. Affective factors (e.g., emotional problems such as anxiety, boredom, and feelings of powerlessness)

4. Interpersonal factors (e.g., family problems, difficulties with fellow workers or colleagues)

5. Sociocultural factors (food selection, food preparation, and food consumption practices)

6. Environmental factors (e.g., salient cues for eating behavior and level of environmental sensitivity)

Although heredity plays a role in predisposition toward excessive weight gain, it is more important to focus on personal (cognitive, affective), interpersonal, sociocultural, and environmental influences (Kikuchi & Watanabe, 2000; Ounpuu, Woolcott, & Greene, 2000).

The primary goal of interventions for weight loss is the permanent alteration of eating patterns and physical activity, rather than weight loss only. Actually, adopting more healthful eating behaviors is directed toward increasing rather than decreasing the pleasures derived from eating. New awareness of taste, texture, and form of foods allows the individual to participate to the fullest in the eating experience, totally involving gustatory, visual, olfactory, and tactile senses. Eating that promotes optimum health can be fulfilling, self-actualizing, and totally enjoyable.

The individual who maintains desired weight has taken a major step toward decreasing the risk for many chronic health problems. Not only does weight loss decrease the risk of chronic disease, but it has been shown to increase self-esteem, perceptions of control, and feelings of social desirability and acceptance. Individuals of normal weight are more active than their overweight counterparts, and this further promotes health and decreases the risk for health problems. Diet modification (wholesome nutrition and low meat) has been associated with an improved lipid profile (Richter et al., 2004). Adipocytes are the fat cells within the body that increase in lipid content with weight gain. Weight reduction is achieved through a decrease in the size of cells. As increased by-products of fat metabolism enter systemic circulation, precautions must be taken to prevent their deposit in the lining of vessels and their detrimental effects to internal organs such as the liver and kidneys. Stability of weight may prevent many of these potential hazards.

Initiating a Weight-Reduction Program

The individual who desires to lose more than 30 pounds should consult with a health care provider before starting an aggressive weight loss program. Consultation with a provider may influence what type of diet the individual selects and the provider will likely determine that the individual should have a health history, physical examination, blood lipid and glucose analysis, and electrocardiogram before beginning a weight-loss program. Whether individuals who desire to lose less than 30 pounds should consult a health care provider is best determined by the individual after studying various diets (books, web sites) and selecting the best one based on lifestyle, costs, and self-knowledge.

Also, careful assessment of current dietary habits is essential in order to develop an individualized, effective program.

Other points to consider include the following:

- Is the person strongly motivated to change?
- Are there health conditions that make weight reduction a high priority?
- If change is desired, are expectations realistic?
- Does the person have a support system within or outside of the family to facilitate weight loss?
- Has the person had past successes in weight loss? If so, what worked? What did not work?

The best weight-loss program will be one that closely mirrors the *Dietary Guidelines* described earlier. Caloric reduction with attention to portion size while maintaining adequate nutrient levels, adequate vitamins and minerals, and adequate fiber is the best way to achieve and maintain desired weight. Thus, radical changes in food consumption patterns are not recommended as a means of weight loss. The nurse should review the many weight loss web sites to help clients determine if a web site program is a practical alternative to in-person diet counseling. The National Heart, Lung and Blood Institute (NIH) has an interesting quiz on its web site about the difference in portion sizes of food today versus 20 years ago, and how long one would have to exercise to lose those extra calories (see web site address at the end of this chapter). A combination of dietary modifications that individuals find palatable and adequate exercise offer the best approach to achieving and maintaining recommended weight. Physical activity promotes expenditure of energy and facilitates weight loss. Exercise is not only useful in burning excess calories; studies have shown that it also prevents the loss of protein from muscle and minerals from bone that frequently occur when attempts at weight loss are accompanied by inactivity. Exercise in combination with restricted calories also assists in reducing undesirable lipoprotein lipids, increasing work capacity, lowering resting heart rate, and decreasing blood pressure. Increased physical activity generally decreases appetite and increases the basal metabolism rate for several hours, offsetting the reduced metabolic rate that accompanies calorie restriction (Zephier et al., 1997).

Further, positive changes in affect and mood that often accompany exercise improve the long-term compliance with newly acquired eating behaviors. Both exercise during leisure time and lifestyle exercise should be increased as a complement to healthy nutritional practices. The reader is referred to Chapter 6 for discussion of further benefits of exercise and how to facilitate exercise adherence.

Directions for Research in Nutrition and Health

Further research is needed to understand the links between nutrition and health. Studies have been conducted on the effects of fats, fiber, and sodium on the development of cardiovascular disorders and cancer. Research has suggested modifications in lifestyle changes and further study is needed. Further research to explore the positive and negative effects of various food components on health as well as on specific disorders is essential to improve health. A better understanding of factors related to undernutrition, particularly eating disorders in adolescents and young adults, and overnutrition is critically needed as a basis for effective nursing interventions.

To promote healthy eating habits across the life span, behavioral theories and models applicable to eating behavior should be tested, and, as warranted, incorporated into intervention studies. Existing theories in nursing, psychology, and public health must be used to design behavioral interventions that focus on the individual, the family, and the community. Studies are needed to apply the most appropriate behavioral model that will test effective tailoring strategies to promote positive eating behaviors of a given client. Further research will provide additional answers concerning the underlying mechanisms through which nutrition improves health and well-being.

Directions for Practice in Nutrition and Health

The responsibility for monitoring the nutritional health of individuals, families, and the community is shared among nurses, nutritionists, and other health professionals. A tremendous gap exists between the knowledge about nutrition and diet and the eating behaviors of the U.S. population. The lack of adoption of positive dietary habits and good nutrition has resulted in a population of children, adolescents, and adults who are overweight and/or obese. The chronic health problems that often follow are costly to the individual and family, as well as the national economy. Dietary counseling and education should be an integral part of nursing practice in all settings. Counseling and follow-up of each client whose BMI is outside the normal range is a challenge the nurse must accept.

Opportunities may be created to engage clients and others in dialogue about their dietary practices and modifications that will improve their health. Nurses are respected professionals who influence their communities and schools. School nurses and occupational health nurses must work with school and industry officials to improve the food choices in cafeterias and vending machines. Internet web sites that focus on nutrition are a quick way to keep current on research findings and practice outcomes as well as to share with clients. Clients need to be encouraged to seek information from the Internet and discuss it with the nurse. One of the most important ways the nurse can influence others is to role model weight management and good dietary habits.

SUMMARY

Professional support of the client by the nurse and suggestions for constructively dealing with barriers to changing eating behaviors facilitate the client's efforts to eliminate or minimize obstacles that block attainment of desired nutritional goals. Promoting good nutrition is a critical concern in illness prevention and health promotion and an important dimension of competent self-care and dependent care. Cultural background influences eating behavior. The family and community should be considered as points for nutritional intervention that may, in the long run, be more productive than individual interventions.

Because much is yet to be learned about nutrition and health, nurses and other health scientists should accept the challenge of exploring eating behavior as an important health promotion activity.

Learning Activities

1. Select one of the factors influencing eating behavior and develop a five-item questionnaire that you might use in evaluating that factor in client's eating behavior.
2. Discuss three major nutritional needs of adolescents and propose how to influence their inclusion in their diet.
3. Develop a plan, as a young adult, to maintain or reduce your weight including an assessment of possible causes of being overweight or points to consider in a weight-reduction program.

Selected Web Sites

Department of Health and Human Services

http://www.dhhs.gov

Food and Fitness Site

http://www.foodfit.com

Food and Nutrition Information Center

http://www.nal.usda.gov/fnic

Healthy People 2010

http://www.health.gov/healthypeople

National Center for Health Statistics

http://www.cdc.gov/nchs

National Heart, Lung and Blood Institute
Clinical Practice Guidelines

http://www.nhlbi.nih.gov/guidelines

National Heart, Lung and Blood Institution Food Portion Size Quiz

http://www.hin.nhlbi.nih.gov/portion

New England Journal of Medicine

http://www.nejm.org

Nutrition and Your Health: Dietary Guidelines

http://www.health.gov/dietaryguidelines

Office of Disease Prevention and Health Promotion

http://www.odphp.osophs.dhhs.gov

REFERENCES

American Dietetic Association. (2004). Position of the American Dietetic Association: Dietary guidance for healthy children ages 2 to 11 years. *Journal of the American Dietetic Association*, 104(4), 660–677.

Ammerman A. S., Lindquist, C. H., Lohr, K. N., & Hersey, J. (2002). The efficacy of behavioral interventions to modify dietary fat and fruit and vegetable intake: A review of the evidence. *Preventive Medicine, 35*, 25–41.

Barnard, N. D., Akhtar, A., & Nicholson, A. (1995). Factors that facilitate compliance to a low fat intake. *Archives of Family Medicine, 4*, 153–158.

Beresford, S. A. A., Curry, S., Kristal, A., Lazovich, D., Feng, Z., & Wagner, E. H. (1997). A low intensity dietary intervention in primary care practice: The eating patterns study. *Am J Public Health, 87*, 610–616.

Bergmann, M. M., & Boeing, H. (2002). Behavioral changes in observational and intervention studies. *J Nutr, 132*(11 Suppl), 3530S–3533S.

Bessesen, D. H. (2002, March). Obesity as a factor. *Nutr Rev, 58*(3 Pt 2), S12–15.

Bingham, S. A., Day, N. E., Luben, R., Ferrari, P., Slimani, N., Norat, T., et al. (2003). Dietary fibre in food and protection against colorectal cancer in the European Prospective Investigation into Cancer and Nutrition (EPIC): An observational study. *The Lancet, 361*(9368), 1496–1501.

Blandford, G. (1998). Eating disorders. In R. Tallis, H. Fillit, & J. C. Brocklehurst (Eds.), *Brocklehurst's textbook of geriatric medicine and gerontology* (5th ed., pp. 1413–1421). New York: Churchill Livingstone.

Blundell, J. E., & Cooling, J. (1999). High-fat and low-fat (behavioral) phenotypes: Biology or environment? *Proc Nutr Soc, 58*(4), 773–777.

Boschi, V., Siervo, M., D'Orsi, P., Margiotta, N., Trapanese, E., Basile, F., Nasti Papa, A., Bellini, O., & Falconi, C. (2003). Body composition, eating behavior, food-body concerns and eating disorders in adolescent girls. *Ann Nutr Metab, 47*(6), 284–293.

Brownell, K. D. (1999). The central role of lifestyle change in long-term weight management. *Clin Cornerstone, 2*(3), 43–51.

Brunner, E., White, I., Thorogood, M., Bristow, A., Curle, D., & Marmot, M. (1997). Can dietary interventions change diet and cardiovascular risk factors? A meta-analysis of randomized controlled trials. *Am J Public Health, 87*, 1415–1422.

Chen, T. C., & Holick, M. F. (2003). Vitamin D and prostate cancer prevention and treatment. *Trends in Endocrinology and Metabolism, 14*(9), 423–430.

Crane, N. T., Hubbard, V. S., & Lewis, C. L. (1998). National nutrition objectives and the dietary guidelines for Americans. *Nutr Today, 33*, 49–58.

Duffy, V. B., & Bartoshuk, L. M. (2000, June). Food acceptance and genetic variation in taste. *J Am Diet Assoc, 100*(6), 647–655.

Flegal, K. M., Carroll, M. D., Ogden, C. L., & Johnson, C. L. (2002). Prevalence and trends in obesity among U.S. adults, 1999–2000. *JAMA, 228,* 1723–1727.

Food and Drug Administration and National Institutes of Health. (2000, January). Nutrition and overweight (Chapter 19). In *Healthy People 2010* (conference edition). Washington, DC: U.S. Government Printing Office.

Fredericks, S. C. (1999). Motivating people to join a weight management program using a creative promotional tool. *Journal of the American Dietetic Association, 99*(9), A40.

Freedman, D. S., Khan, L. K., Serdula, M. K., Galuska, D. A., & Dietz, W. H. (2002). Trends and correlates of class 3 obesity in the United States from 1990 through 2000. *JAMA, 288,* 1758–1761.

Friedman, M. I. (1998, March). Fuel partitioning and food intake . . . proceedings of a symposium held at the University of Texas Southwestern Medical Center, Dallas, April 22–23, 1996. *Am J Clin Nutr, 67*(3S, suppl), 513S–518S.

Gifford, K. D. (2002). Dietary fats, eating guides, and public policy: History, critique, and recommendations. *The American Journal of Medicine, 113*(9B), 89S–106S.

Glanz, K. (1999). Progress in dietary behavior change. *Am J of Health Prom, 14*(2), 112–117.

Goran, M. I. (1998, March). Measurement issues related to studies of childhood obesity: Assessment of body comparison, body fat distribution, physical activity, and food intake. *Pediatrics, 101*(3, suppl.), 505–518.

Gordon, M. (2002). *Manual of nursing diagnosis: Including all diagnostic categories approved by the North American Nursing Diagnosis Association* (10th ed.). St. Louis: Mosby.

Guillen, E. O., & Barr, S. I. (1994). Nutrition, dieting, and fitness messages in a magazine for adolescent women, 1970–1990. *J Adolesc Health, 15,* 464–472.

Gutierrez, Y. M. (1994). *Nutrition in health maintenance and health promotion for primary care providers.* San Francisco: School of Nursing, University of California, San Francisco.

Heitmann, B. L., Harris, J. R., Lissner, L., & Pedersen, N. L. (1999). Genetic effects on weight change and food intake in Swedish adult twins. *Am J Clin Nutr, 69*(4), 597–602.

Hernandez, B., Uphold, C. R., Graham, M. V., & Singer, L. (1998). Prevalence and correlates of obesity in preschool children. *J of Ped Nurs, 13*(2), 68–76. Available at *http://hin.nhlbi.gov/portion*

Kayser-Jones, J., & Schell, E. (1997). The effect of staffing on the quality of care at mealtime. *Nurs Outlook, 45*(2), 64–72.

Keller, H. H. (1995). Weight gain impacts morbidity and mortality in institutionalized older persons. *J Am Geriatrics Society, 43*(2), 165–169.

Kikuchi, Y., & Watanabe, S. (2000). Personality and dietary habits. *J Epidemiol, 10*(3), 191–198.

Kumanyika, S. K. (2001). Minisymposium on obesity: Overview and some strategic considerations. *Ann Rev Public Health, 22,* 293–308.

Kumanyika, S. K., Van Horn, L., Bowen, D., Perri, M. G., Rolls, B. J., Czajkowski, S. M., & Schron, E. (2000). Maintenance of dietary behavior change. *Health Psychol, 19*(1, suppl), 42–56.

MacIntosh, C. G., Andrews, J. M., Jones, K. L., Wishart, J. M., Morris, H. A., Jansen, J. B., Morley. J. E., Horowitz, M., & Chapman, I. M. (1999). Effects of age on concentrations of plasma cholecystokinin, glucagon-like peptide 1, and peptide YY and their relation to appetite and pyloric motility. *Am J Clin Nutr, 69*(5), 999–1006.

Martinez, J. A. (2000). Body-weight regulation: Causes of obesity. *Proc Nutr Soc, 59*(3), 337–345.

Martinez, M. E. (2004). Session 8 prevention of colorectal cancer: Where are we going? S23. Primary prevention of colorectal cancer: Lifestyle, nutrition, exercise. *European Journal of Cancer Supplements, 2*(1), 25.

McCann, B. S., & Bovbjerg, V. E. (1998). Promoting dietary change. In S. A. Shumaker, E. B. Schron, J. K. Ockene, & W. L. McBee (Eds.), *The handbook of health behavior change* (2nd ed., pp. 166–188). New York: Springer.

Morbidity and Mortality Weekly Report. (1996, June). *Guidelines for school health programs to promote lifelong healthy eating.* Atlanta, GA: Centers for Disease Control.

Morbidity and Mortality Weekly Report. (1998, April). *Recommendations to prevent and control iron deficiency in the United States.* Atlanta, GA: Centers for Disease Control.

Myers, S., & Vargas, Z. (2000). Parental perceptions of the preschool obese child. *Ped. Nurs, 26*(1), 23–30.

National Center for Health Statistics. (1997). *Healthy People 2000 review 1998–1999.* DHHS Pub. No. (PHS) 99-1256. Hyattsville, MD: Public Health Service, U.S. Department of Health and Human Services.

Nord, M., Andrews, M., & Carlson, S. (2002). *Household food security in the United States,* 2001. Report No. FANRR-29. Washington, DC: USDA ERS Food Assistance and Nutrition Research, 55.

Ogden, C. L., Flegal, K. M., Carroll, M. D., & Johnson, C. L. (2002). Prevalence and trends in overweight among U.S. children and adolescents, 1999–2000. *JAMA, 288,* 1728–1732.

O'Neil, PM. (2001). Assessing dietary intake in the management of obesity. *Obes Res, 9*(Suppl 5), 361S–366S & 373S–374S.

Osganian, S. K., Hoelscher, D. M., Zive, M., Mitchell, P. D., Snyder, P., & Webber, L. (2003). Maintenance of effects of the Eat Smart school food service program: Results from the CATCH-ON study. *Health Educ Behav, 30*(4), 418–433.

Ounpuu, S., Woolcott, D. M., & Greene, G. W. (2000). Defining stage of change for lower-fat eating. *J Am Diet Assoc, 100*(6), 674–679.

Prochaska, J. O., Redding C. A. & Couers, K. E. (2002). The transtheoretical model and stages of change. In K. Slang, B. F. Riner, & F. M. Leurs (Eds.), *Health Behavior and Health Education* (pp. 99–120). San Francisco: Jossey-Bass.

Purcell, A. C., O'Brien, E., & Parks, P. L. (1996). Cholesterol levels in children: To screen or not to screen. *J Ped Nurs: Care of Children and Families, 11*(1), 40–44.

Ravussin, E., & Bouchard, C. (2000). Human genomics and obesity: Finding appropriate drug targets. *European Journal of Pharmacology, 410*(2-3), 131–145.

Reger, B., Wootan, M. G., & Booth-Butterfield, S. (1999). Using mass media to promote healthy eating: A community-based demonstration project. *Prev Med, 29*(5), 414–421.

Richter, K. P., Harris, K. J., Paine-Andrews, A., Fawcett, S. B., Schmid, T. L., Lankenau, B. H., & Johnston, J. (2000). Measuring the health environment for physical activity and nutrition among youth: A review of the literature and applications for community initiatives. *Preventive Medicine, 31*(2), S98–S111.

Richter, V., Puaschuritz, K., Rassoul, F., Thiery, J., Zunft, H. J., & Leitzmam, C. (2004). Effects of diet modification on wholesome nutritin study. *Asia Pac & Clin nutr.* 13(Suppl): S106.

Rosenberg, I. H. (Ed.). (2000, June). A healthful diet goes beyond this or that food. *Tufts University Health & Nutrition Letter, 18*(4), 8.

Shepherd, R. (1999). Social determinants of food choice. *Proc Nutr Soc, 58*(4), 807–812.

Shintani, T., Beckham, S., Kanawaliwali, H., et al. (1994). The Waianae Diet Program: A culturally sensitive, community-based obesity and clinical intervention program for the native Hawaiian population. *Hawaii Med J, 53,* 136–147.

Shintani, T., Beckham, S., Tang, J., O'Connor, H. K., & Hughes, C. (1999). Waianae diet program: Long-term follow-up. *Hawaii Med J, 58*(5), 117–122.

Sorenson, G., Stoddard, A., Peterson, K., Cohen, N., Hunt, M. K., Stein, E., Palombo, R., & Lederman, R. (1999). Increasing fruit and vegetable consumption through worksites and families in the Treatwell 5-a-day study. *Am J of Public Health, 89*(1), 54–60.

Stewart, K. J., Seemans, C. M., McFarland, L. D., Weinhufer, J. J., & Brown, C. S. (1999). Dietary fat and cholesterol intake in young children compared with recommended levels. *Journal of Cardiopulmonary Rehabilitation, 19*(2), 112–117.

U.S. Congress, Office of Technology Assessment. (1991). *Adolescent health volume II: Background and the effectiveness of selected prevention and treatment services.* Washington, DC: U.S. Government Printing Office. Publication OTA-H-466.

U.S. Department of Agriculture, U.S. Department of Health and Human Services. (1996). *Home and garden bulletin 252. The Food Guide Pyramid.* Washington, DC: U.S. Department of Agriculture, U.S. Department of Health and Human Services.

U.S. Department of Agriculture/U.S. Department of Health and Human Services. (2000). *Home and garden bulletin 232. Dietary Guidelines for Americans* (5th ed.). Washington, DC: U.S. Department of Agriculture/U.S. Department of Health and Human Services, 30.

U.S. Department of Agriculture and U.S. Department of Health and Human Services. (2000). *Dietary guidelines for Americans* (5th ed.). Home and Garden Bulletin.

U.S. Department of Health and Human Services. (2000). *Healthy People 2010* (Conference Edition, in Two Volumes). Washington, DC: U.S. Government Printing Office.

U.S. Department of Health and Human Services, Public Health Service, National Institutes of Health. (2001). *Third report of the expert panel on detection, evaluation and treatment of high blood cholesterol in adults (adult treatment panel III): Executive summary.* NIH Publication No. 01-3670.

U.S. Preventive Services Task Force. (1996). *Guide to clinical preventive services* (2nd ed.). Washington, DC: U.S. Government Printing Office.

Watanabe, H., Yamane, K., Fujikawa, R., Okubo, M., Egusa, G., & Kohno, N. (2003). Westernization of lifestyle markedly increases carotid intima-media wall thickness (IMT) in Japanese people. *Atherosclerosis, 166*(1), 67–72.

Wellman, N. S. (1994). Dietary guidelines and nutrient requirements of the elderly. *Prim Care, 21*(1), 1–18.

Wing, R. R. (2000). Cross-cutting themes in maintenance of behavior change. *Health Psychol, 19*(suppl 1), 84–88.

Zephier, E. M., Ballew, C., Mokdad, A., Mendlein, J., Smith, C., Yeh, J. L., Lee, E., Welty, T. K., & Howard, B. (1997). Intake of nutrients related to cardiovascular disease risk among three groups of American Indians: The strong heart dietary study. *Prev Med, 26*(4), 508–515.

Zhang, X., Shu, X. O., Gao, Y. T., Yang, G., Li, Q., Jin, F., & Zheng, W. (2003). Soy food consumption is associated with lower risk of coronary heart disease in Chinese women. *J Nutr, 133*(9), 2874–2878.

8

Stress Management and Health Promotion

OBJECTIVES

1. Discuss the relationship between stress and health.
2. Describe four approaches to assist clients to prevent stressful situations.
3. Discuss five psychological conditioning strategies to increase one's resistance to stress.
4. Discuss two interventions to prevent physiologic arousal.

OUTLINE

- Stress and Health
- Stress Across the Life Span
- Approaches to Stress Management
  A. Minimizing the Frequency of Stress-Inducing Situations
  B. Increasing Resistance to Stress
  C. Counterconditioning to Avoid Physiologic Arousal
- Directions for Research on Stress Management
- Directions for Practice in Stress Management
- Summary
- Learning Activities
- Selected Web Sites
- References

Stress is of theoretical and practical interest to nurses. Nurse researchers have studied various aspects of stress in attempts to understand the stress–illness relationship as well as how to promote health through fostering stress resistance and overall resilience among individuals and families. It is estimated that 60% to 80% of visits to health care professionals are caused or made worse by stress (Lawrence & Lawrence, 1994). With this high incidence of stress-related health problems, strategies for promoting stress reduction among clients are of critical importance to minimize insults to well-being and maximize positive challenges and realization of personal potential.

Stress is an inevitable human experience in any modern society characterized by rapid and accelerating change. Selye (1977), a pioneer in stress research, defined stress as "the nonspecific response of the body to any demand made on it." Internal and external manifestations of stress are referred to as the General Adaptation Syndrome (GAS) or the "fight-or-flight" response. Specific physiologic or behavioral changes that occur in response to stressors include:

- Dilation of pupils
- Increased respiratory rate
- Increased heart rate
- Peripheral vasoconstriction
- Increased perspiration
- Increased blood pressure
- Increased muscle tension
- Increased gastric motility
- Release of adrenalin
- Increased blood glucose level
- Raising of body hair
- Cold and clammy hands

The major sources of stress experienced by individuals in modern society originate in interpersonal relationships (communication) and performance demands (action) rather than from direct physical threat. Because communication and action represent two basic human processes, the potential for stress is always present (Selye, 1977).

Stressors, or the causes of stress, are defined by Lazarus and Folkman (1984) as "environmental and internal demands and conflicts among them, which tax or exceed a person's resources." The body's response to stress involves the nervous, endocrine, and immunologic systems, which in turn affect all organ systems. Although all individuals experience stress, people interpret and react to it differently, resulting in differing vulnerabilities to the deleterious effects of stress. Some stressors are viewed as challenges, creating stimulation and excitement. Other stressors are viewed negatively, perhaps because they are considered undesirable, uncontrollable, or emotionally distressing. There is much scientific interest in the "resistance resources" that enable some individuals to successfully manage stressors and flourish whereas others find the same stressors debilitating.

Coping strategies assist individuals in managing stress and are described as learned and purposeful cognitive, emotional, and behavioral responses to stressors used to adapt to the environment or to change it (Lazarus & Folkman, 1984). In the coping process, the ability to regulate emotions, behavior, and the environment are critical to successful adjustment. Cognitive appraisal and coping constitute the stress-coping process. Cognitive appraisal consists of two phases. In *primary appraisal*, the person evaluates whether he or she has anything at stake in the encounter. Is there potential harm or benefit to cherished commitments, values, goals, self-esteem, or the health and well-being of a significant other? If an encounter is threatening, primary appraisal serves to reduce its significance for the person experiencing it. For example, if a person receives notice that the results of a laboratory test are "abnormal," the person may discount the validity of the test (Wenzel, Glanz, & Lerman, 2002). In *secondary appraisal*, the person evaluates what, if anything, may be done to overcome or prevent harm, or to improve the prospects of benefit. Various coping options are evaluated, such as altering the situation, accepting it, seeking more information, or holding back from acting in an impulsive way. Primary and secondary appraisals converge to determine if the person–environment transaction is primarily threatening or challenging.

Coping regulates stressful emotions (emotion-focused coping) and alters the person–environment relationship that is causing the distress (problem-focused coping). Both forms of coping occur in stressful encounters. The success of problem-focused coping may in large part depend on the success of emotion-focused coping, because heightened emotions are likely to interfere with the cognitive activity necessary to deal effectively with stressors. Problem-focused coping is likely to be dominant in encounters viewed as changeable, whereas emotion-focused coping often dominates in encounters viewed as unchangeable, with acceptance as the only recourse (Wenzel et al., 2002). Encounters involving threats to self-esteem are often the most difficult to resolve. These threats include the possibility of losing the affection of someone one cares about, losing self-respect or the respect of others, and appearing to be unethical or incompetent.

Disability, absenteeism, decreased productivity, and health-damaging effects of stress and mental illnesses were estimated to cost business and industry more than $150 billion in 1996 (*Healthy People 2010*, 2000). Financial incentives to businesses and health maintenance organizations to help individuals manage stress and avoid its costly, health-impairing effects are considerable.

The goals of *Healthy People 2010* related to mental health are to ensure access to appropriate, quality mental health services and improve mental health. One of the *Healthy People 2010* Mental Health and Mental Disorders community-focused objectives is increasing the number of persons seen in primary health care settings who receive mental health screening. Adults who seek mental health care in primary care settings have fewer visits per year (average of 4) than do those adults who are seen by specialists (average of 14). Because approximately 6% of all the adult population in the United States use their primary care provider for mental health care, it is imperative that nurses and other providers ensure that all adults are screened and treated for mental health disorders (*Healthy People 2010*, 2000). Of the four *Healthy People 2000* objectives that focused on adults with mental health disorders, the least progress was made on controlling stress and seeking treatment for depression. Measures of progress on the objective related to mental health services showed that nurse practitioners inquired less about parent–child relationships and their adult patients' cognitive, emotional, or behavioral functioning than when assessed at baseline (*Healthy People 2010*, 2000) than other health issues.

Professional nurses in community settings including schools, clinics, and work sites have a responsibility to promote and conduct early screening and intervention for stress-related problems.

Stress and Health

Decreased life satisfaction, the development of mental disorders, the occurrence of stress-related illnesses (such as cardiovascular disease, gastrointestinal disorders, low back pain, headaches), and decreased immunologic functioning, which has been implicated in a diagnosis of cancer, are linked to stress. In terms of heart disease, long-term stress is thought to sensitize arterioles to catecholamines, with even short-term stress responses causing overconstriction of the vessels and endothelial damage. Repetitive overconstriction may lead to hypertension, decreased myocardial perfusion, and arrhythmias (Castillo et al., 2000; Öhlin, Nilsson, Nilsson, & Berglund, 2004). Social factors are intimately related to the experience of stress and subsequently to health and disease (Steptoe, Owen, Kunz-Ebrecht, & Brydon, 2004). Social isolation and loneliness increase a person's risk for heart disease and decrease survival following a heart attack. Patients who have a heart attack and live alone are one-and-a-half times more likely to have a second heart attack than are those who live with someone else (Clay, 2001; Underwood, 2000). In other instances, the nature of interpersonal relationships may be detrimental to health. For example, elderly caregivers experienced chronic distress when caring for a family member with a chronic illness, resulting in impairment of their immune system (Bauer et al., 2000). Because both the absence of social relations and certain characteristics of social relations serve as stressors that may have an impact on health, understanding how social relationships affect the brain, physiologic processes, and health is of critical importance (Bauer et al., 2000; Wenzel et al., 2002).

Psychoneuroimmunology examines the effects of social and psychologic phenomena on the immune system as mediated by the nervous and endocrine systems. This arena of science is particularly important because both acute and chronic infections as well as cancer have been linked to compromised immune functioning. In a series of studies, male undergraduate college students with high heart-rate reactivity to stressors (mental arithmetic test with noise superimposed) were compared to low heart-rate reactors on neuroendocrine and immune responses to stressors. High reactors compared to low showed higher stress-related levels of plasma cortisol and increased natural killer (NK) cell lysis. The finding that cortisol was elevated in high reactors is particularly interesting in view of the extensive literature linking cortisol with down-regulation of multiple aspects of cellular immune function. These findings suggest that individual variation in activation of the hypothalamic-pituitary-adrenocortical axis by brief psychologic stressors may explain why daily stressors have greater health consequences for some individuals than for others. Different mediating roles may be played by the hypothalamic-pituitary-adrenocortical axis and the sympathetic adrenomedullary systems. Evidence is growing that the immune system is influenced by central nervous system processes that are shaped by social psychologic factors (Gaab et al., 2003; Witek-Janusek & Mathews, 2000).

The experience of stress may also influence the immune system. Berger and O'Brien (1998) studied the effect of a cognitive-behavioral intervention on salivary immunoglobulin (sIgA; a factor related to host defense), self-reported levels of stress, and the physical health of 57 undergraduate students. The students were randomly assigned to either the intervention or control group. Each group was divided into sections of 10 students. The 5-week intervention period consisted of giving information about stress, the body's response to stress, immunity, relaxation techniques, cognitive restructuring, and assertiveness training. Pre- and postintervention measures included saliva testing, rating of physical symptoms of stress, and self-reported physical problems. Change was measured using the Undergraduate Stress Questionnaire, the Cohen-Hoberman Inventory of Physical Symptoms, the Daily Stress Inventory, and saliva cultures. Stress was reduced for both the control and intervention groups based on changes in the scores of the self-reported instruments. There was no change in the sIgA results. These findings suggest that the intervention reduced reported stress in the participants but did not have any immunoenhancing effect. Other researchers conducted a meta-analysis to review evidence that psychological interventions affect the immune system. Results based on 85 conducted trials revealed only modest support that the immune system is altered by psychological interventions. The authors suggest that conceptual and methodological issues must be addressed in research studies before it is concluded that psychological interventions do not cause changes in one's immune response (Miller & Cohen, 2001). The findings of these two studies support the need for additional research to focus on identifying immune-enhancing interventions.

A number of physiologic systems seem to be highly responsive to life experiences and the psychologic states that accompany them. Further studies of varying human responses to stress are important as a basis for developing effective stress-management techniques, supporting healthy coping mechanisms, and restructuring faulty psychologic defenses (Bower & Segerstrom, 2004; Werner & Frost, 2000). A holistic approach that integrates the mind and body has long characterized nursing. Nurses understand the relationships between stress and health as well as stress and illness as a basis for assessment and nursing care. Nurses are in a key position to identify individuals and families who are coping ineffectively. Coping strategies for stress reduction; perceived controllability, intensity, and duration of stressors; emotional and behavioral regulation skills; and perceived availability of social support should be assessed. Findings will direct the nurse to structure appropriate interventions or make referrals to assist clients in dealing with stressors before they exert health-damaging effects.

Stress Across the Life Span

Children experience stress and develop coping patterns early in life. Children's stress-coping processes must be assessed because of the hazards imposed by prolonged stress. Sources of stress are related to the child's age, gender, and developmental stage. Children and adults identify very different stressors. For example, children are mostly concerned about daily events that relate to school, peers, parents, and self. Environmental and social stressors that place children and adolescents at high risk for poor adjustment include personal safety concerns, community violence, prolonged poverty, increased availability of drugs, homelessness, and AIDS (Carroll & Ryan-Wenger, 1999). The majority of children, regardless of their environment, have a resiliency that allows them to function well in spite of major stressors. This type of competency develops over time (Masten & Coatsworth, 1998). Some children are more affected by stressful situations and need intervention. The potential is present to increase children's well-being and health through constructive stress management. Personal resilience and environmental protective factors that mediate the relationship between risk factors and healthy development need to be identified and incorporated into family, community, and school interventions. Higher stress has been associated with a range of risk-taking behaviors such as smoking and alcohol use in early adolescence. However, use of behavioral coping (information gathering, decision making, problem solving), cognitive coping (minimizing distress, focusing on the positive), adult social support (talking with an adult), and relaxation were found to be inversely related to substance abuse (Millstein, Petersen, & Nightingale, 1993). Nurses and other health professionals may find that the best approach to avoidance of substance abuse and other risky behaviors is to assist children and adolescents in learning effective stress-coping processes to apply across a variety of life circumstances.

Most of the knowledge about stress has been gained from studies of adults. This information may or may not be directly applicable to children. Some factors that are known to be related to stress in children include self-esteem, personality characteristics (type A behavior and temperament), gender, locus of control, social support, parental child-rearing behavior, and previous stressful experiences. The five most frequently occurring stressors identified by children included feeling sick, having nothing to do, not having enough money to spend, being pressured to get good grades, and feeling left out of the group (Ryan-Wenger, Sharrer, & Wynd, 2000). These differed from parents' perceptions of the most distressing events. Research is needed on sources of stress for children, developmental changes in stressors, coping strategies across childhood and adolescence, and how challenging rather than stressful environments may be created for youth. Seiffge-Krenke (1995) found developmental differences in the stressors most strongly related to psychologic symptoms: family-related stressors such as quarrels in mid-adolescence, peer stressors across early and mid-adolescence, and academic concerns in high-school-age youths. Particularly important are studies of the coping strategies used by resilient children who, despite high levels of stress, appear to cope well with adversity. An excellent overview of instruments to measure stressors in children and physiologic and behavioral indicators of acute and chronic stress is provided by Ryan-Wenger and colleagues (2000).

The stresses often experienced in young and middle-age adulthood relate to establishing oneself in a productive career, nourishing enduring relationships in a dyadic unit, child-bearing and child rearing, and creating a sense of self-identity as an independent yet interdependent adult. Work is often cited as a source of stress, and many employers increasingly offer work-site stress-management programs. Sources of work stress include lack of control over job environment or production demands, being "caught in the middle" between supervisors and customers, being underprepared for the job, lack of clarity about job expectations, unexpected transfers across departments or company locations, feeling trapped in a particular job, and lack of positive relationships with coworkers. Stress often causes deterioration in performance, which can further escalate already existing causes of stress and tension. Bond and Bunce (2000) studied the impact of two interventions, an Acceptance and Commitment Therapy (ACT) and an Innovation Promotion Program

(IPP), on employees in a media organization. Improvements in mental health and work-related strain were noted following both interventions. Employees were able to better accept undesirable thoughts and feelings by learning to modify stressors in the workplace.

Support at home can buffer work-related stressors, or the existence of additional stressors at home may have a cumulative effect with those at work and further threaten health. The Double ABCX model of family stress and adaptation (Demarco, Ford-Gilboe, Friedmann, McCubbin, & McCubbin, 2000) describes how families manage stressful events over a period of time. Family demands or accumulation of stressors are referred to as the A factor. Family changes and transitions as well as daily hassles among family members may cause stress. These demands on the family may produce internal tension that requires management. The B factor represents all the assets and resources that a family can draw upon in a time of stress. These include strengths of individual members, strengths of the family unit (open communication, cohesion), and strengths of the community (helpful agencies, supportive social networks). The third factor, C, includes the family's definition and perception of all the demands, the family's stress-meeting resources, and actions that need to be taken to resolve the stress. The result of the interaction between a family's demands and capabilities is its state of adaptation, X. This model is useful to nurses in primary care settings in helping them to conceptualize the stressors and coping capabilities of families as a basis for assessment and intervention.

Constrained finances or arguments between spouses about how to spend limited income may markedly increase tension in the home. Single parents are particularly vulnerable to stress, as they may lack social support and also find that job demands leave them little time for parenting responsibilities. In the absence of authoritative parenting, children may get into difficulties that further stretch limited psychologic resources of parents. Stress-management programs that address changing work and home environments to minimize stress and developing effective coping strategies best meet the needs of young and middle-age adults.

Although some sources of stress may abate in older adulthood, other stressors, particularly those resulting from loss, are more prevalent. The elderly are particularly vulnerable to negative life events such as the death of a spouse, death of a close family member, personal injury or illness, health change of a family member, and retirement. Hassles of daily living may increase as a result of diminished sensory acuity, decreased dexterity and strength, loss of flexibility, and increased fatigue. The elderly may neglect health behaviors that augment their strength and resilience such as proper nutrition, adequate exercise, proper rest, and sleep. Cumulative stress along with depression can compromise immune function, leaving the elderly more vulnerable to acute and chronic infections and chronic disease (Ferraro & Su, 1999; Lenze et al., 2000).

It is in old age when we begin to see the increased morbidity and mortality associated with years of daily hassles and cumulative major life events, particularly where coping strategies have been ineffective. Systemic effects on the cardiovascular, gastrointestinal, neurologic, endocrine, and immune systems may become increasingly apparent. Because of decreased resistance to disease, helping elderly adults to use existing coping techniques productively or learn new ones is of great importance. Nurses familiar with the problems of aging and the capabilities of older adults can equip them to manage the stressors that they encounter more effectively and efficiently, thus conserving valuable personal resources.

Approaches to Stress Management

At any point in time, an individual or family may be subjected to many sources of stress. Multiple stressors combine synergistically, resulting in cumulative stress. A number of nursing diagnoses specific to problems in stress management (defensive coping, ineffective family coping, etc.) are described by Gordon (2002) in the functional health pattern category of Coping-Stress Tolerance Pattern. The nurse and client must assess the level of existing stress as well as the sources of stress and then determine the appropriate interventions to reduce stress. Because there are many forms and techniques of stress management the literature suggests that overall effectiveness of stress management interventions has not been sufficiently studied (Ong, Linden, & Young, 2004).

The primary modes of intervention for stress management consist of the following:

- Minimize the frequency of stress-inducing situations.
- Increase resistance to stress.
- Countercondition to avoid physiologic arousal resulting from stress.

In general, changing the environment to decrease the incidence of stressors should be the "first line of defense." When that is not possible, individual and family coping resources need to come into play to reinterpret stress as a challenge, increase resilience against stress, or decrease the health-threatening effects of stressors.

Minimizing the Frequency of Stress-Inducing Situations

In a technology-rich society, the need for adjustment to externally imposed change is continuous. Approaches to assisting clients in preventing stressful situations include (a) changing the environment, (b) avoiding excessive change, (c) time control, and (d) time management.

Changing the Environment   Widely held values and beliefs shape the environment in any society. Changing the environment, when it is possible, is the most proactive approach to minimizing the frequency of stress-inducing situations. Major changes in societal beliefs, values, and actions are necessary if stress is to be reduced for some vulnerable populations. Sexism, racism, and ageism create stress for selected groups as a result of devaluation of their status and lack of acknowledgment of their contributions to society. Discrimination directed at any group can result in decreased educational and employment opportunities, poverty, and personal devaluation. Kessler argued that the primary causes of racial disparities in disease rates are rooted in differences between races in exposure or vulnerability to pathogenic factors in the physical, social, economic, and cultural environment. The association between perceived discrimination and mental health confirmed that perceived discrimination was a stressor that did not vary on the basis of the minority person's social status (Kessler, Mickelson, & Williams, 1999).

Racial discrimination and blood pressure of young black and white adults showed that differences in blood pressure of the two groups were reduced when the reported experiences of racial discrimination and unfair treatment were accounted for in the blood pressure readings (Krieger & Sidney, 1996). Attempts to improve social environments for low-income African Americans require changes in policies, values, and belief systems.

The work environment is frequently identified as a major source of stress. Changes in the work environment itself can reduce the incidence of stressful events. For example, instituting policies that provide flextime, job sharing, or child-care benefits or facilities can ease the stress on parents who must both maintain a job and care for young children. Protecting workers from job-related hazards, redesigning work assignments, creating pleasant work stations, instituting quality circles, or employing more participatory management styles also can foster lower levels of stress at work. Job-related stresses may also be avoided by becoming more aware of those persons or experiences that create personal stress and minimizing contact to the extent possible. In a study by McKenna and colleagues (2003) the majority of nurses reported that while they had begun smoking before becoming a nurse, stress in the work site contributed to their maintaining the habit. Committee membership in groups that are stress inducing might be better delegated to someone else who experiences less stress from the activity or who obtains actual enjoyment from participation. A study by Giga, Cooper, and Faragher (2003) suggests that the best outcomes for reduction of stress in the workplace occur when a comprehensive framework guides the chosen interventions.

If a job change is required by the client to decrease stress, new employment possibilities should be analyzed to make sure that stress phenomena similar to those already encountered are not an inherent part of the new employment setting. Protective factors in the broader environment that can further decrease stress include a family characterized by warmth and cohesion, culture and ethnic events and customs that promote identity, supportive relationships with others outside the family, and involvement in community structures such as churches and neighborhood organizations that promote competence and support (Friedman, 2002).

Avoiding Excessive Change   When children as young as 8 to 12 years of age were asked to report the coping strategies that they used in anticipation of stressful events, they reported avoidance of the situation, distracting behaviors, and some reported using relaxation behaviors (Ryan-Wenger, Sharrer, & Wynd, 2000). Teaching children when and how to avoid excessive change is important, as coping strategies developed early in childhood often continue into adulthood and affect patterns of behavior throughout the life span.

During periods of significant life change and resulting negative tension states, any unnecessary changes should be avoided. For example, if a family is experiencing the illness of one of its family members and a subsequent job loss, this may not be the time to consider geographic relocation, pregnancy, or any other change in lifestyle. Negative tension created by multiple changes is synergistic. Each time a distressing change occurs, the potency of previous change for upsetting stability is increased. Deliberately postponing changes that result in negative tension assists clients in dealing more constructively with unavoidable change and prevents the need for multiple adjustments all at one point in time.

Any changes that are made in lifestyle during periods of high or moderate stress should be self-initiated and provide challenge to the client rather than threat. Increasing positive sources of tension that promote growth and self-actualization can offset the deleterious effects of negative tension. For instance, learning to play tennis, to swim, or to dance may provide a distracting challenge to counterbalance potentially debilitating stress.

Time Control   Alec Mackenzie (1997) has suggested time control as a technique to set aside specific time for adaptation to various stressors. This period of personal time may be daily, weekly, or monthly. It offers clients time to focus on a specific change and develop strategies for adjustment. The major advantage of time control is that it ensures that important goals or concerns are addressed and critical tasks are accomplished. Mackenzie (1997) encourages individuals to focus on managing time more effectively to prevent most of the stress that time shortages produce. This strategy reduces the sense of urgency and lack of time, the level of anxiety, and associated feelings of frustration and failure.

Time Management   This approach to stress management suggests organizing oneself to accomplish those goals most important in life within the time available. Because lack of time is often given by individuals and families as a reason for not participating in health-promoting activities, assisting clients to manage time better makes a major contribution to their health and fitness. Time-pressured, type A clients with high risk for cardiovascular disease may be particularly in need of time-management skills.

Identifying values and goals and prioritizing goals serve as a framework for time management. Identifying time wasted on activities unrelated to personal goals permits the client to restructure how time is spent. Overcommitment to others or unrealistic expectations of oneself is a frequent source of stress. Time overload may be avoided by learning to say "no" to demands of others that are unrealistic or of low personal or family priority. Overload results in frustration and loss of satisfaction from the work accomplished, because one seldom expends one's best efforts under strain and pressure.

An important approach to time management is the reduction of a task into smaller parts. A task as a whole may appear as an overload; however, if the task is broken down into smaller segments, accomplishment becomes feasible. An example of this for a client may be learning several effective conditioning exercises before learning a complete conditioning routine, or developing skill with a conditioning routine before beginning a walk-jog activity. To take the whole health-promoting behavior as one task may be overwhelming. Breaking it down into component parts allows mastery and feelings of competence.

Avoid overload by delegating responsibilities to others and enlisting their assistance. Making use of others' skills and recognizing their ability to perform assigned tasks provides freedom from the expectation of having to be "all things to all people." Another important aspect of time management is to reduce the perception of time pressure and urgency. Not all perceptions of time urgency are warranted; some are needlessly self-imposed. The client should differentiate between time urgencies that are valid and others that are needlessly created. One may avoid time urgencies by minimizing procrastination. Leaving tasks that need to be completed until the last minute often results in needless pressure and stress (Davis, McKay, & Eshelman, 1995).

Increasing Resistance to Stress

Resistance to stress is achieved through either physical or psychologic conditioning. Physical conditioning for stress resistance focuses on exercise. Psychologic conditioning to increase resistance resources focuses on (a) enhancing self-esteem, (b) enhancing self-efficacy, (c) increasing assertiveness, (d) setting realistic goals, and (e) building coping resources.

Promoting Exercise   Exercise is discussed at length in Chapter 6. However, the relationship between exercise and stress is addressed here briefly. Four processes have been suggested to account for the positive effects of exercise on responses to mental stress. The first is that psychologic changes are the by-product of cardiorespiratory fitness. However, this explanation is weakened by the fact that psychologic responses and fitness are frequently not correlated. A second possibility is that changes in exercise-related self-efficacy and mastery generalize to other situations, resulting in improvements in self-concept and coping ability. A third process that may underlie decreased stress responses following periods of exercise is a blunting of the psychophysiologic responsiveness to stressors (Hong, Farag, Nelseen, Ziegler, & Mills, 2004). The third process suggests that exercise might help the brain deal better with stress by enhancing the body's response. Long-term exercise may increase the efficiency of the body's stress reaction system. Exercise is thought to require that all of the body systems (e.g., cardiovascular, muscular, and kidney) communicate with each other, giving the systems practice in managing stress. This "workout" of the body's systems may make communication between the systems more efficient and reveal the significance of exercise (Sothman & Kastello, 1997). Epidemiologic research suggests that physical activity is positively related to good mental health. In general, people who are inactive are twice as likely to be depressed whereas people who exercise regularly report feelings of well-being. However, increased fatigue, anxiety, and decreased vigor can occur with overtraining. Regular physical exercise contributes to good mental health (Hassman, Koivuta, & Uutela, 2000; Sothern, Loftin, Suskind, Udall, & Blecker, 1999).

Enhancing Self-Esteem   Self-esteem is the value attributed to self or how the person feels about self. This valuation is based on a person's concept of his or her desirable and undesirable attributes, strengths and weaknesses, achievements, and success in interpersonal relationships. Research is limited on the relationship between exercise and self-esteem in older adults (Cousins et al., 1998). Research on self-esteem indicates that it is associated with a history of an active physical lifestyle. However, most studies recruit persons who already have a positive self-esteem so one would expect change to be minimal. Exercise is more likely to increase the self-esteem of persons who have low self-esteem before the intervention and that of women more so than men. Cousins and colleagues (1998) summarized intervention and comparison studies and correlational and epidemiological studies of self-esteem and exercise in older people. Felton, Liu, Parsons, and Geslani (1998) studied self-image in 128 adolescent girls ages 16 to 19 years. Self-image related significantly to positive health-promoting behaviors including exercise. Dubois and colleagues (2002) found that adolescents who have parents and friends who are very supportive tend to achieve higher levels of self-esteem. Nurse practitioners and school nurses have excellent opportunities to promote positive self-concepts and healthy levels of self-esteem for adolescents as a basis for healthy functioning throughout life.

Although self-esteem is developed over time, studies have shown that the level of self-esteem may be changed. One approach is positive verbalization. In using this technique, clients identify positive aspects of self or personal characteristics that they value highly. They should also ask significant others to comment on their positive attributes. Each characteristic, one per day, is placed on a 3×5 index card, and the cards are placed in a conspicuous place. Each card should be read several times a day. This technique helps clients to spend more time thinking positively about self and decreases the amount of time spent in self-devaluation. Increased self-awareness of positive characteristics and their presence in conscious thought result in more frequent behavior that reflects these attributes and more positive responses from significant others.

Enhancing Self-Efficacy   Mastery experiences also appear to positively build a sense of competence to perform effectively and overcome obstacles. Experiencing successful performance of a particular, valued behavior provides positive messages concerning personal skills and abilities. Counseling clients to undertake tasks that are challenging but from which they experience success rather than failure can build a sense of efficacy in a particular domain. Self-beliefs about personal efficacy have wide-ranging ramifications affecting level of motivation, affect, thought, and action. Perceiving oneself to be efficacious has been shown to predict performance better than actual ability. In other words, if people's beliefs in their efficacy are strengthened, they approach situations more assuredly and make better use of the skills that they have (Bandura, 1997).

Persons with high levels of efficacy, compared to those with low levels, mentally rehearse success rather than failure at a task, set high goals, and make a firm commitment to attain them, perceive more control over personal threats, and are less anxious in the face of day-to-day challenges. Highly efficacious persons also tend to be more assertive in accessing the support they need to optimize their chances of success (Seila & Wieiseke, 2000). The nurse should help clients identify areas of skill most important to them and then help them augment their efficacy in these highly valued areas.

Increasing Assertiveness   Substituting positive, assertive behaviors for negative, passive ones increases personal capacity for psychologic resistance to stress. Assertiveness is the appropriate expression of oneself, one's thoughts, and one's feelings and results in greater personal satisfaction in living. Assertiveness is more constructive than aggression and deals more effectively than aggression with most problems. Many books and articles on assertiveness training are available. Assertiveness allows individuals to share their perceptions and feelings with others in a way that facilitates rather than inhibits personal or group productivity. Clients should be encouraged to use the following suggestions for becoming more assertive:

- Making a deliberate effort to greet others and call them by name.
- Maintaining eye contact during conversations.
- Commenting on the positive characteristics of others.
- Initiating conversation.
- Expressing opinions.
- Expressing feelings.
- Disagreeing with others when holding opposing viewpoints.
- Taking initiative to engage in a new behavior or learn a new activity.

The webs and constraints that entangle human beings are frequently self-constructed and disappear easily when efforts are made to become more open, assertive, and self-fulfilling. Although it is possible for clients to become more assertive through the use of simple techniques, very passive and reserved clients might well benefit from more comprehensive assertiveness training by a competent instructor or counselor. The nurse may assist clients in locating such resources for personal development.

Setting Realistic Goals   Clients must not only set goals but understand why accomplishment of those goals is rewarding. Long- and short-term goals help the client stay on course. Long-term goals set the direction for change and short-term goals allow for immediate successes. Goals should be set that can be attained within a reasonable time frame. If goals are met, it may reinforce the client's desire to continue to set health-promoting goals. Another useful rule is to plan to change only one behavior at a time. Flexibility on the part of the client permits achievement of desired outcomes through several approaches. Reward or reinforcement is possible through accomplishment of alternative goals. As a result, lack of success in initial attempts to reach goals becomes much less ominous because of the probability of success in achieving alternative goals that bring similar rewards (Lipson & Steiger, 1996).

Building Coping Resources   Stress results when there is an imbalance between appraised demands and appraised coping capabilities. Hobfoll (1998) suggests that more attention be directed to the resource side of the equation rather than the demand side. He maintains that coping resources are more predictive of reactions to stressors than the actual demands. General coping resources that have been identified to enhance stress resistance include:

- *Self-Disclosure:* Predisposition to share one's feelings, troubles, thoughts, and opinions with others.
- *Self-Directedness*: Degree to which a person respects his or her own judgment for decision making and, therefore, demonstrates assertiveness in interpersonal relationships.
- *Confidence*: Ability to gain mastery over one's environment and to control one's emotions in the interest of reaching personal goals.
- *Acceptance*: Degree to which persons accept their shortcomings and imperfections and maintain a positive and tolerant attitude toward others and the world at large.
- *Social support*: Availability and use of network of caring others.
- *Financial Freedom*: Extent to which persons are free of financial constraints in their lifestyles.
- *Physical Health*: Overall health condition including absence of chronic disease and disabilities.
- *Physical Fitness*: Conditioning resulting from personal exercise practices.
- *Stress Monitoring*: Awareness of tension buildup and situations that are likely to prove stressful.
- *Tension Control*: Ability to lower arousal through relaxation and thought control.
- *Structuring*. Ability to organize and manage resources such as time and energy.
- *Problem Solving*: Ability to resolve personal problems.

The Coping Resources Inventory for Stress measures these stress-coping resources of older adolescents and adults (Matheny, Aycock, Curlette, & Junker, 1993; Siqueira, Diab, Bodian, & Rolnitzky, 2000). After assessing the extent to which the various coping resources are present, nurses should assist clients in maximizing existing strengths and in developing additional resistance resources.

Counterconditioning to Avoid Physiologic Arousal

Research findings have substantiated the ability of individuals to intentionally control autonomic nervous system functions such as respiratory rate, heart rate, heart rhythm, blood pressure, and temperature in the extremities, functions previously thought to be under unconscious control. Training aimed at assisting clients to attain conscious control of physiologic responses to stressful events provides an important set of strategies for the management of stress. The goal of counterconditioning is to replace muscle tension and heightened sympathetic nervous system activity produced by stress with muscle relaxation and increased parasympathetic functioning. The two interventions most frequently used to assist the client in accomplishing this are relaxation training and imagery.

Progressive Relaxation Through Tension-Relaxation Techniques   Progressive Muscle Relaxation (PMR), developed by Edmund Jacobson in 1938, involves decreasing voluntary muscle activity and activity within the sympathetic nervous system while increasing parasympathetic functioning (Clark, 1996). There has been increasing accumulation of evidence in the scientific literature that supports Jacobson's findings that tension levels may be reduced through use of relaxation skills. Relaxation appears to be a way of turning off the body's response to the sympathetic nervous system and decreasing neurohormonal changes that take place in reaction to the experience of negative tension states (Snyder & Lindquist, 2002).

Stress causes change in the body's immune system. The overreaction or underreaction of the immune system to stress may result in disease or illness. Research is mixed on whether PMR has any positive effect on the body's immune system (Potts, 2003; Snyder & Lindquist, 2002; Wimbush & Nelson, 2000). However, positive outcomes have been documented when PMR is used for stress reduction either as the prescribed therapy or as an adjunct therapy. Murphy and colleagues (1999) reported that improvement was seen in migraine headaches when PMR was used to manage this diagnosis. Snyder and Lindquist (2002) also reported changes in blood pressure and anxiety levels after PMR. Although PMR has not been shown to reduce blood pressure in healthy persons, PMR may be a valuable tool to use to maintain health. The reader is referred to *Complementary Alternative Therapies in Nursing* (Snyder & Lindquist, 2002) for further information and precautions in the use of PMR. Murphy and colleagues (1999) effectively argue the need for a national research agenda to evaluate complementary and alternative therapies.

Relaxation is suggested to result in the following changes (Murphy et al., 1999; Snyder & Lindquist, 2002):

- Decrease in the body's oxygen consumption
- Lowered metabolism
- Decreased respiration rate
- Decreased heart rate
- Decreased muscle tension
- Decreased premature ventricular contractions
- Decreased systolic and diastolic blood pressures
- Increased alpha brain waves
- Enhanced immune function

To conduct relaxation training, a very pleasant, quiet, soundproof room in which lighting may be dimmed, with reclining lawn or lounge chairs for clients, provides an optimum setting. Tight clothing should be loosened, glasses removed, shoes removed, and a comfortable position assumed in the chair. Relaxation should never be taught with clients lying flat. Although this is a common position assumed for rest and sleep, it often results in muscle strain in the upper back and neck along with drowsiness, which interferes with training. A reclining position or sitting position is most appropriate.

At the beginning of each session, clients should be encouraged to focus on their own breathing as the air moves gently in and out. The purpose of this focusing activity is to increase awareness of self and the often-imperceptible functions of the human body. Following the focusing activity, clients are moved slowly through tension and relaxation cycles for each of the major muscle groups listed in Table 8–1, maintaining tension for 8 to 10 seconds and releasing tension instantaneously on cue. The entire tension–relaxation cycle should be repeated twice during the first session to increase clients' awareness of the differences in body sensations during tensed and relaxed periods. The tension–relaxation instructions should be given very slowly, allowing clients to enjoy the feelings of relaxation they are experiencing. The guidance provided by the nurse is critical for successful relaxation.

To facilitate daily practice of relaxation techniques, clients at home may use training tapes. Clients should keep a schedule of the frequency and length of time that relaxation is practiced, and are encouraged to "think through" the relaxation procedure and do their own coaching. A "prompt sheet" on the sequence of the muscle groups should be sent home with them for easy reference. This is intended to move clients toward independent practice of relaxation rather than encouraging reliance on the nurse or the coaching tape as a means of providing relaxation cues.

TABLE 8–1   **Muscle Group Sequence for Tension–Relaxation Cycle**

Muscle Group	Abbreviated Instructions
1. Right hand and forearm	Make a fist.
2. Right upper arm	Pull elbow tightly into side.
3. Left hand and forearm	Make a fist.
4. Left upper arm	Pull elbow tightly into side.
5. Forehead	Wrinkle brow.
6. Upper cheeks and nose	Squint eyes and wrinkle nose.
7. Lower cheeks and jaws	Place teeth together and make a "forced" smile.
8. Neck and throat	Pull chin toward chest.
9. Chest, shoulders, and upper back	Take a deep breath. Push shoulder blades toward each other.
10. Upper abdomen	Pull stomach in and hold
11. Lower abdomen	Bear down against the seat of the chair.
12. Right upper leg	Push down against the foot of the chair.
13. Right lower leg and foot	Point toes toward head and body.
14. Left upper leg	Push down against the foot of the chair.
15. Left lower leg and foot	Point toes toward head and body.

Some common problems that clients report include:

- Overly rapid self-pacing through the relaxation sequence.
- Distraction by environmental noise.
- Difficulty keeping attention on own monologue.
- Interruption of distracting thoughts during relaxation.
- Residual tension in some muscles after tension–relaxation.

Encouraging clients to slow down internal speech or coaching pace usually solves the problem of overly rapid self-pacing. Autogenic phrases such as "I feel calm," "I feel very relaxed," and "my arms and legs feel heavy" may be interspersed throughout self-instruction. Encouraging family members to join in the relaxation practice sessions often fosters stress-management skills among the entire family unit.

Progressive Relaxation Without Tension   While tension–relaxation techniques result in high levels of voluntary muscle relaxation, clients may be taught how to relax without first tensing muscles. Relaxation through counting down and relaxation through imagery are frequently used strategies. The major advantage of these techniques is that tension is no longer required. This is particularly important for clients with hypertension or coronary heart disease, because elevations in blood pressure caused by prolonged or extensive muscle tensing may be contraindicated. Deep relaxation without tension is the goal. Phrases that might be repeated to facilitate relaxation include:

- I feel quiet.
- I am beginning to feel quite relaxed.
- My feet feel heavy and relaxed.
- My ankles, my knees, and my hips feel heavy.
- My solar plexus and the whole central portion of my body feel relaxed and quiet.
- My hands, my arms, and my shoulders feel heavy, relaxed, and comfortable.
- My neck, my jaw, and my forehead feel relaxed. They feel comfortable and smooth.
- My whole body feels quite heavy, comfortable, and relaxed.
- I am quite relaxed.
- My arms and hands are heavy and warm.
- My whole body is relaxed and my hands are warm—relaxed and warm.
- My hands are warm.
- Warmth is flowing into my hands. They are warm, warm.
- I can feel the warmth flowing down my arms into my hands.
- My hands are relaxed and warm.
- My whole body feels quiet, comfortable, and relaxed.
- My mind is quiet.
- I withdraw my thoughts from the surroundings, and I feel serene and still.
- My thoughts are turned inward, and I am at ease.
- Deep within my mind, I can visualize and experience myself as relaxed, comfortable, and still.

- I am alert, but in an easy, quiet, inward-turned way.
- My mind is calm and quiet.
- I feel an inward quietness.

These phrases were suggested as a result of work in biofeedback at the Menninger Foundation. Such phrases result in physiologic imagery that decrease both sympathetic nervous system activity and tension in voluntary muscles.

Relaxation through the countdown procedure initially focuses on each of the muscle groups used previously. The client is encouraged to relax each muscle group progressively as the count proceeds from 10 down to 1. When the client has practiced and becomes skilled with this procedure, total body countdown is used, relaxing the entire body while silently counting down from 10 to 1. This is a particularly useful procedure for the office or when facing stressful social situations. In 2 to 3 minutes, the skilled client can achieve total body relaxation while in a sitting position with eyes open and focused on a specific object. This is one of the shortest procedures through which relaxation is accomplished. Mini-relaxation sessions several times throughout the day promote generalization of relaxation training to everyday life.

Relaxation Through Yoga   Yoga techniques involve the use of both physical exercise and meditation. Breathing techniques, various postures, and spinal flexibility are the focus of the physical exercises. The mental exercises consist of imagery and mantras. Deep relaxation without sleep and drowsiness are the results of yoga. The practice of yoga requires a warm, quiet environment and relaxing music.

Relaxation Through Imagery   Imagery is an intervention in which the interrelationship of the body and mind is used to influence physiologic responses. The benefits of imagery include its influence on physiological and immunological responses of the autonomic nervous system that result in stress reduction. Research supports imagery as an effective intervention for stress reduction in many situations including the birth process, pain management, and changing health behaviors. However, it is difficult to determine if the outcomes are directly related to imagery or a combination of interventions. The reader is referred to *Complementary Alternative Therapies in Nursing* (Snyder & Lindquist, 2002) for further information and precautions in the use of imagery.

Using imagery to relax requires that the client passively concentrate on pleasant scenes or experiences from the past to facilitate relaxation. Recalling the warmth of the sun, the feeling of warm sand, the sensations of a gentle breeze, the vision of palm trees swaying, or the sounds of ocean waves may be comfortable and pleasant for clients. Such recall promotes muscle relaxation.

Each client will vary in scenes or images that result in actual changes in muscle tension. For some clients, visualizing specific colors, shapes, or patterns are as effective as visualizing landscapes or scenes. If clients initially have difficulty using imagery or visualization for relaxation, the nurse may use one of the following techniques:

- Have the client, with eyes closed, visualize a particular room of his or her house (living room, bedroom, kitchen), focusing on colors, shapes, and specific objects. The client's mind should wander about the room, with the client describing verbally what is seen in as much detail as possible.

- Have the client focus on a particular piece of clothing that is a personal favorite. The client should describe the color, texture, design, and trim of the piece of clothing and how it feels when worn (e.g., soft, loose, fitted, light, warm).

As individuals become more vivid in descriptions of concrete objects, their ability to use less concrete imagery for purposes of relaxation increases. Imagery is a highly useful relaxation technique in many settings in which muscle tension or biofeedback equipment would be obtrusive.

Directions for Research on Stress Management

Major advances in understanding the effects of stressors on the neuroendocrine and immune systems have offered new possibilities for managing the brain–body interface to promote health. However, more research is needed to test stress-reducing interventions and their effect on these systems. More research is needed concerning the profile of stressors most likely to occur at different developmental stages and the best way to match stressors with targeted coping processes. A research challenge is to discover how to build coping resources, resilience, and personal competence in the early childhood years so that patterns of successful adaptation manifest themselves throughout adolescence and adulthood.

Research that suggests how to decrease environmental and family stressors for vulnerable populations is a priority. Human tolerance for stress is finite, as people can manage only so much stress. What are the changes in social policies, social structures, and relationships across cultures that need to be addressed to get at the root of the problem: the social injustice, discrimination, and inequity that are the unfortunate experience of many? Through the efforts of scientists from multiple disciplines, the phenomenon of stress pervasive in our society will be addressed. Applied research findings will create a less stressful world for all.

Directions for Practice in Stress Management

Everyone experiences stressors and yet individuals who experience the same stressors often respond differently. Stress-related illnesses are very common and require appropriate interventions or referrals to assist the client to manage stress before negative outcomes present. The promotion and conduct of early screenings and developmentally specific interventions are necessary because children, adolescents, young adults, and older adults develop and use different coping strategies. Awareness of these differences ensures that the nurse intervenes at the appropriate time and with the appropriate strategy to achieve stress reduction. While the techniques of stress management discussed in this chapter are within the nurse's scope of practice, one should gain expertise in the use of them by working with an experienced provider. Research into the relationship between stress and health is offering new insights into the causes and treatments of stress-related illnesses. This rapidly growing field of research in nursing and other disciplines mandates that each practitioner stay abreast of advances in practice.

SUMMARY

A number of different approaches for assisting individuals and families in managing stress have been presented in order to familiarize the reader with the range of strategies available. Some approaches suggested are relatively unstructured, whereas others are more formally defined and require instrumentation. The client and the nurse must make the decision regarding which strategies to use collaboratively. This decision should be based on the characteristics of the client, sources of stress experienced by the client, and general patterns of response to stressful events. The reader is encouraged to consult the references at the end of this chapter for further information on the use of stress-management strategies as nursing interventions.

LEARNING ACTIVITIES

1. Develop a list of strategies to manage stress for children, young and middle adults, and the elderly.
2. Select one approach to preventing stressful situations and develop a written guide (i.e., formulate questions and/or age-related issues) for use with a client.
3. Select one of the psychologic conditioning focus areas that has personal significance to you, a family member, or friend, and together set three goals to address how to strengthen resistance to stress.
4. Practice progressive relaxation without tension using the suggested phrases until you feel comfortable saying them and you identify a difference in your relaxation state. Then apply the technique with a friend.

SELECTED WEB SITES

American Academy of Pediatrics

http://www.aap.org/

American Psychological Association

http://www.apa.org/

Department of Health and Human Services

http://www.dhhs.gov

Healthy People 2010

http://www.healthypeople.gov

The National Center for Complementary and Alternative Medicine

http://www.nccam.nih.gov

Office of Disease Prevention

http://odp.od.nihi.gov

REFERENCES

Bandura, A. (1997). Exercise of personal and collective efficacy in changing societies. In A. Bandura (Ed.), *Self-efficacy in changing societies*. New York: Cambridge University Press.

Bauer, M. E., Vedhara, K., Perks, P., Wilcock, G. K., Lightman, S. L., & Shanks, N. (2002). Chronic stress in caregivers of dementia patients is associated with reduced lymphocyte sensitivity to glucocorticoids. *Journal of Neuroimmunology, 103*(1), 84–92.

Berger, J. A., & O'Brien, W. H. (1998). Effect of a cognitive-behavioral stress management intervention on salivary IgA, self-reported levels of stress, and physical health complaints in an undergraduate population. *Int J Rehabil Health, 4*(3), 129–152.

Bond, F. W., & Bunce, D. (2000). Mediators of change in emotion-focused and problem-focused worksite stress management interventions. *Journal of Occupational Health Psychology, 5*(1), 156–163.

Bower, J. E., & Segerstrom, S. C. (2004). Stress management, finding benefit, and immune function: Positive mechanisms for intervention effects on physiology. *Journal of Psychosomatic Research, 56*, 9–11.

Carroll, M. K., & Ryan-Wenger, N. A. (1999). School age children's fears, anxiety, and human figure drawings. *J Ped Health Care, 13*, 24–31.

Castillo, R. A., Schneider, R. H., Alexander, C. N., Cook, R., Myers, H., Nidich, S., Haney, C., Rainforth, M., & Salerno J. (2000, March). Effects of stress reduction on carotid atherosclerosis in hypertensive African Americans. *Stroke, 31*(3), 568–573.

Clark, C. C. (1996). *Wellness practitioner: Concepts, research and strategies* (2nd ed.). New York: Springer.

Clay, R. (2001) Bringing psychology to cardial care. *Monitor on Psychology*, 32(1), 1–3.

Cousins, S. O., et al. (1998). *Active living among older adults: Health benefits and outcomes*. Faculty of Physical Education and Recreation, University of Alberta, Edmonton, AB, Canada, and Well Quest Consulting, LTD in Canada.

Davis, M., McKay, M., & Eshelman, E. (1995). *The relaxation and stress reduction workload* (2nd ed.). Oakland, CA: New Harbinger.

Demarco, R., Ford-Gilboe, M., Friedmann, M. L., McCubbin, H. I., & McCubbin, M. A. (2000). *Handbook of stress, coping, health: Implications of nursing research theory and practice*. Thousand Oaks, CA: Sage Publications.

DuBois, D. L., Burk-Braxton, C., Swenson, L. P., Tevendale, H. D., Lockerd, E. M., & Moran, B. L. (2002). Getting by with a little help from self and others: Self-esteem and social support as resources during early adolescence. *Development Psychology, 38*(5), 822–839.

Felton, G. M., Liu, Q., Parsons, M. A., & Geslani, G. P. (1998). Health promoting behaviors of rural adolescent women. *Women and Health, 27*(4), 67–77.

Ferraro, K. F., & Su, Y. (1999). Financial strain, social relations, and psychological distress among older people: A cross-cultural analysis. *J Gerontol B Psychol Sci Soc Sci, 54*(1), 53–55.

Friedman, M. N. (2002). *Family nursing: Research theory and practice* (5th ed.). New York: Prentice Hall.

Gaab, J., Blättler, N., Menzi, T., Pabst, B., Stoyer, S., & Ehlert, U. (2003). Randomized controlled evaluation of the effects of cognitive-behavioral stress management on cortisol responses to acute stress in healthy subjects. *Psychoneuroendocrinology, 28*, 767–779.

Giga, S. I., Cooper, C. L., & Faragher, B. (2003). The development of a framework for a comprehensive approach to stress management interventions at work. *International Journal of Stress Management, 10*(4), 280–296.

Gordon, M. (2002). *Manual of nursing diagnosis: Including all diagnostic categories approved by the North American Nursing Diagnosis Association* (10th ed.). St. Louis: Mosby.

Hassman, P., Koivula, N., & Uutela, A. (2000, January). Physical exercise and psychological well-being: A population study in Finland. *Prev Med, 30*(1), 17–25.

Healthy People 2010 (Conference Edition). (2000). *Mental health and mental disorders.* Washington DC: U.S. Public Health and Human Services publications PHS 91-50212.

Hobfoll, S. E. (1998). Stress, culture and community: The psychology and physiology of stress. Kluwer Academics/Plesure Publishers.

Hong, S., Farag, N. H., Nelseen, R. A., Ziegler, M. G., & Mills, P. J. (2004). Effects of regular exercise on lymphocyte subsets and CD62L after psychological vs. physical stress. *Journal of Psychosomatic Research, 56*(3), 363–370.

Kessler, R. C., Mickelson, K. D., & Williams, D. R. (1999). The prevalence, distribution, and mental health correlates of perceived discrimination in the United States. *J Health Soc Behav, 40*(3), 208–230.

Krieger, N., & Sidney, S. (1996, October). Racial discrimination and blood pressure: The CARDIA study of young black and white adults. *Am J Public Health, 86*(10), 1370–1378.

Lawrence, A., & Lawrence, L. (1994). *Stress-related disorders. Illness: An intelligent act of the body.* Tarzana, CA: ALLME Publications.

Lazarus, R. S., & Folkman, S. (1984). *Stress, appraisal and coping.* New York: Springer.

Lenze, E. J., Mulsant, B. H., Shear, M. K., Schulberg, H. C., Dew, M. A., Begley, A. E., Pollock, B. G., & Reynolds, C. F. (2000). Comorbid anxiety disorders in depressed elderly patients. *Am J Psychiatry, 157*(5), 722–728.

Lipson, J. G., & Steiger, N. H. (1996). *Self-care nursing in a multi-cultural context.* Thousand Oaks, CA: Sage Publications.

MacKenzie, A. (1997). *The time trap* (3rd ed.). New York: AMACOM.

Masten, A. S., & Coatsworth, J. D. (1998). The development of competence in favorable and unfavorable environments: Lessons from research on successful children. *Am Psychol, 53*, 205–220.

Matheny, K. B., Aycock, D. W., Curlette, W. L., & Junker, G. N. (1993, November). The coping resources inventory for stress: A measure of perceived resourcefulness. *J Clin Psychol, 49*(6), 815–830.

McKenna, H., Slater, P., McCance, T., Bunting, B., Spiers, A., & McElwee, G. (2003). The role of stress, peer influence and education levels on the smoking behavior of nurses. *International Journal of Nursing Studies, 40*, 359–366.

Miller, G. E., & Cohen, S. (2001). Psychological interventions and the immune system: A meta-analytic review and critique. *Health Psychology, 20*(1), 47–63.

Millstein, S. G., Petersen, A. C., & Nightingale, E. O. (Eds.). (1993). *Promoting the health of adolescents: New directions for the twenty-first century.* New York: Oxford University Press.

Murphy, P. A., Kronenberg, F., & Wade, C. (1999). Complementary and alternative medicine in women's health: Developing a research agenda. *Journal of Nurse-Midwifery, 44*(3), 192–204.

Öhlin, B., Nilsson, P. M., Nilsson, J. Å., & Berglund, G. (2004). Chronic psychosocial stress predicts long-term cardiovascular morbidity and mortality in middle-aged men. *European Heart Journal, 25*(10), 867–873.

Ong, L., Linden, W., & Young, S. (2004). Stress management. What is it? *Journal of Psychosomatic Research, 56*, 133–137.

Potts, J. M. (2003). Alternative approaches to the management of prostatitis: Biofeedback, progressive relaxation and the concept of functional somatic syndromes. *European Urology Supplements, 2*(2), 34–37.

Ryan-Wenger, N. A., Sharrer, V. W., & Wynd, C. A. (2000). Stress, coping and health in children. In V. H. Rice (Ed.), *Handbook of stress, coping, health: Implications of nursing research theory and practice* (pp. 295–333).Thousand Oaks, CA: Sage Publications.

Seiffge-Krenke, I. (1995). *Stress, coping, and relationships in adolescence.* Mahwah, NJ: Lawrence Erlbaum Associates, Publishers.

Seila, D., & Wieiseke, A. W. (2000). Stress, self-efficacy, and health. In V. R. Rice (Ed.), *Handbook of stress, coping, health: Implications of nursing research theory and practice* (pp. 495–516). Thousand Oaks, CA: Sage Publications.

Selye, H. (1977). Introduction. In D. Wheetley (Ed.), *Stress and the heart.* New York: Raven Press.

Siqueira, L., Diab, M., Bodian, C., & Rolnitzky, L. (2000). Adolescents becoming smokers: The roles of stress and coping methods. *Journal of Adolescent Health, 27*(6), 399–408.

Snyder, M., & Lindquist, R. (2002). *Complementary alternative therapies in nursing* (4th ed.). New York: Springer.

Sothern, M. S., Loftin, M., Suskind, R. M., Udall, J. N., & Blecker, U. (1999, April). The health benefits of physical activity in children and adolescents: Implications for chronic disease prevention. *Eur J Pediatr, 158*(4), 271–274.

Sothman, M., & Kastello, G. K. (1997). Simulated weightlessness to induce chronic hypoactivity of brain norepinephrine for exercise and stress studies. *Med Sci Sports Exerc, 29*(1), 39–44.

Steptoe, A., Owen, N., Kunz-Ebrecht, S. R., & Brydon, L. (2004). Loneliness and neuroendocrine, cardiovascular, and inflammatory stress response in middle-aged men and women. *Psychoneuroendocrinology, 29,* 593–611.

Underwood, P. A. (2000). Social support: The promise and the reality. In V. H. Rice (Ed.), *Handbook of stress, coping, and health: Implications for nursing research, theory, and practice.* Thousand Oaks: Sage Publications.

U.S. Department of Health and Human Services. (1996). *Physical activity and health: A report of the surgeon general* (pp. 31–32, 136–140). Atlanta, GA: U.S. Department of Health and Human Services, Centers for Disease Control and Prevention, National Center for Chronic Disease Prevention and Health Promotion.

Wenzel, L., Glanz, K., & Lerman, C. (2002). Stress, coping, and health behavior. In K. Glang, B. K. Rimer, F. M. Lewis (Eds.), *Health behavior and health education* (3rd ed., pp. 210–240) San Francisco: Jossey-Bass.

Werner, J. S., & Frost, M. H. (2000). Major life stressors and health outcomes. In V. H. Rice (Ed.), *Handbook of stress, coping, health: Implications of nursing research theory and practice* (pp. 97–124). Thousand Oaks, CA: Sage Publications.

Wimbush, F. B., & Nelson, M. L. (2000). Micro-stressors and health outcomes. In V. H. Rice (Ed.), *Handbook of stress, coping, health: Implications of nursing research theory and practice.* Thousand Oaks, CA: Sage Publications.

Witek-Janusek, L., & Mathews, H. L. (2000). Stress, immunity, and health outcomes. In V. H. Rice (Ed.), *Handbook of stress, coping, health: Implications for nursing research, theory, and practice.* Thousand Oaks, CA: Sage Publications.

9

Social Support and Health Promotion

OBJECTIVES

1. Differentiate between social networks and social support.
2. Describe components that need to be assessed to elucidiate an individual's social network.
3. Discuss the major subcategories of social support that need to be assessed in a social systems review.
4. Identify three major sources of support for an individual.
5. Discuss strategies to enhance social support systems.

OUTLINE

- Social Networks
- Social Support
  - A. Functions of Social Support Groups
  - B. Family as the Primary Support Group
  - C. Community Organizations as Support Groups
  - D. Peers as a Source of Support
  - E. Self-Help Groups
- Reviewing Social Support Systems
- Social Support and Health
  - A. Social Networks, Social Support, and Use of Prevention Services
  - B. Social Support and Health Behavior

Understanding the social context in which individuals live and work is critically important in health promotion. In human interactions, individuals and groups both give and receive social support, a reciprocal process and interactive resource that provides comfort, assistance, encouragement, and information. Social support fosters successful coping and promotes satisfying and effective living. The amount and type(s) of social support needed fluctuates across the life span and across situations. Individuals and families usually call on personal resources first to cope with unanticipated, difficult, or threatening circumstances. Contacts with others in the support system may then be initiated only when self-reliance fails. All individuals need a system of sustaining support to realize their full potential. However, it is important to note that many choose not to ask for or accept support. Given that social support is a basic human need, its multiple dimensions have been explored, defined, and measured in various ways. In addition the relationship between social support and health has been studied extensively. Social support is considered to be a person–environment interaction that decreases the occurrence of stressors, buffers the impact of stress, and decreases physiologic reactivity to stress.

Much of our understanding of the relationship between social support and health has come from multiple disciplines, including sociology, anthropology, psychology, medicine, and nursing (Uchino, 2004). Results of research in these disciplines indicate that social support is related to decreased stress during times of life crisis. Continued advances in our understanding of the pathways by which social support affects mental and physical health are essential to be able to design interventions to promote mental, social, and physical well-being. Relationships among social support, health behaviors, and health are addressed in this chapter. In addition, the nurse's role in assisting clients to assess, modify, and develop effective social support systems that meet their needs are described.

Social Networks

Although the terms *social networks* and *social support* are often used interchangeably, they are not the same (Berkman, Glass, Brissette, & Seeman, 2000). Social networks refer to the web of social relationships that surround an individual. Social networks are defined as the objective, structural components of support, whereas social support is considered the qualitative or perceived functional component (Heaney & Isreal, 2002; Uchino, 2004).

A *social network* is made up of persons an individual or family knows and with whom he or she interacts. These interactions may occur frequently or infrequently and may include a large number of individuals. *Social support* refers to the social interactions within the network that are sensed as being available and supportive (perceived) or that actually provide support (received). The social support system for any given individual or family is usually much smaller than the social network or number of contacts. Social networks are linkages between people. To illustrate, each individual is a node in the social network and each exchange is a link. An individual influences the environment at any point in time through network links, and links provide pathways through which the environment influences the individual.

Social networks can be defined with the following terms (Uchino, 2004).

- *Size*: Actual number of individuals.
- *Composition*: Types of persons in the network, such as spouse or friends.
- *Geographic Dispersion*: Distances separating network members.
- *Intensity*: Frequency and extent of contact with network members.
- *Density*: Extent to which members know and interact with each other.
- *Homogeneity*: Similiarity of network members on various characteristics.

Social network has been considered a static concept, as it refers to relationships across the life span. Social convoy, a term suggested by Antonucci (2003), is considered a more dynamic concept to describe an individual's social network. The nature of an individual's relations can be depicted using a hierarchical mapping technique that has three progressively enlarging concentric circles around an inner circle. The inner circle consists of one's closest, intimate relationships such as family and long-time friends. Individuals in the middle circle may be close relatives, friends, and neighbors. The outer circle reflects contacts who are somewhat close, such as coworkers. Throughout the life span the middle and outer circles are more likely to change, whereas the inner circle tends to be more stable. Inner circle members are difficult to replace; when they are no longer available, there is a sense of grief and loss.

Social networks are important to individuals and families to the extent that they fulfill members' needs. In addition, knowledge of the interactions of network members shed light on how they influence the quantity and quality of social support. The size of the network is the major component in social support (Underwood, 2000). However, the types of persons in the network who provide the support, not the network size, have been associated with satisfaction. For example, voluntary social network ties may be more important for well-being than obligatory social network ties, such as the family, because one usually chooses social network ties that are rewarding. Research has shown that voluntary network ties, such as friends and church membership, are related to greater self-esteem and less psychological distress (Berbrier & Schulte, 2000). Characteristics of an individual social network that need to be assessed include the following (Berkman, Glass, et al., 2000).

- *Frequency of Contact*: Number of visual (face to face) and nonvisual (telephone or e-mail) interactions with network members.
- *Duration*: Length of time an individual knows another.
- *Reciprocity*: Extent to which exchanges are mutual.

Social Support

The functions provided by social relationships are considered to be social support. Social support can be defined as a network of interpersonal relationships that provide companionship, assistance, and emotional nourishment. Four broad categories of social support have been described: emotional, instrumental, informational, and appraisal support (Antonucci et al., 2003; Berkman et al., 2000; House, 1981). Emotional support refers to the demonstration of caring, empathy, love, and trust. Instrumental support includes tangible support or actions, including goods or services. In informational support, advice is provided as well as personal information or suggestions. Last, appraisal support refers to the provision of affirmation support or constructive feedback that is useful for self-evaluation. The type of support that is beneficial at any given time may differ, depending on the nature and stage of the confronting situation. Emotional support may help in a crisis circumstance, whereas informational support may be more useful in assisting individuals to understand how to relate effectively with their peers. Instrumental or tangible assistance or aid provides help with specific tasks, such as the preparation of nutritious meals or transport of children to recreational activities. Appraisal or affirmation support consists of constructive feedback to help individuals realize their own strengths and potential.

Understanding social support within the context of culture requires knowledge of cultural characteristics that shape receiving and giving support. Cultural boundaries define the various subgroups of American society, such as African Americans, Asian Americans, Hispanic–Latinos, and Native Americans. Within these cultural boundaries, social support operates uniquely within each social context. For example, based on the history of slavery in the African American community and group effort needed for survival, the family and church have been the major providers of social support (Dilworth-Anderson & Marshall, 1996). Hispanic–Latino Americans and Asian Americans are similar in that the core of their social support systems is familism or the family that reflects close and distant kin. Asian Americans have rules regulating gender hierarchies (patrilineage) and respect for older adults, and use shame and harmony in giving and receiving support. In the Native American culture, social support is less well understood, as the term is not defined in many tribal languages. However, Native Americans live in relational networks that foster mutual assistance and support, and the extended family is a core feature of their network. Opportunities for affiliation and attachment enable support to be provided within cultures in spite of transitions or disruptions such as migration.

Although many similarities in social support exist among the various American cultures, the influence of the sociohistorical context differs greatly across the different populations (Dilworth-Anderson & Marshall, 1996). Culturally sensitive theoretical views are needed to understand the role of social support as well as gender and life-span differences in these populations.

Several social support systems relevant to health have been identified and described in the literature: natural support systems (families), peer support systems, organized religious support systems, organized professional support systems, and organized self-help support groups not directed by health professionals. Peer and professional support can now be provided through the Internet. However, in most instances, the family (natural support system) remains the primary support group. Families, in order to provide appropriate support, must be sensitive to the needs of their members, establish effective communication, respect the unique needs of family members, and establish expectations of mutual help and assistance.

Peer support systems consist of people who function informally to meet the needs of others. These persons maintain a reputation of helpfulness because of the support they provide. Many of these individuals have encountered an experience that has had a major influence in their own life and achieved successful adjustment and growth. Because of personal insight, their advice is sought primarily in relation to resolving a problem of immediate concern with which they are familiar. Examples include the avid runner, the health-food enthusiast, or the individual who has lost a large amount of weight.

Organized religious support systems such as churches, temples, mosques, or other religious meeting places constitute a support system for individuals because the congregation shares a similar value system, a common set of beliefs about the purpose of life, traditions of worship, and a set of guidelines for living. Even highly mobile individuals may find a support system in the local church or synagogue. The church takes primary responsibility for support to enhance the spiritual dimension of health, which has been defined as the ability to develop one's inner nature to its fullest potential (Chuengsatiansup, 2003). This includes the ability to discover and articulate one's basic purpose in life; to learn how to experience love, joy, peace, and fulfillment; and how to help oneself and others achieve full personal potential.

A third type of support system is composed of professional helpers with a specific set of skills and services to offer clients. Interestingly, many questions have been raised about the effectiveness of their role in social support (Heaney & Isreal, 2002). Although professionals have access to information and resources that might not otherwise be available, they are seldom the first source of help for an individual. Family and close friends or peers are sought for advice and support initially. Health professionals are rarely included as members of an individual's social network in an assessment and become the support system only when other sources of help are unavailable, interrupted, or exhausted. Professionals are usually unable to provide support over long periods of time. In addition, these relationships are not characterized by reciprocity, they usually involve a power differential, and they offer limited empathic understanding due to lack of intimacy. In spite of these limitations, professional helpers have a role to play in offering short-term support as well as in playing a major role in providing informational support.

Organized support systems not directed by health professionals include voluntary service groups and self-help groups. These types of groups do not have an expert leader, as distinguished from support groups, which are led by a trained facilitator. Self-help groups (e.g., Alcoholics Anonymous, Take Off Pounds Sensibly [TOPS], and Recovery, Inc.) attempt to change the behaviors of members or promote adaptation to a life change such as chronic illness or a disabled family member. The number of self-help groups continues to increase in the United States. Some have sprung up because of disenchantment with the health care system. Others are a result of attempts to manage problems uncommon in the general society. Service groups and self-help groups play a significant role in social support relevant to health.

All support systems of a given individual or family are synergistic. In combination, they represent the social resources available to the client to facilitate stability and actualization. Various systems will be dominant at different points in the life cycle, depending on the stage of development and the stressors or challenges at hand. For example, in preadolescence and early adolescence, parents are the greatest source of support. The network shifts to a greater reliance on peers for lifestyle choices during middle adolescence with a decreased perception of parental support. Friends remain dominant in young adults, whereas the family network as well as friends are important sources of support for the elderly.

Functions of Social Support Groups

The primary functions of social support groups are to augment personal strengths of members and promote achievement of life goals. The functions of social support groups in promoting health can be conceptualized in four ways, as depicted in Figure 9–1. Social groups can contribute to health by (a) creating a growth-promoting environment that supports health-promoting behaviors, self-esteem, and high-level wellness; (b) decreasing the likelihood of threatening or stressful life events; (c) providing feedback or confirmation that actions are leading to anticipated and socially desirable consequences; and (d) buffering or mediating the negative effects of stressful events through influencing interpretation of events and emotional responses to them, thus decreasing their illness-producing potential. Support groups function to share common social concerns, provide intimacy, prevent isolation, respect mutual competencies, offer dependable assistance in crises, serve as a referral agent, and provide mutual challenge.

Internet or online support groups are increasing in popularity because of their ability to be a resource for ongoing information, emotional support, and encouragement (Eastin & LaRose, 2004). Internet social support activities have been found to improve self-care through the provision of information, support in decision making, and connections to

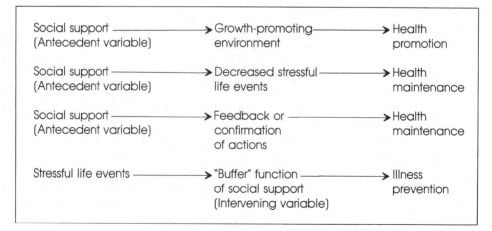

FIGURE 9–1 Possible Impact of Social Support on Health Status

experts as well as peers (Leung & Lee, 2004). However, evidence indicates that although Internet use may increase social interaction and support, in some cases it may lead to decreased interactions and social isolation (Swickert, Hittner, Harris, & Herring, 2002). More research is needed to clarify the controversial findings.

Internet technology has been shown to be acceptable across ethnically diverse groups. However, access continues to be determined by socioeconomic status (Bowen, 2003; Wong, 2004). Many elders continue to exhibit a strong aversion to computers, pointing to the need to improve user interface in this group (Cutler, Hendricks, & Guyer, 2003). This is significant, as online social support groups among the elderly have the potential to overcome many of the barriers that prevent elders from participating in groups, such as mobility changes, lack of available transportation, and finances. (See Chapter 12 for a more detailed discussion of the positive aspects and limitations of Internet technology.)

Family as the Primary Support Group

The family is the primary context for learning to give and receive social support. Family cohesion, expressiveness, and lack of conflict are reflected in the supportive behaviors that family members provide to one another. Low family support and poor child–parent interactions influence the life course trajectories of young people (Butters, 2002). Family stressors, such as unemployment, welfare dependence, change in family structure such as a divorce, and crime and substance use may decrease family cohesion and increase conflict, as well as adolescent behavioral and mental problems (Goebert et al., 2000).

In a long-term study of children raised in adverse conditions (poverty, perinatal stress, parental substance abuse, and family discord), competent parenting styles that were supportive enhanced self-esteem and fostered resilience (Werner, 1997). The results of this 40-year study suggest that the effects of risk factors on children can be buffered by the existence of protective factors such as social competencies, communication skills, and social support. Those who grew to be competent, caring adults were more likely to have had a supportive caregiving environment with more parental attention and less parental conflict. Other studies attribute resilience to the presence of a family environment that provides cohesion, encourages positive coping, and helps children develop feelings of competence and self-efficacy.

Family social support exerts complex effects on the physical and mental health of its members. The well-known Alameda County California study provided initial information about the association of social networks and support and mortality (Berkman & Syme, 1979). Men who are single or widowed have consistently shown higher mortality rates than married men. However, the mechanisms underlying this relationship are not well understood. Depressive symptoms have been associated with an adverse family environment that offers low levels of social support. Men who remain alone after losing their partners are at higher risk of developing symptoms of chronic depression, while having a supportive spouse and relatives has been associated with a decreased risk for major depression (Wade & Kendler, 2000). Having a marital partner, or if unmarried having social support, significantly reduces the incidence of depression in community-living elders (Schoevers et al., 2000). Using the convoy model (Antonucci et al., 2003), two

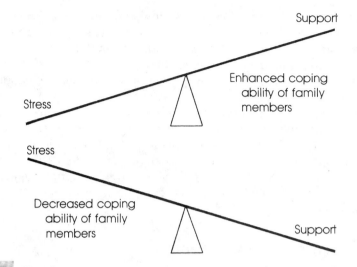

FIGURE 9–2   **Family as a Source of Support or Stress**

aspects of social support networks—a greater proportion of kin and the presence of family members in the inner circle—significantly reduces distress, especially in young adults (Peek & Lin, 1999). The interplay between family stressors and family support is depicted in Figure 9–2.

Within families, both positive and negative interactions occur. Negative interactions can be viewed as stressors, whereas positive, helpful interactions constitute support. A family's ability to foster positive interactive styles among its members may also relate to the extent to which the family has its own social network of long-term supportive relationships, and the extent to which the family is accorded respect within the community. Positive emotional bonds of the family with its social network buttress the family's competence and effective functioning.

Community Organizations as Support Groups

Characteristics of a community and its organizations have a direct bearing on the level of well-being of individuals and families that reside in it. The quality of social interaction and the life experiences of residents can contribute positively to health or negatively, resulting in social disorganization and illness. Stability within a community tends to promote close-knit ties among residents that mitigate the effects of crises on community members. Stable communities are characterized by value similarity, mutual assistance, shared trust, and concern for members.

Organizations, particularly churches, are viewed as a source of support in the community for health and healing. This is especially true for African Americans, as the church has been the most important institution in the community, for reasons mentioned earlier. Churches represent miniature, dynamic communities that may provide supportive programs through the provision of child care, meals, transportation, counseling, and other resources. In addition, volunteer helpers are readily available. A sense of affiliation has been shown to be an important factor in promoting adherence to an exercise program in an African American church (Izquierdo-Porrera, Powell, Reiner, & Fontaine, 2002). Nurses are also beginning to function in the role of parish nurses in churches to support health promotion and well-being through screening and targeted programs, such as physical activity or nutrition.

Peers as a Source of Support

Informal support from one's peers has consistently been shown to have powerful stress-buffering effects and health-promoting influences, which are greater than formal support services. Support from peers is important when there is a breakdown in an individual's usual support network. The peer is a source of support who shares salient similarities and possesses specific concrete knowledge that is pragmatic and derived from personal experiences rather than formal training. Peer support can be provided through one-to-one sessions, self-help groups, or online computer groups in diverse settings. All peer interactions include some degree of informational, appraisal, and emotional support (Dennis, 2003). Peer support primarily occurs without the provision of instrumental support. Peers are a valuable source of support with whom the individual can identify and share common experiences. The more similar the peer relationship, the more likely the support will lead to understanding, empathy, and mutual help. Evidence is accumulating to suggest that peer support positively affects physical and mental health outcomes (Cohen, Gottlieb, & Underwood, 2000).

Two related concepts are natural lay helpers and paraprofessionals. Natural lay helpers are individuals in the community to whom members naturally turn to for advice, counselling, and aid (Dennis, 2003; Heaney & Isreal, 2002). Natural lay helpers are different from peers in that their usual helping is embedded in their daily lives and they do not have the mutual experiences of the individual seeking support. *Paraprofessional* refers to a peer who has been trained by health care professionals to perform a specific support role. When professionals train peers their accountability is shifted to the health care system, decreasing their mutual identification and commonality with clients (Dennis, 2003).

Peers need to be skilled in communication, active listening, and problem solving (Cowie, Naylor, Chauhan, & Smith, 2002). In addition peers need empathy with the person's difficulties and must be willing to take a supportive role. The common forms of peer support include befriending, mediation/conflict resolution, mentoring, and counseling (Cowie et al., 2002). Peer support systems are being developed in schools and colleges to decrease aggressive acts and social isolation as well as to teach skills and promote health. Gender is an issue, as males are greatly underrepresented as peer supporters. Telephone peer support has been used successfully to help support low-income women to stop smoking (Solomon, Scharoun, Flynn, Secker-Walker, & Sepinwall, 2000).

Self-Help Groups

Self-help or nonprofessional, peer-operated groups are an important source of assistance within most communities. Self-help groups have also been called "mutual help groups" to reflect the fact that group members give and receive advice, encouragement, and support (Humphreys et al., 2004). Self-help groups may not charge fees. Examples of self-help groups include Narcotics Anonymous, Alcoholics Anonymous, Mended Hearts, Compassionate Friends, and physical fitness clubs. Characteristics of self-help groups include a critical mass sufficient to form a group, a form of publicity or recruitment to attract members, and a central goal or activity that gives the group purpose and sustains the investment of its members. The question has been raised as to why individuals use self-help groups rather than other resources, such as professional services. Two possible reasons are offered: (a) Self-help groups fulfill a need for services not being offered, or (b) self-help groups arise because of disappointment with or lack of meaningful resources within the community.

Self-help groups are an important resource, as they enable group members to expand their social networks as well as receive informational, instrumental, emotional, and appraisal support from others. Self-help groups as well as lay health-promotion programs empower individuals by increasing hope, support, and affirmation. The helping transactions that occur in these groups are thought to be an important therapeutic mechanism to increase self-efficacy (Rogers, Oliver, Bower, Lovell, & Richards, 2004). As noted in Chapter 2, self-efficacy refers to the strength of an individual's belief in the capability to perform a specific task or achieve a certain result. A self-help group offering continuing care for obesity has been shown to produce long-term weight loss (Latner, Wilson, Stunkard, & Jackson, 2002). Tailored self-help interventions have also been successful in promoting dietary changes in yonger and older adults (Kristal, Curry, Shattuck, Feng, & Li, 2000).

Self-help groups are a valuable source of support. Their records of success in assisting individuals to cope with a variety of different life experiences attest to their continuing viability as an integral part of community health resources. Self-care may be particularly effective for individuals who do not receive support from other relationships (Heaney & Isreal, 2002).

Reviewing Social Support Systems

It is important for both clients and health care providers to be aware of available sources of social support. Two approaches for reviewing the social support networks of clients are described in Chapter 4. These approaches can be useful in giving both the client and nurse insight into existing support resources. When assessing the adequacy of a client's support systems, it is important to be cognizant of factors that may cause the assessments to vary. Such things as the client's culture, stage of life-span development, social context (school, home, work), and role context (parent, student, professional) need to be considered for their influence on perceived and received support.

Social Support and Health

The importance of social support to mental and physical health is now well established. Lower levels of support are consistently linked to higher rates of morbidity and mortality. However, the actual mechanisms linking social support to health are still not well understood. Several different processes have been proposed. First, social support may be directly linked to health by promoting healthy or unhealthy behaviors, by supplying information, or by making available tangible resources (child care, opportunities for work). Psychologically, social support may foster a sense of meaning in life or be associated with more positive affective states, such as an enhanced sense of self-worth and increased sense of control. Individuals may appraise events as less threatening, resulting in less physiologic arousal. Biologically, social support may intensify positive neuroendocrine and immunologic responses despite the presence of stressors (DeVries, Glasper, & Detillion, 2003; McDade, 2001). All of these possible mechanisms present challenging topics for social support research.

The second way in which social support may contribute to health is by buffering the effects of stress on an individual. The buffering model of support has been most widely researched (Uchino, 2004). Social support is thought to be beneficial because it decreases the negative effects of stress on one's mental and physical health. Even when faced with extremely stressful events, having individuals who provide support can reduce the intensity of stress. However, the long-term effects of the buffering model have not been thoroughly tested.

Social support interventions have been categorized as (a) the nature of the relationship between the support provider and the participant (professional or peer), (b) unit of support (individual or group intervention), and (c) the type of intervention (building social skills or increasing network size) (Antonucci et al., 2003; Heaney & Isreal, 2002; Uchino, 2004). When developing social support interventions, it is important to consider exactly the type of social support that will be the target of the intervention. Will it be emotional or informational support or an increase in social contacts? Perceived support is a function of an individual's personality characteristic, the social environment, and an interaction between the perceiver and supporter (Hogan, Linden, & Najarian, 2002). The kind of support, who provides the support, and contextual issues all play a role. Interventions to increase perceived support need to focus on helping persons recruit supportive others into their social network by teaching them relationship-building skills.

Although the relationship between social support and health is well known, a review of interventions that have been tested to improve some type of social support reveals varying long-term results (Antonucci et al., 2003; Heaney & Isreal, 2002; Uchino, 2004). While many studies on this topic have been conducted, many suffer from weaknesses that limit the ability to generalize the findings. In addition, studies that were well designed showed no effects of the intervention or improvement in support. In other words, while the intervention may have improved health or well-being, if the client's naturally occurring social support did not change, the desired outcomes would not last when the intervention was completed. Social support is complex and includes characteristics of the person who needs or desires support (perceiver), characteristics of the person who gives the support (supporter), characteristics of the situation, and the interaction of these factors. All of these factors need to be taken into consideration when designing interventions to improve social support.

Social Networks, Social Support, and Use of Prevention Services

It is widely accepted that social networks function as conduits for information and as links to broader societal contacts, such as health care providers. For example, social networks have been shown to be a major factor in predicting participation in cancer screening for Hispanic women (Suarez et al., 2000). In a multiethnic Asian population, women who reported ever having a Pap screening were more likely to have close friends with whom they could discuss their health (Seow, Huang, & Straughan, 2000).

The mechanisms linking social support and use of preventive services need to be better understood. Understanding how beliefs about personal vulnerability to disease or illness and cultural beliefs interact with the level and type of social support necessary to motivate the use of screening services is particularly important.

Social Support and Health Behavior

Social support systems also influence health behavior. It is well known that significant others function as an important lay referral system for individuals in making decisions to seek professional care for health promotion, illness prevention, or care in illness. The resultant effects can be negative or positive. When a client is a member of a culture that differs markedly from that of health professionals, an extended lay-consultant structure may be available, which delays seeking professional care. In contrast, when the client's culture is similar to that of health professionals, the lay system is usually bypassed, and contact with health providers is made early in the course of a problem or concern. Individuals use their lay referral system not only when deciding whether to seek care, but also when making decisions about adherence. Diagnostic decisions, prescriptions for medication, and life changes recommended by health professionals frequently are discussed with significant others who constitute the individual's lay referral system. Concurrence by the lay referral system often determines the extent to which advice from health professionals is actually followed.

Social support from spouses or partners is related to health behaviors. This relationship may be due to the encouragement and support of the health behavior, including giving approval and disapproval, having control over aspects of the proposed change such as food shopping and preparation, and participating in the behavior change, such as joining the exercise program. High levels of warmth, encouragement, and assistance occur in spousal and partner support. In a review of 51 studies that looked at the relationship between marital status and adherence, persons who were married were more likely to adhere than persons who were unmarried (Dimatteo, 2004). Functional social support has a stronger effect on adherence than structural support (social networks), indicating that the presence of people does not matter as much as the quality of the relationship. However, a nonsupportive network can interfere with successful alteration of health habits by limiting the client's time and energy available for health behavior or introducing stress that compromises healthy behaviors.

Social support has been correlated with adoption of other health behaviors or cessation of negative behaviors. Adult smokers who had attended at least one meeting of a smoking cessation program reported that both family and peer support were positively associated with behavior change (Wagner, Burg, & Sirois, 2004). Having the trust, acceptance, and support of a family member or friend increased the individual's use of the transtheoretical model process of change for smoking cessation. In a community-based smoking cessation intervention, smokers who had supportive people attend at least one of the support group sessions had higher cessation rates at 3, 6, and 12 months compared to those without a support person in attendance (Carlson, Goodey, Bennett, Taenzer, & Koopmans, 2002). In an international study of physical activity, the strongest predictor of being physically active was the social environment (Stahl et al., 2001). Those with low perceived social support were twice as likely to be sedentary than those who reported high social support. There is also strong evidence that social support interventions in community settings are effective in increasing levels of physical activity (Kahn et al., 2002).

Adoption and maintenance of health-behavior change over time is difficult unless the behavior is encouraged through support from family members and friends. This points to the importance of naturally occurring support and connectedness or long-term formal or informal support systems if natural ones are not available. Many retrospective studies have described the effect of social support on health behavior. However, more prospective studies are needed to identify networks of social support that promote health-promotion and illness-prevention behaviors.

Identifying Social Support Strengths and Needs

Functional health patterns relevant to social support include self-perception–self-concept pattern, role–relationship pattern, and coping–stress tolerance pattern. Each functional health pattern contains a number of diagnoses relevant to social support problems or needs such as altered family processes, hopelessness, self-esteem disturbance, and chronic low self-esteem (Gordon, 2002). The diagnostic taxonomy, while facilitating problem identification, does not provide for a description of social support assets and resources. This gap has been addressed by proposing that nurses diagnose for wellness to clearly identify and support client strengths. Inclusion of the assets and strengths of clients as phenomena relevant to nursing care is extremely important if nurses are to provide leadership in developing positive strategies to enhance the health of populations.

Enhancing Social Support Systems

Support-enhancing strategies have three goals: assisting individuals and families to strengthen existing supportive relationships, helping individuals and families to establish satisfying interpersonal ties, and preventing disruption of ties from evolving into mental or physical illness.

Facilitating Social Interactions

Social skills training represents one approach to changing the characteristics of clients to enable them to develop supportive interpersonal relationships with others. Training can be conducted with individuals or with groups who have similar skill deficits, such as dysfunctional families (Lakey & Lutz, 1996). Social skills training is based on the belief that socially competent responses can be learned just like other behaviors.

Initially, training is directed toward assessing and modifying perceptions of appropriate behavior in social situations. In addition, persons are taught to reevaluate their thoughts about themselves in a more positive manner. Attempts are made to improve social interaction patterns through modeling, role-playing, performance feedback, coaching, and homework assignments. Skills to be taught might include initiating conversations, giving and receiving compliments, handling periods of silence, enhancing physical attractiveness, nonverbal methods of communication, and handling criticism and conflict (Lakey & Lutz, 1996). Within the school setting, training in social skills and problem solving can be provided in the classroom to prevent the acquisition of socially alienating behaviors. To complement such work, the broader aspects of the school environment should be assessed to determine the extent to which they facilitate or inhibit students' opportunities for and skills in developing social ties (Cowie et al., 2002).

Enhancing Coping

A lack of social ties may result in serious psychologic and physical problems during developmental or situational transition periods. Support seminars or groups for widows, children of separated or divorced parents, parents who have lost a child, or relatives of imprisoned persons can assist such persons to learn to cope effectively with life stress. Benefits from such programs include help in understanding puzzling and disturbing emotional reactions, reducing feelings of alienation, and assisting people to move ahead into the future. It is important that programs be tailored to the unique needs of individuals, as clients desire different types of support from different members in their networks (Carpenter, Van Haitsma, Ruckdeschel, & Lawton, 2000).

Preventing Loss of Support and Loneliness

Preventing loneliness or social isolation is a more desirable approach than treatment of loneliness and isolation after they have occurred. Two approaches to prevention include the identification of high-risk groups and educational interventions that focus on developing social support ties for persons of all ages (Bonin, McCreary, & Sadava, 2000; Holmen & Furukawa, 2002). Young, unmarried, unemployed, and low-income persons are particularly vulnerable to lack of support and loneliness. Obstacles to social participation, such as lack of transportation for the elderly or constant caretaking responsibilities for middle-age women with elderly parents, create populations at risk for loneliness. When such groups are identified, programs can be planned to decrease aloneness and isolation. Possible programs include transportation vehicles staffed by volunteers for those in need, respite programs to provide relief for caretakers, community support groups for families with disabled or impaired members, and Internet support groups that can be accessed at home. Reports indicate that the social behavior of lonely individuals is enhanced when online, and they report making friends and satisfaction with their online friends (Morahan-Martin & Schumacher, 2003).

Educational approaches to prevent loss of social support and subsequent loneliness include classroom experiences for schoolchildren that help them gain experience in making friends, working cooperatively with others, and resolving differences or conflict. A growing body of evidence over the past 30 years has substantiated that poor social functioning of children often leads to serious personal adjustment problems in later life. Most experts would agree that children require the security of positive reciprocal relationships with their peers, parents, and teachers for maximum growth and development (Barrera & Li, 1996).

For older adults, media campaigns, such as public service announcements about resources for formal support or the health benefits of staying connected with relatives and friends, may provide cues to initiate support-enhancing behaviors. In addition, pamphlets, community programs, and neighborhood activities can be designed to help persons build relationships or to reach out to others who may need emotional or instrumental support. Older adults report great loneliness at night and on the weekends, so activities need to be planned during these times (McInnis & White, 2001). The elderly also need assistance in developing positive relationships with others in their environment, especially if they are in low-cost senior housing. If computer support is not an option, telephone support should be considered.

Other general suggestions for enhancing social support include:

- Mutual goal setting with significant others to achieve common needs for support.
- Constructively resolving conflict between oneself and support network members.
- Offering assistance to individuals within the social network to show concern and promote trust.
- Seeking counseling, if needed, to enhance marital and/or family adjustment.
- Making use of the nurse and other health professionals as community support resources.
- Increasing ties to organized social groups to expand growth opportunities.

Clients should be encouraged to identify specific goals to enhance personal support networks. By focusing on one or two realistic changes relevant to the goals of highest priority, clients can alter the breadth and depth of social support available to them.

Directions for Research in Social Support

Evidence from research supports the relationship between social networks, social support, and health. However, there are inconsistencies in this body of research and many questions remain to be answered. For example, theory development is needed to identify and test antecedents and consequences of social support. The specific mechanisms by which social support enhances health are not known and need further investigation. Interventions that enhance social support need to be refined and tested. The amount or "dosage" of social support necessary to promote health also needs to be explored. Culturally sensitive interventions as well as interventions across the life span to enhance support need to be developed and tested in subgroups of the population. Additionally, culturally sensitive, reliable, and valid measures need further development and testing. Research is also needed on immune function and its relationship to social support. Finally, investigations are needed to understand the relationship between Internet support participation and health outcomes. Nurse scientists play a major role in social support research and should lead interdisciplinary teams to investigate these issues, as nursing research on social support is limited.

Directions for Practice in Social Support

Although research findings are available that provide important information about social support and health, many of these findings have not been incorporated into practice. Utilization of research findings from nursing as well as other disciplines should become part of the nursing practice to learn better ways to intervene to enhance social networks and social support. Assessment of social support systems needs to be a basic component of the initial nursing assessment, using strategies such as those described in this chapter. In these assessments, nurses should know how to obtain culturally sensitive information from diverse populations. If the social network needs to be enhanced, the nurse needs to develop programs to teach clients the skills needed to develop supportive relationships. Finally, nurses need to incorporate sources of social support such as families, self-help groups, Internet groups, and community organizations in their interventions to increase the potential for success in health promotion and lifestyle change.

SUMMARY

Social support plays an important role in the health and well-being of clients. The nurse must consider the client as well as the social environment in order to facilitate comprehensive health promotion. Social support groups assist clients to cope with everyday hassles and major stressful life experiences and enhance emotional and physical well-being. The extent to which stressful events threaten health may well depend on the support available from core (family) or extended (peer, community, and professional) social networks. The design and evaluation of nursing interventions to increase social support is critical. These interventions will contribute to scientifically sound nursing care interventions that will enhance the quality of human social transactions across the life span.

Learning Activities

1. Perform a social network review with a young adult and an elderly client, using the six components described in the chapter.
2. Design a plan to establish a self-help group for adolescents who are overweight. Incorporate both face-to-face and Internet group meetings into your plan.
3. Detail three strategies to increase your client's social support, based on the previous assessment, taking current sources as well as potential sources of support into consideration.

SELECTED WEB SITES

Health Plus: Relationships and Social Support

http://vanderbiltowc.wellsource.com/dh/center.asp?id=32470

Tools for Coping with Life Stress

http://www.coping.org

The Self-Help Connection

http://www.selfhelpconnection.ca

Self-Help Group Sourcebook

http://mentalhealth.net/self-help

eSupport Groups

http://esupportgroups.com

Support Path

http://www.supportpath.com

Pediatric and Women's Health Support Programs

http://www.levindale.com

REFERENCES

Antonucci, T. C., Ajrouch, K. J., & Janevic, M. R. (2003). The effect of social relations with children on the education-health link in men and women aged 40 and over. *Social Science & Medicine, 56,* 949–960.

Barrera, M., Jr., & Li, S. A. (1996). The relation of family support to adolescents' psychological distress and behavior problems. In G. R. Pierce & B. R. Sarason (Eds.), *Handbook of social support and the family* (pp. 313–343). New York: Plenum Press.

Berbrier, M., & Schulte, A. (2000). Binding and nonbinding integration: The relational costs and social ties on mental health. *Research in Community and Mental Health, 11,* 3–27.

Berkman, L. F., Glass, T., Brissette, I., & Seeman, T. E. (2000). From social integration to health: Durkheim in the new millennium. *Social Science & Medicine, 51,* 843–857.

Berkman, L., & Syme, S. L. (1979). Social networks, host resistance, and mortality: A nine-year follow-up study of Alameda County residents. *Am J Epidemiology, 115,* 684–694.

Bonin, M. F., McCreary, D. R., & Sadava, S. W. (2000, June). Problem drinking behavior in two community-based samples of adults: Influence of gender, coping, loneliness, and depression. *Psychol Addict Behav, 14*(2), 151–161.

Bowen, D. (2003). Predictors of women's Internet access and Internet health seeking. *Health Care Women Int, 24*(10), 940–951.

Butters, J. E. (2002). Family stressors and adolescent cannabis use: A pathway to problem use. *Journal of Adolescence, 25*, 645–654.

Carlson, L. E., Goodey, E., Bennett, M. H., Taenzer, P., & Koopmans, J. (2002). The addition of social support to a community-based large-group behavioral smoking cessation intervention: Improved cessation rates and gender differences. *Addictive Behaviors, 27*, 547–559.

Carpenter, B. D., Van Haitsma, K., Ruckdeschel, K., & Lawton, M. P. (2000). The psychosocial preferences of older adults: A pilot examination of content and structure. *Gerontologist, 40*(3), 335–348.

Chuengsatiansup, K. (2003). Spirituality and health: An initial proposal to incorporate spiritual health in health impact assessment. *Environmental Impact Assessment Review, 23*, 3–15.

Cohen, S., Gottlieb, B., & Underwood, L. G. (2000). Social relationships and health. In S. Cohen, B. Gottlieb, & L. G. Underwood (Eds.), *Social support measurement and intervention* (p. 3). Toronto: Oxford University Press.

Cowie, H., Naylor, P., Chauhan, L. T. P., & Smith, P. K. (2002). Knowledge, use of and attitudes towards peer support: A 2-year follow-up to the Prince's Trust survey. *Journal of Adolescence, 25*, 453–467.

Cutler, S. J., Hendricks, J., & Guyer, A. (2003). Age differences in home computer availability. *Journal of Gerontology, 58B*, S271–S280.

Dennis, C. L. (2003). Peer support within a health care context: A concept analysis. *International Journal of Nursing Studies, 40*, 321–332.

DeVries, A. C., Glasper, E. R., & Detillion, C. E. (2003). Social modulation of stress responses. *Physiology & Behavior, 79*, 399–407.

Dilworth-Anderson, P., & Marshall, S. (1996). Social support in its cultural context. In G. R. Pierce, B. R. Sarason, & I. G. Sarason (Eds.), *Handbook of social support and the family* (pp. 67–79). New York: Plenum Press.

DiMatteo, M. R. (2004). Social support and patient adherence to medical treatment: A meta-analysis. *Health Psychology, 23*(2), 207–218.

Eastin, M. S., & LaRose, R. (2005, in press.) Alt.support: Modeling social support online. *Computers in Human Behavior,* available online 4/24/2004.

Goebert, D., Nahulu, L., Hishinuma, E., Bell, C., Yuen, N., Carlton, B., Andrade, N. N., Miyamoto, R., & Johnson, R. (2000). Cumulative effect of family environment on psychiatric symptomatology among multiethnic adolescents. *Journal of Adolescent Health, 27*, 34–42.

Gordon, M. (2002). *Manual of nursing diagnosis*, 10th edition. St. Louis: Mosby Year Book.

Heaney, C. A., & Isreal, B. A. (2002). Social networks and social support. In K. Glanz, B. K. Rimer, & F. M. Lewis (Eds.), *Health behavior and health education* (3rd ed., pp. 185–209). San Francisco: Jossey-Bass.

Hogan, B. E., Linden, W., & Najarian, B. (2002). Social support interventions: Do they work? *Clinical Psychology Review, 22*, 381–440.

Holmen, K., & Furukawa, H. (2002). Loneliness, health and social network among elderly people—A follow-up study. *Archives of Gerontology and Geriatrics, 35*, 261–274.

Humphreys, K., Wing, S., McCarty, D., Chappel, J., Gallant, L., Haberle, B., Horvath, A. T., Kaskutas, L. A., Kirk, T., Kivlahan, D., Laudet, A., McCrady, B. S., McLellan, A. T., Morgenstern, J., Townsend, M., & Weiss, R. (2004). Self-help organizations for alcohol and drug problems: Toward evidence-based practice and policy. *Journal of Substance Abuse Treatment, 26*, 151–158.

Izquierdo-Porrera, A. M., Powell, C. C., Reiner, J., & Fontaine, K. R. (2002). Correlates of exercise adherence in an African American church community. *Cultural Diversity and Ethnic Minority Psychology, 4*, 389–394.

Kahn, E. B., Ramsey, L. T., Brownson, R. C., Heath, G. W., Howze, E. H., Powell, K. E., Stone, E. J., Rajab, M. W., & Corso, P. (2002, May). The effectiveness of interventions to increase physical activity—A systematic review. *American Journal of Preventive Medicine, 22*(4:1), 73–107.

Kristal, Curry, S. J., Shattuck, A. L., Feng, Z., & Li, S. (2000). A randomized trail of a tailored, self-help dietary intervention: The Puget Sound Eating Patterns Study. *Preventive Medicine, 31*, 380–389.

Lakey, B., & Lutz, C. J. (1996). Social support and preventive and therapeutic interventions. In G. R. Pierce, B. R. Sarason, & I. G. Sarason (Eds.), *Handbook of social support and the family* (pp. 435–465). New York: Plenum Press.

Latner, J. D., Wilson, G. T., Stunkard, A. J., & Jackson, M. L. (2002). Self-help and long-term behavior therapy for obesity. *Behavior Research and Therapy, 40*, 805–812.

Leung, L., & Lee, P. S. N. (2004, in press). Multiple determinants of life quality: The roles of Internet activities, use of new media, social support, and leisure activities. *Telematics and Informatics*, available online June 1, 2004.

McDade, T. W. (2001). Lifestyle incongruity, social integration, and immune function in Samoan adolescents. *Social Science and Medicine, 53*, 1351–1632.

McInnis, G. J., & White, J. H. (2001). A phenomenological exploration of loneliness in the older adult. *Archives of Psychiatric Nursing, 15*(3), 128–139.

Morahan-Martin, J., & Schumacher, P. (2003). Loneliness and social uses of the Internet. *Computers in Human Behavior, 19*, 659–671.

Peek, M. K., & Lin, N. (1999, September). Age differences in the effects of network composition on psychological distress. *Soc Sci Med, 49*(5), 621–636.

Rogers, A., Oliver, D., Bower, P., Lovell, K., & Richards, D. (2004). Peoples' understandings of a primary care-based mental health self-help clinic. *Patient Education and Counseling, 53*, 41–46.

Schoevers, R. A., Beekman, A. T., Deeg, D. J., Geerling, M. I., Jonke, C., & Van Tilbur, W. (2000, August). Risk factors for depression in later life: Results of a prospective community based study (AMSTEL). *J Affect Disord, 59*(2), 127–137.

Seow, A., Huang, J., & Straughan, P. T. (2000, March). Effects of social support, regular physician and health-related attitudes on cervical cancer screening in an Asian population. *Cancer Causes Control, 11*(3), 223–230.

Solomon, L. J., Scharoun, G. M., Flynn, B. S., Secker-Walker, R. H., & Sepinwall, D. (2000). Free nicotine patches plus proactive telephone peer support to help low-income women stop smoking. *Preventive Medicine, 31*, 68–74.

Stahl, T., Rutten, A., Nutbeam, D., Bauman, A., Kannas, L., Abel, T., Luschen, G., Rodriguez, J. A., Vinck, J., & van der Zee, J. (2001). The importance of the social environment for physically active lifestyle—Results from an international study. *Social Science and Medicine, 52*, 1–10.

Suarez, L., Ramirez, A. G., Villareal, R., Marti, J., McAlister, A., Talavera, G. A., Trapido, E., & Perez-Stable, E. J. (2000). Social networks and cancer screening in four U.S. Hispanic groups. *American Journal of Preventive Medicine, 19*(1), 47–52.

Swickert, R. J., Hittner, J. B., Harris, J. L., & Herring, J. A. (2002). Relationships among Internet use, personality, and social support. *Computers in Human Behavior, 18*, 437–451.

Uchino, B. N. (2004). *Social support & physical health*. New Haven: Yale University Press.

Underwood, P. (2000). Social support: The promise and the reality. In V. H. Rice (Ed.), *Handbook of stress, coping and health: Implications for nursing research, theory, and practice* (pp. 367–391). Thousand Oaks, CA: Sage Publications.

Wade, T. D., & Kendler, K. S. (2000). The relationship between social support and major depression: Cross-sectional, longitudinal, and genetic perspectives. *J Nerv Ment Dis, 188*(5), 251–258.

Wagner, J., Burg, M., & Sirois, B. (2004). Social support and the transtheoretical model: Relationship of social support to smoking cessation stage, decisional balance, process use, and temptation. *Addictive Behaviors, 29*(5), 1039–1043.

Werner, E. E. (1997, July). Vulnerable but invincible: High-risk children from birth to adulthood. *Acta Paediatr Suppl, 422*, 103–105.

Wong G. (2004). Internet access is a socioeconomic issue. Accessed July 27, 2004 at *http://bmj.bmjjournals.com/cgi/full/328/7449/1200-b*

Part 4

Evaluating the Effectiveness of Health Promotion

10

Measuring Outcomes of Health Promotion and Prevention Interventions

OBJECTIVES

1. Define health outcomes and their significance for nursing.
2. Describe the major categories of nursing-sensitive outcomes and give examples of each.
3. Discuss two factors to consider when deciding to measure outcomes.
4. Differentiate between cost effectiveness, cost utility, and cost-benefit analysis.
5. Describe the major challenges in measuring health outcomes.

OUTLINE

- Defining Health Outcomes
  A. Nursing-Sensitive Outcomes
  B. Significance of Nursing-Sensitive Outcomes
- Deciding Which Health Outcomes to Measure
  A. Client, Provider, and Community Outcomes
  B. Short-Term, Intermediate, and Long-Term Outcomes
  C. Economic Outcomes
- Developing a Plan to Measure Health Outcomes
- Challenges in Measuring Health Outcomes
- Directions for Nursing Research in Outcomes Measurement
- Directions for Nursing Practice in Achieving Health Outcomes

- Summary
- Learning Activities
- Selected Web Sites
- References

The goal of nursing in health promotion is to maintain or enhance the client's health status and well-being. Nurses in all types of settings have implemented interventions that promote health and prevent disease. However, until recently, assessment of outcomes of health promotion received less attention by most practicing nurses. Today's emphasis on the use of outcome measures to demonstrate the effectiveness of health-promotion interventions challenges nurses in all settings to describe the effects of their practice on client–patient outcomes.

Florence Nightingale (1858), recognized as the first person who used outcome measures in health care, used morbidity and mortality statistics to measure the quality of care for British soldiers during the Crimean War. These traditional outcomes have continued to be used in medicine and epidemiology. In today's health care environment, outcomes measurement is much more comprehensive and complex and takes into account all factors that influence health outcomes, including client, provider, and system characteristics, as well as the process of delivering the health-promotion interventions.

Increased emphasis on outcomes measurement in this country has occurred as a result of the need to determine the most appropriate and cost-effective interventions in the current competitive health care market with its fiscal restraints. Substantial variations in practice exist in different settings, irrespective of the same organizational and financial arrangements, with resulting variations in outcomes (Kahn, Malin, Adams, & Ganz, 2002). This lack of uniformity has prompted questions about the relationship between the use of clinical services (process) and their end results (outcomes). Policy makers and purchasers of health care are also interested in sources of costs that do not result in benefits to clients in order to select cost-effective interventions. All of these factors have resulted in an emphasis on the measurement, monitoring, and management of outcomes to improve the quality of care. Nurses are responding by evaluating their contribution to outcomes of health care and health-related interventions.

Defining Health Outcomes

Outcomes, or patient–client outcomes, refer to the consequences of a treatment or intervention (Whitman, 2002a). In this definition, the consequences or results of care may be intended or unintended changes in individuals and populations. Intended changes are desired results of interventions, whereas unintended changes are unanticipated outcomes that may occur as a result of the intervention. Health outcomes are the effects of interventions manifested by changes in any dimension of health or resolution of the problem targeted by the intervention (Whitman, 2002b). Health outcomes focus on the health status of individuals, families, or communities. The health outcomes of health-promotion interventions will vary with the purpose, complexity, and strength of the intervention (Whitehead & Russell, 2004). For example, a physical activity intervention that involves weekly monitoring and supervision over a 6-month time period is anticipated to result in significant changes in the client's level of activity, as compared to a physical activity intervention that provides minimal monitoring and supervision over a 3-month period of time. Thus, outcomes differ according to the structure of the intervention, as well as the process of implementing the intervention.

Client choice is important when defining outcomes of health-promotion interventions. The client's view, as well as the health care provider's view, is needed to determine appropriate outcomes. Clients may have very different preferences for outcomes, depending on factors such as health status or age, or where there are important trade-offs between survival and quality of life. The nurse needs to know what the client wants and expects from the intervention in order to define achievable and acceptable health outcomes.

Health outcomes have traditionally included the five "Ds": death, disease, disability, discomfort, and dissatisfaction (Lohr, 1988). In the past, patient preferences were seldom used to evaluate health services, as they were considered subjective and unreliable. However, this has changed as individuals have become active participants in decision making related to their care. Health outcomes have now been expanded to include subjective health perceptions and appraisals, functional measures, preferences, and satisfaction with services (Kahn et al., & Ganz, 2002). Many consider these outcomes broad measures of health-related quality of life.

Sidani and Braden (1998) divide health outcomes into four major categories: clinical endpoints related to the client's response to health interventions; functional status related to the maintenance or improvement in physical, mental, and social functioning; perceptual outcomes related to clients' well-being and satisfaction with the care received; and financial outcomes or the use of resources and costs.

Two additional terms that need to be understood are outcomes monitoring and outcomes management. *Outcomes monitoring* is the repeated observation, description, and quantification of outcome measures for the purpose of improving care or practice. Outcomes may be monitored intermittently or continuously during a health-promotion intervention. *Outcomes management* refers to all activities in which nurses use data collected from measuring and monitoring outcomes to continuously improve nursing practice. In outcomes management, costs and quality are measured and examined to improve the quality of care and health status of clients. Information is used to continuously reexamine practice in outcomes management.

Nurses need to demonstrate the effectiveness of their practice in achieving desired health outcomes by individuals, families, and communities. However, assessment of outcomes that result from nursing treatments and interventions is considered rudimentary in most health care settings. Although quality of care has always been a concern for nursing, quality improvement programs have focused on structure and process. The shift to outcomes poses a major issue for nursing, because nurses often practice in an interdisciplinary role, whereby health outcomes are influenced by more than one discipline. For example, nurses, along with nutritionists, psychologists, and exercise physiologists, may be involved in many health-promotion programs. The challenge is to identify and measure nursing-sensitive outcomes, or outcomes that are influenced by nursing activities, to document nursing's contributions. Dependent, independent, and interdependent nursing activities need to be differentiated in order to determine outcomes that nurses are accountable for in their practice.

Several sources are available to assist in identifying health outcomes. For example, the Agency for Healthcare Research and Quality (AHRQ), a federal agency that funds research on health care outcomes, provides information on outcomes that have been documented across populations. Its web site is listed at the end of this chapter. Specialty organizations have also begun to publish outcomes relevant to specific populations.

Nursing-Sensitive Outcomes

The American Nurses' Association as well as several nurse authors have identified nursing-sensitive outcomes (Head, Maas, & Johnson, 2003; Ingersoll, McIntosh, & Williams, 2000; Lewin-VHI, 1995). Categories of these outcomes are summarized in Table 10–1. Physiological outcomes are the most common and include such things as weight, skin-fold thickness, blood pressure, and cholesterol values. Psychosocial outcomes measure patterns of behavior, communication, and relationships. Psychosocial measures may include attitude, mood, emotions, coping, and social functioning. Functional measures include activities of daily living, mobility, and self-care ability. Behavioral outcomes are concerned with the client's activities and actions. For example, a behavioral outcome may be regular physical activity. Knowledge, the cognitive level of understanding, is a common nursing-sensitive outcome, because teaching is a major component of nursing practice.

TABLE 10–1   **Categories of Nursing-Sensitive Interventions**

Category	Examples
Physiological	Blood pressure
	Weight
	Laboratory values
Psychosocial	Attitudes
	Emotions
	Moods
	Social functioning
Functional	Activities of daily living
	Mobility
	Self-care
Behavioral	Actions
	Activities
Cognitive	Knowledge
Home functioning	Family support
	Family roles
Safety	Noise-free environment
Symptom control	Smoking withdrawal
Goal attainment	Behavior change
Satisfaction	Program/service contentment
Costs	Cost effectiveness

Home-functioning outcomes focus on the performance of the client and family in the home environment. Measures of this outcome may include family support, family functioning, and role function. Safety is a nursing-sensitive outcome, as nurses implement interventions to promote safe home environments. For example, the nurse may work with clients in work sites to promote safe work environments that prevent hearing loss.

Symptom-control outcomes are concerned with the management of symptoms. For example, health-promotion interventions for smoking cessation may need to manage symptoms associated with smoking withdrawal. Alternatively, symptoms of low self-esteem or depression as a result of unsuccessful health behavior change may need attention.

Goal-attainment outcomes refer to the accomplishment of program objectives at designated intervals. Client satisfaction, as an outcome, is a global measure of contentment with the services provided to the client. For example, measures of satisfaction or dissatisfaction with health-promotion programs provide valuable information for potentially needed changes in the program.

Cost outcomes are also considered sensitive to nursing practice. However, the nursing profession has just begun to seriously focus on the cost effectiveness of nursing interventions. Health-promotion and risk-reduction interventions offer an exciting opportunity to assess the cost effectiveness of their counseling and teaching activities.

The Nursing Outcomes Classification (NOC) is a standardized classification of patient–client outcomes developed to evaluate the effects of nursing interventions (Moorhead, Johnson, & Maas, 2004). Seven categories have been identified: physiological health, functional health, psychosocial health, family health, health knowledge and behavior, perceived health, and community health. The NOC system has been linked to the North American Nursing Diagnosis Association (NANDA) diagnoses, to Gordon's functional patterns, Omaha System problems, resident admission protocols used in nursing homes, the OASIS system used in home care, and the Nursing Intervention Classification (NIC) (Moorhead et al., 2004). NOC is also one of the standardized languages recognized by the American Nurses Association (ANA). Information about the NOC system is available on its web site (see end of chapter listing).

The ANA (2002) published a list of nursing-sensitive outcomes for acute care in 1996, and in 2000 a document was published identifying 10 nursing-sensitive outcomes for community-based settings. The reports have enabled nurses to document these outcomes following interventions. The National Database of Nursing Quality Indicators (NDNQI), an ANA project, serves as a repository for data from national efforts to implement nursing's quality indicators. Within this project the Center for Nursing Quality was created to promote and facilitate the standardization of information on nursing quality and patient outcomes.

Health outcomes that reflect nursing's contribution to health promotion and risk reduction need to be identified and measured. Some of these include lifestyle behaviors (e.g., dietary and physical activity behaviors), knowledge, attitudes, values, coping behaviors, physiological changes (e.g., weight, blood cholesterol values, blood pressure), self-esteem, self-efficacy, and empowerment. Nursing's focus on positive lifestyle change and wellness places an emphasis on positive health-promoting behaviors. In addition, nurses create environments conducive to health, which presents a challenge in identifying and measuring community health outcomes.

Valid and reliable measures are needed to measure the health-promotion outcomes that are identified. Although multiple measures are available, many do not fully capture the effects of nursing practice for health promotion. Nurses have begun to develop and test new measures. The Health Promoting Lifestyle Profile developed by Pender and colleagues (1998) is an example.

Significance of Nursing-Sensitive Outcomes

All health care providers are being challenged to demonstrate their contributions to patient outcomes as a result of the high costs of health care, increasing health care competition, and the need to balance quality and costs. Nursing has been challenged to provide information about which nursing interventions are the most effective and efficient. Although it is known that clients benefit from nursing actions, nursing's effectiveness must be demonstrated to employers, consumers, and health policy makers. Health outcomes that occur as a result of nursing interventions are a measure of nursing's contribution. Documentation of nursing's contribution enhances our visibility and ensures that we are not overlooked by health care organizations, health care purchasers, consumers, and health policy makers (Sidani & Braden, 1996). Nurses are key players in implementing health-promotion interventions and measuring their effectiveness. Our view of the total situation and the holistic view of the individual and family is unique, and this contribution needs to be made explicit.

Deciding Which Health Outcomes to Measure

The choice of which health-promotion outcomes to measure depends on the goals to be attained, the type of program or intervention, and the ability to access the information needed to measure the results of the program. The challenge is to select health outcomes that are comprehensive, comparable, meaningful, and accurate in reflecting the effects of the health-promotion intervention.

Client, Provider, and Community Outcomes

Three categories of outcomes can be measured: Client-focused, provider-focused, and community-focused outcomes. These are described in Table 10–2 (Jennings, Staggers, & Brosch, 1999; Kleinpell, 1997).

Client-focused outcomes measure the end results of health care interventions. These outcomes have been further classified into diagnostic-specific and holistic (Jennings et al., 1999). Diagnostic-specific outcomes focus on a specific client problem and are measured as a subelement within the patient, such as laboratory values or other physiologic measures. These outcomes are discrete and limited in scope. However, it is important to measure the physiologic effects of health-promotion or risk-reduction interventions. For example, health-promotion outcomes as a result of a nutritional intervention for weight reduction might include weight or body mass index, blood pressure, and triglycerides, as these reflect changes in health status.

TABLE 10–2 **General Classification of Outcomes**

Category	Types of Outcomes
Client focused	
Diagnostic specific	Physiologic measures
	Weight
	Body mass index
Holistic	Lifestyle change
	Functional status
	Perceptions
	Self-care
	Quality of life
Provider focused	
Health care provider	Appropriate interventions
	Expertise
	Client outcomes
Family	Support
Community focused	
	Costs
	Service use
	Health of community

Holistic outcomes extend beyond the diagnosis or client problem to measure the overall functioning and health of the individual, family, or community (Jennings et al., 1999). Holistic outcomes include knowledge, lifestyle change, functional status, psychosocial functioning, perceptions, self-care, and health-related quality of life. A major issue in measuring these types of outcomes is lack of clarity in the definitions, which results in lack of clarity in measures of the outcomes. For example, quality of life has been defined and measured differently in many studies, such as symptoms, physical health, mental health, or ability to return to work. Consistent definitions are needed in health-promotion outcomes with measures that accurately reflect the definitions. Monitoring holistic outcomes is important in health-promotion efforts, as these outcomes may detect changes before physiologic effects are measurable. When measuring client-focused outcomes, both problem-specific and holistic measures may be needed to capture the effects of the interventions.

Provider-focused outcomes address aspects of health care practice that affect client outcomes. The provider may refer to the health care professional or family member. Outcome measures in this category may include the appropriateness of the intervention and the technical expertise of the provider, such as the number of physical activity programs the health care provider has conducted. Negative outcomes may also be measured, such as the number of persons who continued to smoke after a smoking cessation program. Provider-focused outcomes are an issue as many nurses practice in teams or groups. However, work to classify nursing interventions and link outcomes to these interventions is ongoing to solve this problem. More work is needed to identify the contributions of nurses in health promotion at the individual, family, and community levels.

Community outcomes are the most global types of measures in health promotion, as they focus on results of community- or organizational-level interventions and the quality of services and care delivered by community organizations (Jennings et al., 1999; Kleinpell, 1997). Community outcomes include costs of care and use of services as well as other measures to evaluate the services provided by the community organizations. These outcomes also measure aggregates or groups of clients rather than individual clients. This type of measurement poses multiple challenges, but has great potential for communities and community-based systems.

Short-Term, Intermediate, and Long-Term Outcomes

The lack of effectiveness of health-promotion interventions may be due to inappropriate timing of outcome measures (Breslin, Burns, & Moores, 2002). The timing of measurement of outcomes is critical to the result obtained. If information is collected immediately following the intervention, it may be too soon to capture the change in lifestyle behaviors. If the nurse waits too long, other factors may have intervened to influence the expected results. Therefore, the timing of measurement of health outcomes needs to be planned carefully to capture the anticipated effects. Measurement at multiple time points is usually necessary. Short-term outcomes are measured immediately following the intervention. Examples of appropriate short-term outcomes are knowledge, coping behaviors, and readiness to change. Intermediate outcomes are those targeted at a period of time following the intervention when a change is expected to have occurred. Intermediate outcomes are measured soon enough following the intervention so that its effects can be isolated from other possible reasons. Intermediate interventions may be useful in reflecting attitude changes or attempts to change, although lifestyle change has not yet occurred. Long-term outcomes are the ultimate outcomes, as they are the final or end results of the health-promotion intervention. Long-term outcomes include behavior change, longevity, and improved quality of life. These long-term outcomes may also be used to assess intermediate outcomes. When measured at a greater distance from the intervention, the nurse is able to document long-term change. However, the intervening factors mentioned earlier must be considered when interpreting the results of long-term measurement.

Economic Outcomes

The role of economic outcomes in health promotion is becoming increasingly important because of the high costs of health care in this country. Several types of analyses currently exist, including cost effectiveness, cost utility, and cost benefit (Muennig, 2002).

A simple way to describe the different types of analyses is by the questions they answer. Cost-effective analysis answers the question, "What is the most inexpensive way to achieve a given outcome?" In cost–utility analysis, the question answered is, "What is the cost per quality-adjusted life years?" Finally, in cost–benefit analysis, the question answered is, "What is the net benefit of a given alternative?" Economic outcomes began with merely reporting the cost of the illness or problem being addressed (Buerhaus, 1998). This was followed by cost–benefit analysis, which placed a monetary value on a health outcome. However, cost–benefit analysis requires that all outcomes have a dollar value, and this was met with issues, as many were uncomfortable placing monetary values on human life or quality of life (Kaplan & Groessl, 2002). Cost-effective analysis has emerged as an alternative.

Cost-effective analysis (CEA) reflects the amount of benefit a treatment or intervention provides relative to alternatives (Kaplan & Groessl, 2002). The purpose of CEA is to evaluate the comparative potential of expenditures on different health care interventions. CEA does not determine whether an intervention is worth its cost in some absolute sense. It provides a relative measure of which services afford the highest health benefit per dollar. The cost-effective ratio (C/E), the central measure used in CEA, is the incremental price of obtaining a unit of health effect from a given health intervention when compared to an alternative intervention. Implicit in the C/E ratio is a comparison between alternatives: the intervention under study with either another intervention or no intervention. The two intervention outcomes must have a common unit of measurement to be compared. CEA is meant to be informative and identify interventions that produce the greatest health using the resources available. It is meant to provide additional information for a decision; however, it is not meant to be the sole determinant of the decision to use or eliminate an intervention. A sensitivity analysis needs to be conducted after the cost-effectiveness analysis to evaluate how the error sources in the data might affect the cost or effectiveness of the intervention (Muennig, 2002). In a cost-effectiveness study of brief interventions to reduce alcohol consumption, results indicated that a primary-care-based brief intervention was more effective and less costly than more intensive strategies (Wutzke, Shiell, Gomel, & Conigrave, 2001). A sensitivity analysis was performed, varying the screening rate, the detection rate (postintervention alcohol consumption), and the reach of the program. Findings indicated that increasing each of these factors increased the total cost of the intervention, but the average cost-effectiveness remained the same, as well as the average cost per life year saved.

Examples of CEA studies are available in the literature. For example, a cost-effective analysis was performed on the Community Trial of Mammography Promotion, a collaborative effort to increase the use of breast cancer screening (Anderson, Hager, Su, & Urban, 2002). Cost effectiveness was assessed for three different interventions that were implemented: individual counseling, community activities, and a combination of both. The community activities intervention was found to be the most cost effective. However, further exploratory analysis indicated that the most cost-effective method of promoting mammography use may vary with the target population.

Cost-utility analysis is a special case of cost-effectiveness analysis that uses the expressed preference (utility) of a health state as the unit of outcome (Kaplan & Groessl, 2002). The outcome units reflect the preferences of the population. For example, quality-adjusted life years (QALYs) are commonly used in cost–utility analysis. A study to examine the effects of screening for Type 2 diabetes mellitus provides an example of the use of both cost-effectiveness analysis and cost–utility analysis (Hoerger et al., 2004). Targeted screening (only persons with risk factors for diabetes) and universal screening (all persons) were compared. Findings showed that at all ages, targeted screening was more cost effective than universal screening. Screening was also more cost effective for persons over age 55 than for younger ages. The cost per quality-adjusted life year (QALY) for target screening was significantly less than universal screening.

Several issues need to be taken into consideration when deciding to perform cost-effectiveness analysis on an intervention (Ramsey, McIntosh, & Sullivan, 2001). First, intervention studies usually include groups that are not representative of the general population. Second, intervention studies and cost-effectiveness analyses are designed for different purposes, and the distinction creates several issues. The outcomes needed for the two are usually different, sample size needs may be different, and the time frame needed may also differ. Last, adding cost–effectiveness analysis to an intervention study can be quite burdensome, in terms of increased sample size, data collection, periods of observation, and staff and expertise needed. These issues need to be addressed in the design phase of the intervention.

Cost-effective analysis and other economic evaluations are increasingly assuming an important role in health care policy decisions. The approach has been standardized with principles and procedures for reporting the results. Regulatory bodies now consider cost effectiveness to be a part of the approval process for new medications and technologies. However, the analytic techniques are not simple and have many pitfalls, so only those who have the background to do so should use them. In addition, although consensus-based recommendations have been published to guide CEA and a standard set of methods have been developed, the techniques are still evolving. Nurses need to understand CEA and other types of economic analyses, as these methods have important implications for practice.

Developing a Plan to Measure Health Outcomes

Developing a plan to measure health outcomes begins with thinking about health-promotion interventions in terms of desired outcomes (Oermann & Huber, 2003). Nurses and all health care providers continually need to ask if their interventions are achieving the most effective outcomes. First, select the specific health-promotion intervention. The choice is based on the client's lifestyle area that either is of interest for change or one in which change is needed. Decide what needs to be achieved with the intervention and how these outcomes can be most effectively attained. Next, identify the most effective strategies to manage the problem or the most effective method to implement the intervention by reviewing the literature. A literature search will shed light on how the problem has been approached successfully by others. For example, if planning to intervene with a client to improve nutrition, a literature review of nutritional programs will help to identify aspects that work and aspects that should be avoided. Findings from the literature facilitate tailoring the intervention to the specific needs of the client or family. In the outcomes literature, this step is also known as identifying *best practices*, or the most effective way to solve the problem.

The fourth step is to identify factors that might affect the client's response to the intervention. For example, characteristics of the client, such as weight, the values placed on foods, eating habits, any symptoms that are occurring as a result of poor nutrition, and motivation to change eating behaviors will affect the success of the intervention. Demographic characteristics that may influence the outcomes also need to be identified, as factors such as age, education, and socioeconomic status may be significant. Family characteristics might also play a role. For example, if others in the home practice unhealthy nutritional behaviors, it may be more difficult to get support to change.

TABLE 10–3	Steps in Developing a Plan to Measure Outcomes

1. Select health protection—health promotion area of interest.
2. Identify most effective intervention for defined area.
3. Tailor intervention to client.
4. Identify potential factors that may influence outcomes.
   - Client characteristics
   - Demographic factors
   - Family characteristics
5. Select outcomes to measure effects of intervention.
   - Short term
   - Intermediate
   - Long term

Environmental factors may also influence outcomes and need to be identified. All factors that may potentially influence the outcomes need to be specified and addressed before the intervention begins.

In the fifth step, outcomes are selected to measure the success of the intervention and decisions are made about how and when they will be measured. For example, in the nutrition program, although the long-term outcome may be sustained weight loss or normal blood sugar or cholesterol, short-term outcomes may be a change in attitude toward eating and significant other support to change dietary behaviors. Intermediate outcomes might be a decrease in the number of high-fat foods consumed per day. The client needs to be involved to establish realistic outcomes that will enable success. Identification of reliable and valid measures of selected health outcomes is critical to ensure accurate measurement of the results. Measures that have been tested beforehand should be used whenever possible.

Additional resources may be needed to measure outcomes and analyze the data for complex interventions with groups of clients, families, or communities. Costs, time, and effort must always be considered when deciding which outcomes to measure, as well as the number of outcomes to measure. Attention also needs to be given to the burden placed on clients when measuring outcomes. Too many measures at multiple time points may result in a low participation rate. The five steps are easy to follow when planning to measure outcomes. Each step should be carefully considered and completed before moving to the next one. By following this type of plan, information about the outcomes of health-promotion interventions implemented by nurses will begin to accumulate. Table 10–3 reviews the steps in developing a plan to measure outcomes of health-promotion interventions.

Challenges in Measuring Health Outcomes

Many challenges confront nurses and other health care providers in the measurement of health outcomes. Several have already been described. For example, separating the contribution of nursing from other health care providers remains a challenge. This challenge has increased with the proliferation of paraprofessional groups in school settings, the workplace, and the community, as many of these groups focus on health promotion and health education in their practice (Davies, 2003). The interdisciplinary emphasis is expected to continue, so it is more important than ever to clearly define nursing's role in health promotion and identify health outcomes that reflect the contribution of nursing.

Finding measures that are sensitive to change remains a challenge when assessing many health-promotion outcomes. Sensitivity refers to the ability to detect small differences in behaviors, attitudes, values, and other outcomes of interest in health promotion. For example, many quality-of-life measures do not detect changes in life quality at multiple time points although other information may indicate that life quality is indeed changing dramatically. Lack of sensitivity means that important changes may be missed or thought to be insignificant. The challenge is to find measures that are sensitive to the anticipated change and to measure outcomes at multiple time points to be able to detect the change.

The choice of measures for holistic-focused outcomes is another challenge. Although these types of measures enable comparison of clients across interventions and populations, they often lack the sensitivity to detect clinically important changes. Measures that are specific to a particular problem may be more sensitive but may not be usable across groups of clients or settings. A novel approach is to focus on individual specificity in outcomes measurement, which is client centered, rather than generic or condition specific (Bilsbury & Richman, 2002). The challenge is to decide if it is important to compare across populations or focus on a specific group or problem.

Another challenge is the measurement of community- or organizational-focused outcomes, when the data are aggregated instead of reported for individual clients. For example, when measuring community level outcomes for smoking cessation, measures report cessation rates of the total community. Individual rates within a practice setting or a smoking cessation program are not known. Because most measures have been developed to measure individual outcomes, few aggregate measures are available. Measurement of community-focused outcomes means that more attention is needed to develop instruments to assess community outcomes accurately.

Deciding on the perspective to use is another challenge in measuring outcomes (Dickey, 2000). For example, the client's perspective may be best for changes related to certain aspects of the intervention, while the health care provider's perspective is more valid when assessing changes in physiological markers. In addition the perspective of family members may be considered in the measurement of outcomes, if the interest is change within the family that might influence the client outcomes, such as social support.

Directions for Nursing Research in Outcomes Measurement

The science related to the measurement of outcomes sensitive to health-promotion nursing interventions is limited due to several factors. First, because the emphasis on outcomes research began in the 1990s, nurse scientists have only recently begun to implement studies to identify and evaluate health-promotion outcomes. Second, the challenges that have been discussed in this chapter pose issues for research as well as practice. All of these challenges create many opportunities for research in health promotion. Exploratory studies are needed to identify holistic outcomes that reflect nursing's contribution as a member of the health care team. Exploratory studies are also needed to learn patient preferences. Experimental research needs to be designed to test health-promotion interventions that are evaluated with client outcomes at multiple points in time. Sensitive measures of health-promotion outcomes that reflect nursing's influence need to be developed and tested. Community-level outcome measures also need to be designed and tested for use in community interventions. Nurse scientists need to learn how to measure economic outcomes, such as cost-effective outcomes, and implement studies to evaluate the costs of health-promotion and risk-reduction interventions. The science of outcomes for health promotion has created opportunities for collaboration in research across disciplines. Nurse scientists have opportunities to work with other disciplines on research projects to understand how clients change their lifestyle practices as well as how to measure the outcomes of these changes effectively.

Directions for Nursing Practice in Achieving Health Outcomes

The outcomes movement in health care has challenged nurses to reflect on the value of their practice. The mandate of health care environments to deliver the most effective, cost-efficient care means that nursing must delineate its contribution to health outcomes. Outcomes of care should continually be assessed to identify the most effective approaches for health promotion. Identification of best approaches means that familiarity with the current literature will become more and more important for nurses in practice. Prior to implementing health-promotion interventions, detailed assessments need to be conducted that take into account client, family, and environmental factors that may influence the outcomes of the intervention. It is also important to learn about the standardized outcome taxonomies that are available to be able to choose appropriate outcomes for health-promotion and risk-reduction interventions. In addition nurses are being called upon to identify specific health outcomes that are relevant for their practice and to document these outcomes. Documentation of interventions and outcomes is critical to assess nursing's contribution to health care. Measuring outcomes that are sensitive to change is often a challenge. However, nurses can seek expertise to assist in identifying accurate and sensitive outcomes that are easily implemented in practice. Finally, nurses need to play a major role as members of interdisciplinary health care teams, as they view the totality of factors that influence the client's health. These teams are expected to continue to play a major role in health care delivery to enhance client outcomes. The nurse needs to be a contributing member of the team by being credible and competent in outcomes measurement, monitoring, and management.

SUMMARY

Changes in health care have resulted in a mandate to measure the outcomes of health-promotion interventions. In the current competitive, cost-conscious environment, nurses and other health care providers must document the effectiveness and efficiency of their care. Payers of health care are demanding accurate information about the costs of provider services and the effects of these services on the quality and costs of health promotion. Nurses are challenged to document the value of their practice to health care for payers and consumers of care. Nurses are key players in health promotion and must continue to validate their contribution by identifying outcomes of their interventions that are sensitive to the holistic wellness perspective. Although much work remains for both practicing nurses and nurse scientists, evidence of nursing's contribution is being documented as health outcomes sensitive to nursing interventions are identified, refined, and measured.

LEARNING ACTIVITIES

1. Develop a plan to measure health outcomes for a client intervention of your choice (weight loss, physical activity, stress reduction, etc.).
   a. Describe the rationale for your choice of intervention based on a description of the most recent literature about the effectiveness of the proposed intervention.
   b. Discuss how the intervention would be tailored differently for a 16-year-old girl versus a 50-year-old man.
   c. Identify one short-term, two intermediate, and one long-term outcome to measure the effectiveness of the intervention.
2. Describe the factors you would need to consider to perform a cost-effectiveness analysis as well as a cost–utility analysis for the previous intervention.

SELECTED WEB SITES

Agency for Healthcare Research and Quality (AHRQ)

http://www.ahrq.gov

American Nurses Association

http://www.nursingworld.org

Joint Commission on Accreditation of Healthcare Organizations

http://jcaho.org

National Association for Healthcare Quality

http://www.nahq.org

National Center for Nursing Quality

http://www.nursingquality.org

National Commission for Quality Assurance

http://www.ncqa.org

University of Iowa Nursing Outcome Classification System

http://www.nursing.uiowa.edu/centers/cncce

REFERENCES

American Nurses Association (2002, February) Nursing-Sensitive Indicator for Community-Based Non-Acute Care Settings and ANA's Safety & Quality Initiative. *Nursing Facts*, Silver Spring, MD: ANA.

Anderson, M. R., Hager, M., Su, C., & Urban, N. (2002). Analysis of the cost-effectiveness of mammography promotion by volunteers in rural communities. *Health Education and Behavior*, *29*(6), 755–770.

Bilsbury, C. D., & Richman, A. (2002). A staging approach to measuring patient-centered subjective outcomes. *Acta Psychiatrica Scandinavica*, *106*(414), 5–40.

Breslin, E., Burns, M., & Moores, P. (2002, March). Challenges of outcomes research for nurse practitioners. *J Am Acad Nurse Pract*, *14*(3), 138–143.

Buerhaus, P. I. (1998). Milton Weinstein's insights on the development, use and methodologic problems in cost-effectiveness analysis. *Image: Journal of Nursing Scholarship*, *30*(3), 223–227.

Davies, C. (2003). Introduction: A new workforce in the making? In C. Davies (Ed.), *The future health workforce* (pp. 1–13). Great Britain: Antony Rowe Ltd.

Dickey, B. (2000, July/August). Outcome assessment in women's mental health. *Women's Health Issues*, *10*(4), 192–201.

Head, B. J., Maas, M., & Johnson, M. (2003). Validity and community-health-nursing sensitivity of six outcomes for community health nursing with older clients. *Public Health Nursing*, *20*(5), 385–398.

Hoerger, T. J., Harris, R., Hicks, K. A., Donahue, K., Sorensen, S., & Engelgau, M. (2004). Screening for Type 2 diabetes mellitus: A cost-effectiveness analysis. *Annals of Internal Medicine*, *140*(9), 689–E710.

Ingersoll, G. L., McIntosh, E., & Williams, M. (2000). Nurse-sensitive outcomes of advanced practice. *Journal of Advanced Nursing*, *32*(5), 1272–1281.

Jennings, B. M., Staggers, N., & Brosch, L. R. (1999). A classification scheme for outcome indicators. *Image: Journal of Nursing Scholarship*, *31*(4), 381–388.

Kahn, K. L., Malin, J. L., Adams, J., & Ganz, P. A. (2002). Developing a reliable, valid and feasible plan for quality-of-care measurement for cancer—How should we measure? *Medical Care, 40*(6), III-73–III-85.

Kaplan, R. M., & Groessl, E. J. (2002). Applications of cost-effectiveness methodologies in behavioral medicine. *Journal of Consulting and Clinical Psychology, 70*(3), 482–493.

Kleinpell, R. M. (1997, September). Whose outcomes patients, providers, or payers? *Nursing Clinics of North America, 32*(3), 513–521.

Lewin-V. H. I., Inc. (1995). *Nursing report card for acute care.* Pub. No. NP-101, Washington, DC: American Nurses Association.

Lohr, K. N. (1988). Outcome measurement: Concepts and questions. *Inquiry, 25*(1), 37–50.

Moorhead, S., Johnson, M., & Maas, M. (2004). *Nursing Outcomes Classification (NOC)* (3rd ed.). St. Louis, MO: Mosby.

Muennig, P. (2002). *Designing and conducting cost-effectiveness analyses in medicine and health care.* San Francisco, CA: Jossey-Bass.

Nightingale, F. (1858). *Notes on matters affecting the health, efficiency, and hospital administration of the British Army.* London: Harrison & Sons Nightingale.

Oermann, M. H., & Huber, D. (1999). Patient outcomes. *American Journal of Nursing, 99*(9), 40–47.

Pender, N. J. (1998). Motivation for physical activity among children and adolescents. *Annu Rev Nurs Res, 16*, 139–172.

Ramsey, S. D., McIntosh, M., & Sullivan, S. D. (2001). Design issues for conducting cost-effectiveness analyses alongside clinical trials. *Annu. Rev. Public Health, 22*, 129–141.

Sidani, S., & Braden, C. J. (1998). Outcomes-related factors. In Sidani S & Braden C, *Evaluating nursing interventions: A theory-driven approach* (pp. 138–160). Thousand Oaks, CA: Sage Publications.

Whitehead, D., & Russell, G. (2004). How effective are health education programmes–resistance, reactance, rationality and risk? Recommendations for effective practice. *International Journal of Nursing Studies, 41*, 163–172.

Whitman, G. R. (2002a, September). Outcomes research: Getting started, defining outcomes, a framework, and data sources. *Crit Care Nurs Clin North Am, 14*(3), 261–268.

Whitman, G. R. (2002b, September). Outcomes research in advanced practice nursing selecting an outcome. *Crit Care Nurs Clin North Am, 14*(3), 253–260.

Wutzke, S. E., Shiell, A., Gomel, M. K., & Conigrave, K. M. (2001). Cost effectiveness of brief interventions for reducing alcohol consumption. *Social Science and Medicine, 52*, 863–870.

11

Evaluating Individual and Community Interventions

OBJECTIVES

1. Describe the purpose of evaluation for health promotion.
2. Compare three approaches to evaluation and provide examples of each.
3. Describe the evidence for continuing to implement programs for individuals.
4. Describe the evidence for continuing to promote community-level interventions.
5. Discuss strategies to implement in order to effectively evaluate health-promotion interventions.

OUTLINE

- Purpose of Evaluation
- Approaches to Evaluation for Health-Promotion Interventions
  - A. Efficacy or Effectiveness of Interventions
  - B. Process or Outcome Evaluation
  - C. Collecting Evidence for Practice
- Evaluation of Interventions with Individuals and Communities
  - A. Individuals
  - B. Community
- Strategies for Evaluation of Health-Promotion Interventions
  - A. Designing the Intervention
  - B. Selecting Outcomes

A scientific knowledge base to guide health-promotion interventions is established by evaluating the accumulating results of health-promotion programs and interventions. Improvements are made in the quality of health-promotion activities when their effectiveness has been clearly demonstrated. Evaluation information can be used to select and implement health-promotion programs that provide the most favorable outcomes for clients. Our knowledge of the effectiveness of health promotion is based on research and program evaluations that have been conducted and published. Nurses and other health care professionals are continually being asked about the effectiveness of their health-promotion and risk-reduction efforts. This question can be answered by carefully examining the research and evaluation evidence that has accumulated about a specific type of health-promotion intervention or program.

Purpose of Evaluation

Evaluation, the process of collecting and analyzing information, is undertaken to learn the value of a health-promotion program or intervention. Evaluations are considered decision-oriented, while research is concerned with generating theoretically valid knowledge (Eriksson, 2000). Evaluations serve many purposes: to assess if program objectives were achieved, to improve program implementation, to contribute to the scientific knowledge of health promotion, to provide accountability to funding agencies, and to inform policy makers (McKenzie & Smeltzer, 2001). Evaluations also provide information to enable nurses to make decisions about resource allocation, as ineffective programs can be eliminated and replaced with cost-effective programs that have been shown to promote change. Health-promotion evaluations enable the nurse to improve the design of the program, to make choices between health-promotion activities, to learn how a particular health-promotion program might be repeated elsewhere, and to test whether a new idea will work in practice (Powell, 1999).

Evaluation needs to be part of the program development process, as this enables appropriate, accurate information to be collected. Planning for evaluations is especially important in order for initial or baseline information to be obtained before the program or intervention is implemented and to be able to train those who will collect the evaluation information. Questions that can be answered by a comprehensive evaluation include the following (Ovretveit, 1998):

- Is the health-promotion intervention effective in an ideal situation (efficacy)?
- Is the health-promotion intervention effective in clinical practice (efficiency)?
- How does the health-promotion intervention work?

- What are the intended and unintended effects (outcomes)?
- How long-lasting are the effects?
- What resources are needed to implement the intervention or program?
- Is it cost effective?
- Are clients satisfied?
- Who will benefit from the intervention?
- How can the program or intervention be improved?

Cost, time, and resources pose limitations on evaluations. In addition, performing an evaluation requires knowledge, skills, and administrative support (Powell, 1999). If these things are not present, the evaluation is unlikely to be performed successfully and produce useful results.

 # Approaches to Evaluation for Health-Promotion Interventions

A growing body of evidence supports the belief that health-promotion programs have a positive effect on health and health care costs (Whitehead & Russell, 2004). Identifying and evaluating evidence for health promotion can be a challenge for clinicians. Evaluation approaches provide the roadmap for the systematic collection, analysis, and reporting of information. Knowledge of differences in efficacy and effectiveness studies and differences in process and outcome evaluations is needed to design an appropriate plan to evaluate evidence for one's practice. Other approaches, such as systems analysis, goal-based evaluations, and decision-making evaluations, will not be covered in this chapter.

Efficacy or Effectiveness of Interventions

Efficacy refers to improvements in health outcomes of interventions achieved in a special setting, under ideal circumstances, by experts (Robey, 2004). In other words, the health-promotion intervention is studied and evaluated under controlled or ideal conditions to demonstrate that the outcomes are due to the intervention and not to chance or other factors unrelated to the intervention. Efficacy is best demonstrated by a phase III clinical trial, when clients are randomly assigned to the intervention or a comparison condition.

The *effectiveness* of an intervention is the result it achieves in the real world, with limited resources, in entire populations or specified subgroups of a population. In other words, effectiveness addresses the clinical usefulness of the intervention, as the intervention is implemented and evaluated in a typical community setting, where it will eventually be applied. Effectiveness studies have also been called phase IV clinical trials. They are implemented in large populations and are expected to have an immediate effect on clinical practice (Piantadosi, 1997).

Both approaches are useful in testing and evaluating interventions. Efficacy studies are considered less applicable to the general population because they are tested under ideal circumstances with a targeted group of clients. However, both types of evidence need to be evaluated. Efficacy studies test the usefulness of interventions, followed by effectiveness studies in which the findings are applied to real-life settings for feasibility, costs, effectiveness of the intervention in actual practice, and acceptance of the intervention by differing groups of clients. For example, if the efficacy of a health-promotion intervention has been scientifically tested, clinicians can take the evidence and evaluate its effectiveness in their client population or clinical setting. In the practice setting, it is difficult to control implementation of the intervention, which often leads to inconsistent delivery across clients. Some clients may receive all of the intervention, whereas others may receive less of the intervention, leading to inaccurate evaluation results. It is important for the nurse to implement the intervention or program plan as faithfully as possible and keep good records of the extent to which the intervention reached the intended audience.

Process or Outcome Evaluation

Process evaluations of health-promotion interventions refer to verifying the content of the intervention and whether it was delivered as intended, whereas outcome evaluations focus on the results of the intervention. Process evaluations provide information to help refine the intervention or delivery of the program and define the needs and preferences of the targeted group. Evaluation of the health outcomes of interventions is critical. However, process evaluations provide valuable information about how the program is being implemented. Variations in delivery among sites and clients are identified as well as "breakdowns" between what was intended and what was actually delivered. Process evaluations provide feedback on the quality of delivery of the intervention and who received the intended intervention. Process evaluation answers the questions: Is the intervention being implemented as planned? Is the intervention reaching its target audience? And are the participants satisfied with the intervention? Process evaluations should involve a feedback loop, so that the intervention can be revised based on the information obtained (Pirie, 1999).

Process evaluations provide insights into what factors might hinder or facilitate achievement of program goals. They provide information about whether the intended "dosage" of the program was delivered. Dosage refers to the amount of exposure to the program or intervention (Sidani & Braden, 1998; Stewart, 2000). In other words, was the exposure strong enough to produce the desired outcomes? Dosage is evaluated by examining the amount, frequency, and total length of time of the program. Process evaluations are important tools for health promotion, as they help explain how and why interventions achieve their effects. Baranowski and Stables (2000) reviewed process evaluations from nine 5-a-Day for Better Health Programs instituted nationwide by the National Cancer Institute to promote consumption of fruits for primary prevention of cancer. Initially they identified the essential components of the program to review. Although all programs did not include all components, they found that process evaluation helped to explain some of the weaker aspects of the programs. The results of their review found that process evaluations can be implemented in diverse community settings and also shed light on how the program was related to outcomes.

Outcomes evaluations focus on the results or changes brought about by the program, intended or unintended. The choice of outcomes to measure is determined by the program goals. For example, if the goal is to achieve weight loss, weight will need to be measured prior to the initiation of the program and at the end of the program. If the goal of the program is primary prevention of cancer, long-term outcomes will be needed to follow clients to learn if and when a diagnosis of cancer is made. Multiple outcomes should be measured to capture the intended changes of a program.

In outcome evaluations, the size of the effect of the intervention is an important question to ask (Wellings & MacDowall, 2000). The size of the effect depends on multiple factors, including the size of the population who received the intervention, the sensitivity of the measures, the time points measured, and the scope of the intervention. Small effects may be important in public health terms when large numbers of people are involved.

Collecting Evidence for Practice

In the current health care environment, health care practitioners can no longer rely solely on their clinical experiences, tradition, and opinion-based processes to guide their health-promotion interventions (Agency for Healthcare Research and Quality, 2002). Instead, the current best evidence must be used to make decisions about their clients and interventions. Current best evidence is obtained from many sources: a synthesis of relevant literature; international, national, and local standards of practice; cost-effectiveness analysis; clinical expertise; and patient preferences. First, a search of the literature is necessary to see if adequate information is available to evaluate the intervention. The literature (evidence) then needs to be critically evaluated and the evidence synthesized. This process has given rise to a new term in health care, *evidence-based practice.*

Evidence-based practice is defined as the integration of clinical expertise with the best-available clinical research findings (Dobrow, Goel, & Upshur, 2004). The aim of evidence-based practice is to reduce wide variations in practice, eliminating worst practices and enhancing best practices to improve quality and decrease costs. Evidence-based clinical practice builds on research utilization as research results, along with other evidence previously mentioned, are transformed into practice.

In evidence-based health-promotion practice the nurse looks for existing evidence as well as new evidence, evaluates the evidence, and then acts on the evidence (Perkins, Simnett, & Wright, 1999). Questions to ask are:

Can I trust this information (validity)?

Will the information make an important difference in my practice (significance)?

Can I use the information in my practice (applicability)?

Evidence-based practice involves assessing if a change is needed in practice, identifying the type of information needed, conducting a literature search, critically appraising the literature using the principles of evidence-based practice, identifying clinically meaningful results, designing a practice change, and applying the change to one's practice (Rosswurm & Larrabee, 1999). Table 11–1 reviews the steps to help establish evidence for a practice intervention. After an evidence-based practice change is implemented, plans are made to evaluate both the process for carrying out the change as well as the expected outcomes.

The process to examine the evidence does not replace clinical expertise, as the nurse has to evaluate new knowledge in light of its applicability to the target population. Although intuition and unsystematic clinical experiences are de-emphasized, the process is not a cookbook approach to nursing and health care. For example, the clinical problem might be the inability to promote physical activity interventions in a rural setting and the potential of using a telehealth intervention to promote physical activity in adults in this setting. The literature about telehealth interventions to promote physical activity is reviewed and evaluated to see if it is applicable to clients in rural settings. In addition, the sociocultural environment of the targeted population, prior experiences with health promotion

TABLE 11-1 Steps in Evidence-Based Practice
Identify what evidence is needed
1. Assess the need for change in practice.
Retrieve and evaluate the evidence
2. Conduct literature search.
3. Critically evaluate literature.
Decide and design what to implement
4. Identify results applicable to practice.
5. Develop practice change to implement results.
Implement
6. Apply change to practice.
Evaluate
7. Evaluate outcomes of new change.

in rural settings, and available resources are considered. If the nurse finds that the evidence is applicable and relevant, based on all of the factors considered, plans are made to implement the new intervention.

Evidence for health interventions may be useful to policy makers and payers, as well as practitioners. Policy makers can use the information in more rational resource allocations or in the development of priorities for health promotion and risk reduction. Payers will use the information to eliminate interventions that are not effective, and practitioners will be able to use the results to make informed decisions about the most effective programs for their clients.

The use of evidence to guide health-promotion activities is the ideal. However, community-based programs place a high value on the community's role in defining the health problem and participating in the solution. In this case, the research evidence is only one component in the decision-making process to define the program. In addition, criteria to evaluate community-based programs are often difficult to define and measure. Therefore, the intervention chosen may not be the most effective even though it is strongly supported by the community. Last, a rapid response to a problem may be needed, or the government may take the opportunity to pursue a policy when time does not allow evidence to be established. For example, public education has been implemented to promote abstinence from drug use, without evidence of the effectiveness of media campaigns to promote abstinence. These issues show how research can be applied in varying ways, despite the availability or lack of evidence. This points to the need for flexibility in order to match the evidence with the type of approach needed.

Evaluation of Interventions with Individuals and Communities

Changes in the conceptualization of health have resulted in different approaches to promoting and evaluating wellness. One difference focuses on whether health-promotion strategies concentrate on individual lifestyle changes or community-wide changes. Individual approaches identify a finite number of lifestyle areas that can be targeted for intervention. McKinlay (1975) coined the term *downstream* to describe interventions that are aimed at individuals. *Midstream* interventions describe community-based interventions and are aimed at schools, work sites, health plans, and other organizational channels, as well as entire communities or specific populations. *Upstream* health-behavior interventions are those that address policy and environmental changes. For example, upstream strategies may include protection from environmental hazards such as asbestos in old buildings or nuclear wastes, changes in advertising of unhealthy behaviors such as antismoking campaigns, food labeling, and economic incentives such as excise taxes on liquor and cigarettes. Table 11–2 describes the three levels of interventions and suggested activities and outcomes for the three levels. Wellness behaviors are a result of individual attitudes, beliefs, and values as well as conditions in the community. Because the three types of interventions are interrelated, success is more likely to be achieved if all are taken into consideration when planning and evaluating health-promotion programs.

Individuals

Programs that target individuals provide clients with strategies for wellness and/or lifestyle change. These individuals must then maintain their new behaviors in the larger social environment that often rewards at-risk behaviors or provides barriers to the maintenance of healthy behaviors (Orleans, 2000). Low-income and disadvantaged individuals are at greatest risk for not sustaining the change because of a lack of resources in their social and physical environments (Jeffery et al., 2000; Ockene et al., 2000). A challenge for nurses and health care professionals is to develop, test, evaluate, and implement models of health promotion that incorporate the influences of community factors (work sites, schools, etc.), environmental factors, and sociocultural factors with individual behaviors to promote wellness.

TABLE 11–2 Levels and Types of Interventions

Level	Target	Types of Interventions
Downstream	Individuals	Education
		Counseling
		Support
Midstream	Communities	Work site programs
		School programs
		Community-based programs
Upstream	Public policy	Tax incentives or deterrents
	Environment	Policy changes
		Local ordinances
		Laws
		Media campaigns

(Based on McKinlay's model for health behavior change, McKinlay J. and Marceau L. 2000, *U.S. Public Health and the 21st Century: Diabetes Mellitus*, The Lancet, *356*, 757–761.)

Individual models of health behavior were described in Chapter 2. These models focus on attitudes, beliefs, or other characteristics within the individual that are amenable to change. Interventions promote knowledge and skills needed to change individual behaviors. Impressive gains have been made in the science and practice of health-behavior change at the individual level (Orleans, 2000). Bandura's social learning theory (1986) and Prochaska and DiClemente's stages of change model (1983) have had major effects on the design and delivery of individual health-promotion interventions. Effective short-term changes (6 to 24 months) have occurred as a result of cognitive–behavioral interventions. A recent review on stage-based lifestyle interventions in primary care based on the transtheoretical model showed strong evidence for the use of the model on fat intake, but limited or no evidence was found for an effect of the stages of change on smoking and quitting rates or physical activity (van Sluijs, van Poppel, & van Mechelen, 2004). This review points to the limited scientific evidence for the usefulness of this model, particularly for long-term change.

Individual strategies for health promotion that warrant continued use based on evaluation results include contests and competition to recruit and maintain participants in programs (Whitlock, Orleans, Pender, & Allan, 2002). Contests promote attention and excitement and the costs are modest, so they are recommended to promote awareness and participation. Self-help and minimal but repeated contact programs for individuals are also effective, relatively easy to implement, inexpensive, and they may reach persons who are not easily accessed by other means.

Screening for health education, as well as case finding, has also been found to be a successful intervention at the individual level. Health education provided to every person who is screened, regardless of risk, to improve lifestyle has been shown to change lifestyle patterns. However, screening is expensive and requires a high level of professional competence. In addition, strategies to promote screening need to be tailored to the target population. What may motivate an urban group of men to participate in prostate cancer screening may be very different from motivational strategies needed for rural men.

Community

Community-based programs build on existing community structures to promote wellness and behavior change. These types of interventions consider broader factors that influence health other than individual beliefs and attitudes. Instead, the system in which the individual lives and works is targeted. This approach necessitates the collaboration of individuals and organizations within the community and often demands considerable resources, including time and money.

Community settings that have most commonly been the site of health-promotion programs include the workplace, churches, and schools. The work site is appealing because of the ability to implement comprehensive programs that may result in cost savings. Process evaluations indicate that work site interventions reported in the literature vary in comprehensiveness, intensity, and duration in providing health education to employees. Evaluation results suggest that providing opportunities for counseling employees within the context of a comprehensive program may be the critical component (Pelletier, 2001). Work site programs for smoking cessation consistently show positive benefits (Janer, Sala, & Kogevinas, 2002). Organizational factors have been shown to either facilitate or hinder the implementation of work-site health-promotion programs (Sorensen, Linnan, & Hunt, 2004). Specifically, leadership characteristics are key to acceptance and implementation.

Churches and other places of worship have been used as sites for health promotion (Peterson, Atwood, & Yates, 2002). In these settings there is a higher level of volunteer involvement to assist with program implementation, so less professional involvement is needed. Religious organizations have access to large numbers of people, effective communication channels, and adequate meeting facilities, all factors that have been shown to facilitate successful delivery of health education.

Another popular site for health promotion is the school, where the focus is on children and adolescents. Schools are appealing because of the amount of time students spend in this environment, and it is possible to involve the parents in health-promotion activities. This approach is based on the premise that the family, as well as peers, play an important role in the adoption and maintenance of healthy behaviors (Michaud, 2003). A comprehensive school-based health-promotion program consists of health instruction, health services, social support services, health education curricula, extracurricular activities that meet the needs and interests of the students, and involvement of the family. Additional program components have focused on specific behaviors, such as food service changes to promote a healthy diet, or physical activity instruction and programs.

Community health promotion relies on coalitions to address the targeted health behaviors, so community activation is a critical component in implementing community programs (von dem Knesebeck, Joksimovic, Bandura, & Siegrist, 2002). Activation of the community is also very difficult because of the need to coordinate many agencies and develop actions that will not reflect the interests of a particular group or agency. Because of the difficulty, successful, sustained community activation to promote health has been a commonly unfulfilled goal in community-based health-promotion interventions. Factors have been identified in process evaluations that facilitate community activation. These include the ability of the community coalition to provide its own vision, members who have the skills and time to work together, frequent and productive communication, and a sense of cohesion (Pluye, Potvin, & Denis, 2004; von dem Knesebeck et al., 2002). Barriers to communication and coalition building include staff who lack organizational skills, staff turnover, difficulty recruiting members, and reluctance of community members to conduct activities.

Media campaigns have been found to be useful as an adjunct to both individual- and community-based interventions. Message repetition is important and presentations must be of high quality, which means that media campaigns can be expensive. However, some media programs are inexpensive, such as bill inserts, grocery bag flyers, television feature news stories, and community newspapers. Modern technology has resulted in media-based interventions that are delivered in personalized, interactive formats. Media campaigns that use print and/or telephone have been found to be effective in changing short-term behavior (Reger, Wootan, & Booth-Butterfield, 2000). Repeated contact media tailored to target audiences have also been found to be more effective than one-shot, broad messages.

In summary, intervention approaches at the individual and community levels have resulted in behavior change, which is cause for optimism in health promotion. Effective individual-based programs have mainly used cognitive–behavioral theories to guide the interventions. Growing awareness of the role of the context in which the individual works and lives points to the need for an approach that balances individual and community strategies. Community health-promotion programs have the potential to improve health because of their ability to target large segments of the population through broad-based interventions. Because of the broad base, community health promotion also offers many challenges in the evaluation of these programs.

Strategies for Evaluation of Health-Promotion Interventions

Strategies have been identified that increase the likelihood of effective health-promotion programs based on the results of evaluation. Program strategies need to be addressed in designing the intervention, selecting outcomes to measure the intervention, deciding on the time frame to implement the intervention, and evaluating the outcome of the intervention. Knowledge about long-term maintenance of behavior change, the last step in the change process of health promotion, is limited, as this area has not received adequate attention. However, strategies to increase sustainability of community-based programs have been identified.

Designing the Intervention

Health-promotion interventions are complex and usually involve multiple components. When designing programs, the nurse needs to assess the appropriateness of the intervention or intervention components for the target population. This can be accomplished by applying specific criteria (Morley & Farewell, 2000). First, the intervention has to be affordable to individuals, agencies, or communities. Needless to say, a program that is too expensive will result in poor participation. If the intervention is too expensive or resource intensive for community-based systems, commitment by the agency will be lacking and participation will be poor. The intervention must also be manageable and compatible with existing programs in the community. Programs that are less complex and fit with existing programs have a greater chance of being successfully implemented. Evidence should be available to document the effectiveness of the intervention in the targeted setting and population. If the effectiveness of the intervention has not been tested with different socio-cultural groups, results of implementing the intervention in the new group or community need to be evaluated carefully.

Selecting Outcomes

Realistic, quality outcomes need to be chosen when designing the evaluation phase of health-promotion interventions to appropriately measure the program results. The outcomes of many health-promotion interventions may not be known for many years. In addition, community-level outcomes are complex and often very expensive, so the decision of which endpoints and outcomes are realistic is a critical one. The outcome evaluation component needs careful planning so that the results, while realistic and affordable, are meaningful. Once a decision is made about which outcomes to use based on program goals, the nurse needs to decide how to measure them. Self-report measures are used in many health-promotion programs (Hardeman, Griffin, Johnston, Kinmonth, & Wareham,

2000). However, objective measures need to be used whenever possible, as they are more precise and sensitive to change for many health-promotion interventions, such as physical activity and dietary changes. Measurement of community-level outcomes has not received as much attention as individual outcomes and they are less well developed because of their complexity. This issue also needs to be considered when deciding on outcome measures. One strategy is to also measure improvements in the community, such as the number of new public physical activity facilities or the number of restaurants that provide healthy choices. These broader outcomes provide information about how the program has improved the community, independent of the behavior change of individual members.

Potential outcomes that can be measured when behavioral long-term outcomes may not be realistic include program participation rates. Although participation does not measure effectiveness, it provides information about the acceptance of the intervention and its implementation, as the program cannot be successful if it is not well attended. Process measures are also useful to assess the effectiveness of implementing the intervention. Measurement of the "delivered dose," or an assessment of aspects of the program that were delivered, and "received dose," or the number of people who participated in the program, are useful aspects of process evaluation (Sidani & Braden, 1998).

Deciding Time Frame

A realistic time frame is necessary to properly conduct the program and evaluate the results. What is realistic depends on the type, comprehensiveness, and complexity of the program and the target population. In a straightforward, individual-focused intervention targeted to a small group, 6 months may be a realistic period to implement and evaluate short-term results. However, 5 years may be needed to implement and evaluate a complex community-based program targeted to primary schools. The time frame for a community-based program is related to acceptance and action by the community, as it may backfire if it is rushed.

Maintaining Behavior Change

Most of the progress in health-promotion research has been in promoting health-behavior change, while less progress has been seen in promoting maintenance of these changes. Maintenance of healthy behaviors is now seen as a process that needs exploration, rather than an end state (Wing, 2000). Psychological processes that underlie the decision to adopt health behaviors have, until recently, been assumed to generalize to behavior-maintenance decisions (Rothman, 2000). This is evident in most of the current models of health behavior that stress how people decide to adopt health behaviors. Two exceptions are Bandura's cognitive theory, which states that self-efficacy beliefs are a critical determinant of both the initiation and maintenance of behavior change, and Prochaska and DiClemente's transtheoretical model, which includes maintenance as a stage in the model. However, neither of these theories offers guidance about the process of maintenance and how it differs from the initiation and adoption of behaviors (Rothman, 2000). The distinction between initiation and maintenance of behavior change has opened new challenges for health-promotion practice and research because the process is not well understood. Understanding the theoretical and behavioral processes that guide successful behavioral maintenance will enable interventions to be developed to address long-term behavior change.

Collaboration is key to successful maintenance of health-promotion programs in the community. Models have been developed to link schools of nursing to communities to provide culturally competent, evidence-based health-promotion interventions (Lundeen, 1999; Marcus, 2000). A holistic approach that continually assesses community needs, nurtures collegial relationships, and supports the health of community residents has been shown to be effective (Lundeen, 1999). Maintenance of these collaborations is a challenge, as they are dependent on funding and the ability to balance multiple agendas and missions. However, barriers need to be confronted, as community collaborative partnerships are essential in promoting the health of the community.

Sustainability or institutionalization of community-based programs is determined by many factors (von dem Knesebeck et al., 2002). The intervention program needs to be transferred from outside agencies to the community to have a sustained effect. Sustainability is influenced by the design of the intervention and implementation factors, facilitators and barriers within the targeted community setting, and factors in the broader community environment. Sustainability is more likely to be successful when capacity building has occurred in the community and program goals have included long-term maintenance. Sustainability needs to be conceptualized as an ongoing process that is ever-changing as new knowledge is gained. An infrastructure that integrates resources needs to be established to support the program. These resources might include state health department units, universities, professional societies, and federal organizations. Attention to sustainability is important for the program to continue to promote health behaviors.

Directions for Research in Evaluating Health Promotion

The results of evaluation of health-promotion activities offer many avenues for research. First, it is evident that our current theories of health promotion need to be expanded and tested, as most theories have not paid much attention to long-term behavior change. Innovative models of health promotion that identify determinants of behavior maintenance need to be developed and tested. Socioecological models of health promotion, which integrate strategies of behavior change with social and physical environmental enhancements, need further development and testing.

Second, more accurate and sensitive measures of behavior change are needed to evaluate individual and community outcomes. Self-report measures of behavior change need to be developed that are reliable, valid, and sensitive to both short-term and long-term change. Objective measures of behavior change also need to be developed to more precisely measure changes, such as dietary behaviors and physical activity. Outcome measures also need to be standardized across studies of health behaviors, such as physical activity, to enable researchers and practitioners to compare findings. Additional outcomes that measure community-level behavior change need to be identified, and measures developed to assess these large-scale outcomes.

Research is needed to describe, predict, and intervene to promote long-term maintenance. This opens possibilities for all types of research. Exploratory studies are needed to answer such questions as, "What factors promote successful maintenance of healthy behaviors?" "What factors promote relapse?" "What are the greatest difficulties encountered in maintenance?" Descriptive studies are necessary to describe factors associated with maintenance of behaviors over long periods of time as well as differences in factors that predict success in various age groups. For example, what role do parents play in the maintenance of physical activity by children? Experimental studies that evaluate interventions to promote long-term maintenance are also needed. These studies need to be implemented for individuals as well as in schools and work sites in the community.

As can be seen from this brief discussion, opportunities for research to evaluate individual- and community-based interventions are not lacking. Interdisciplinary teams, which capitalize on the expertise of all members, are encouraged to ensure successful funding and rigorous studies to address the issues.

Directions for Practice in Evaluating Health Promotion

Evaluation of health-promotion interventions provides nurses and other health care providers evidence on which to base their practice. Health care professionals are mandated to base their practice on current research findings, as well as other factors, so it is important to understand the criteria used to evaluate the evidence. Courses that teach these skills can be offered in the clinical setting or through collaboration with local chapters of professional organizations or universities. Knowledge of evaluation criteria will enable the nurse to accurately review the literature and make informed decisions about the evidence.

Knowledge of effective health-promotion interventions and programs provide the nurse with information to refer clients to successful programs or deliver aspects of either individual- or community-based interventions that have been successful. An interdisciplinary approach has been shown to be more effective in the delivery of complex or community-based interventions.

Nurses in clinical settings need to implement and evaluate new models of delivery of health-promotion interventions. For example, telephone counseling and follow-up is a relatively low-cost intervention that can be effectively used to provide ongoing contact, social support, and expertise to answer questions. Telephone and telehealth interventions need to become a standard component of self-help interventions and follow-up, especially for elderly and rural populations.

Maintenance continues to be a major problem in health-behavior change, so nurses need to follow clients carefully to identify early relapse and provide these individuals with ongoing interventions. Counseling can be used to identify problems related to relapse. Although little is known about successful strategies to promote long-term maintenance, nurses can identify individual strategies based on counseling and discussions with clients and their families. New strategies should be implemented and evaluated with realistic long-term follow-up, if feasible.

SUMMARY

Evaluation of health-promotion programs sheds light on what is most effective in promoting wellness and behavior change as well as what does not work. Evaluating health-promotion interventions facilitates the development of a knowledge base on which to make decisions about programs that are most effective for behavior change for clients and communities. The evaluation process is complex and time consuming, and requires advanced knowledge not previously applied in practice. However, learning to evaluate the literature provides valuable information about the usefulness of individual- and community-based interventions.

LEARNING ACTIVITIES

1. Select a health-promotion intervention of interest, such as physical activity in the elderly, and, using the steps in Table 11–1, establish whether or not there is evidence on which to base your planned intervention.

2. Develop an evaluation plan for a health education program to teach adolescents proper nutrition.

   a. What factors would you consider in designing the program?

   b. Develop a process evaluation plan, describing how you will evaluate the dosage of the intervention received by the participants.

   c. Describe your outcome evaluation plan. Which outcomes will be appropriate to measure, and how will you measure them? Consider both short-term and intermediate outcomes.

   d. Describe the time frame you will use to evaluate the results of the program and the rationale for choosing the particular time points.

   e. What factors do you need to consider to promote sustainability of the change, and how will you monitor sustainability?

SELECTED WEB SITES RELEVANT TO EVALUATION OF HEALTH PROMOTION

ACT Health Promotion–Evaluation

http://www.healthpromotion.act.gov.au/howto/evaluation

The Health Communication Unit

http://www.thcu.ca/infoandresources/evaluation.htm

National Network for Health

http://nnh.org

REFERENCES

Agency for Healthcare Research and Quality. (2002). *Systems to rate the strength of scientific evidence.* U.S. Department of Health and Human Services. Publication No-02-EO15, 47 pp. 1–11.

Bandura, A. (1986). *Social foundations of thoughts and actions.* Upper Saddle River, NJ: Prentice Hall, Inc.

Baranowski, T., & Stables, G. (2000). Process evaluations of the 5-a-day projects. *Health Educ Behav, 27*(2), 157–166.

Dobrow, M. J., Goel, V., & Upshur, R. E. G. (2004). Evidence-based health policy: Context and utilisation. *Social Science & Medicine, 58,* 207–217.

Eriksson, C. (2000). Learning and knowledge-production for public health: A review of approaches to evidence-based public health. *Scand J Public Health, 28,* 298–308.

Hardeman, W., Griffin, S., Johnston, M., Kinmonth, A. L., & Wareham, N. J. (2000, February). Interventions to prevent weight gain: A systematic review of psychological models and behaviour change methods. *Int J Obes Relat Metab Disord, 24*(2), 131–143.

Janer, G., Sala, M., & Kogevinas, M. (2002). Health promotion trials at worksites and risk factors for cancer. *Scand J Work Environ Health, 28*(3), 141–157.

Jeffery, R. W., Drewnowski, A., Epstein, L. H., Stunkard, A. J., Wilson, G. T., Wing, R. R., & Hill, D. R. (2000). Long-term maintenance of weight loss: Current status. *Health Psychol, 19*(1)(Suppl), 5–16.

Lundeen, S. P. (1999). An alternative paradigm for promoting health in communities: The Lundeen community nursing center model. *Fam Community Health, 21*(4), 15–28.

Marcus, T. (2000, May-June). An interdisciplinary team model for substance abuse prevention in communities. *J Prof Nurs, 16*(3), 158–168.

McKenzie, J. F., & Smeltzer, J. L. (2001). Evaluation—An overview. In J. F. McKenzie, B. L. Neiger, & J. L. Smelter (Eds.), *Planning, implementing, and evaluating Health promotion programs. A primer* (3rd ed., pp. 269–280). Needham Heights, MA: Allyn & Bacon.

McKinlay, J. B. (1975). A case for re-focusing upstream: The political economy of illness. In A. J. Enelow & J. B. Henderson (Eds.), *Applying behavioral science to cardiovascular risk* (pp. 7–18). Seattle, WA: American Heart Association.

Michaud, P. A. (2003). Prevention and health promotion in school and community settings: A commentary on the international perspective. *Journal of Adolescent Health, 33,* 219–225.

Morley, R., & Farewell, V. (2000). Methodological issues in randomised controlled trials. *Semin Neonatol, 5,* 141–148.

Ockene, J. K., Emmons, K. M., Mermelstein, R. J., Perkins, K. A., Bonollo, D. S., Voorhees, C. C., & Hollis, J. F. (2000). Relapse and maintenance issues for smoking cessation. *Health Psychol, 19*(1)(Suppl.), 17–31.

Orleans, C. T. (2000). Promoting the maintenance of health behavior change: Recommendations for the next generation of research and practice. *Health Psychol, 19*(1)(Suppl), 76–83.

Ovretveit, J. (1998). Evaluation purpose, theory and perspectives. In *Evaluating health interventions* (pp. 24–47). Bristol, PA: Open University Press.

Pelletier, K. R. (2001). A review and analysis of the clinical- and cost-effectiveness studies of comprehensive health promotion and disease management programs at the worksite: 1998–2000 update. *American Journal of Preventive Medicine, 16*(2), 107–116.

Perkins, E. R., Simnett, I., & Wright, L. (1999). Creative tensions in evidence-based practice. In E.R. Perkins, I. Simnett, & L. Wright (Eds.), *Evidence-based health promotion* (pp. 2–21). Chichester: John Wiley & Sons.

Peterson, J., Atwood, J. R., & Yates, B. (2002). Key elements for church-based health promotion programs: Outcome-based literature review. *Public Health Nursing, 19*(6), 401–411.

Piantadosi, S. (1997). *Clinical trials: A methodologic perspective.* New York: John Wiley & Sons.

Pirie, P. L. (1999). Evaluating community health promotion programs. In N. Brach (Ed.), *Health promotion at the community level* (2nd ed., pp. 127–134). Newbury Park, CA: Sage Publications.

Pluye, P., Potvin, L., & Denis, J. L. (2004). Making public health programs last: Conceptualizing sustainability. *Evaluation and Program Planning, 27*, 121–133.

Powell, J. (1999). Monitoring and evaluation in cardiac rehabilitation. In E. R. Perkins, I. Simnet, & L. Wright (Eds.), *Evidence-based health promotion* (pp. 377–385). Chichester: John Wiley and Sons.

Prochaska, J. O., & DiClemente, C. C. (1983). Stages and processes of self-change of smoking: Toward an integrative model of change. *Journal of Consulting and Clinical Psychology, 51*, 390–395.

Reger, B., Wootan, M. G., & Booth-Butterfield, S. (2000). A comparison of different approaches to promote community-wide dietary change. *American Journal of Preventive Medicine, 18*(4), 271–275.

Robey, R. R. (2004). A five-phase model for clinical-outcome research. *Journal of Communication Disorders, 37*(5), 401–411.

Rosswurm, M. A., & Larrabee, J. H. (1999). A model for change to evidence-based practice. *Image: Journal of Nursing Scholarship, 31*(4), 317–322.

Rothman, A. J. (2000). Toward a theory-based analysis of behavioral maintenance. *Health Psychol, 19*(1)(Suppl), 64–69.

Sidani, S. & Braden, C. (1998). Intervention variables. In *Evaluating nursing interventions—A theory-driven approach* (pp. 105–137). Thousand Oaks, CA: Sage Publications.

Sorensen, G., Linnan, L., & Hunt, M. K. (2004). Worksite-based research and initiatives to increase fruit and vegetable consumption. *Preventive Medicine;* in press.

Stewart, W. (2000). Use of process evaluation during project implementation: Experience from the CHAPS project for gay men. In M. Thorogood & Y. Coombes (Eds.), *Evaluating health promotion: Practice and methods* (pp. 84–98). Oxford: Oxford University Press.

van Sluijs, E. M., van Poppel, M. N., & van Mechelen, W. (2004). Stage-based lifestyle interventions in primary care. Are they effective? *American Journal of Preventive Medicine, 26*(4), 330–343.

von dem Knesebeck, O., Joksimovic, L., Bandura, B., & Siegrist, J. (2002). Evaluation of a community-level health policy intervention. *Healthy Policy, 61*, 111–122.

Wellings, S., & Macdowall, W. (2000). Evaluating mass media approaches. In M. Thorogood, & Y. Coombes (Eds.), *Evaluating health promotion: Practice and methods* (pp. 113–128). Oxford: Oxford University Press.

Whitehead, D., & Russell, G. (2004). How effective are health education programmes–resistance, reactance, rationality and risk? Recommendations for effective practice. *International Journal of Nursing Studies, 41*, 163–172.

Whitlock, E. P., Orleans, C. T., Pender, N., & Allan, J. (2002). Evaluating primary care behavioral counselling interventions—An evidence-based approach. *American Journal of Preventive Medicine, 22*(4), 267–284.

Wing, R. (2000). Cross-cutting themes in maintenance of behavior change. *Health Psychol, 19*(1)(Suppl), 84–88.

Part 5

Health Promotion in Diverse Populations

12

Self-Care for Health Promotion Across the Life Span

OBJECTIVES

1. Describe the role of families and schools in the development of self-care health behaviors in children and adolescents.
2. Contrast the focus of self-care in young and middle-age adults and older adults.
3. Discuss the steps in the self-care empowerment process to promote health.
4. Identify the positive and negative aspects of the Internet in self-care.

OUTLINE

- The Role of the Professional Nurse
- Self-Care for Health Promotion Throughout the Life Span
  A. Children and Adolescents
  B. Young and Middle-Age Adults
  C. Older Adults
- Goals of Health Education for Self-Care
- The Process of Empowering for Self-Care to Promote Health
  A. Mutually Assessing Self-Care Competencies and Needs
  B. Determining Learning Priorities
  C. Identifying Long-Term and Short-Term Objectives
  D. Facilitating Self-Paced Learning
  E. Using Positive Reinforcement to Increase Perceptions of Competence and Motivation for Learning

The self-care movement has become a big business targeting consumers as a result of changes in health care financing and the proliferation of managed care. Self-responsibility and self-care are major themes in health policy (Boote, Telford, & Cooper, 2002). In addition, the consumer movement has resulted in individuals, families, and communities expending greater energy in self-care activities to promote and maintain health. Self-care, a universal requirement for sustaining and enhancing life and health, is an area of competence to be developed. Self-care directed toward health promotion can be defined as the practice of activities initiated or performed by an individual, family, or community to achieve, maintain, or promote maximum health and well-being (Orem, 1995). Care of self and others to maximize health includes actions to minimize threats to personal health, self-nurturance, self-improvement, and continued personal growth. Self-care approaches embody the notion of individual rights and accountability. Self-care changes the balance of power in health promotion by challenging the "top down" approach to promote health (Boote et al., 2002). Active involvement in self-care is widely acknowledged as an important strategy for achieving national health goals. *Healthy People 2010* recognizes that one of the greatest opportunities to achieve its goals is to empower individuals to make informed health care decisions and become active participants in improving their health (U.S. Department of Health and Human Services, 2000).

Self-care is considered the predominant and basic form of primary care. It is the universal and predominant form of health care and includes health promotion, disease prevention, diagnosis, treatment, and long-term management of health and illness (Mulatu & Berry, 2001). Self-care includes eating a healthy diet, exercising, adequate rest, use of nutritional supplements, and avoidance of harmful substances and environments. Self-care within chronic illness is defined as the practice of activities to manage the illness, such as self-management of side effects of treatments or symptoms of the disease (Lenoci, Telfair, Cecil, & Edwards, 2002). In chronic illness, self-care activities may include taking medication, eating special foods, or taking direct action, such as making a doctor's appointment.

Self-care for health promotion goes beyond illness self-care and requires that clients gain knowledge and competencies that can be used to maintain and enhance health independently of the medical system (Coulter, 2003). In health promotion, self-care is primary, with professional care secondary. Self-care approaches to promote health extend beyond traditional strategies in medicine, nursing, and other health professions to those previously considered complementary or alternative. Self-care to promote health across the life span will continue to gain significance as consumers challenge the superiority of the traditional paternalistic medical model in health care and health policy.

The Role of the Professional Nurse

Professional nurses have a major responsibility for enhancing clients' capacity for self-care throughout their life span. Nurses have long recognized the right of individuals and families to be informed and active participants in their own care.

In Orem's Self-Care Nursing Model, three types of self-care requisites are described: universal, developmental, and health deviation requirements (Orem, 1995). Universal self-care requirements include sufficient air, water, food, elimination, a balance between activity and rest, a balance between solitude and social interaction, protection from hazards, and protection of human functioning and development. Developmental self-care requirements fall within two categories:

1. Maintenance of living conditions that support life processes and promote development or progress toward higher levels of organization of human structure and maturation.

2. Provision of care either to prevent the occurrence of deleterious effects of conditions that can affect human development or to mitigate or overcome these effects from various conditions.

Self-care activities develop in everyday life through learning and can be affected by genetic and constitutional factors, culture, life experiences, and health state. The nurse is concerned with universal and developmental requirements, although health deviation requirements, such as knowledge and skill needs for self-care in illness, must be attended to if they arise.

In Orem's model, individuals perform self-care to meet the needs and demands consistent with their age, maturation, experience, resources, and sociocultural background. In her model, three systems are described within professional practice: a compensatory system, a partially compensatory system, and an educative-developmental system. In the compensatory system, the nurse provides total care for the client. This care is most common in acute-care settings, such as hospitals during acute illness episodes. Partially compensatory care is implemented when the nurse and the client share the responsibility for care. Care during rehabilitation from illness or in advanced chronic illness is partially compensatory. In contrast, the *educative-developmental* system gives the client primary responsibility for personal health, with the nurse functioning as a consultant. The educative-developmental system is compatible with self-care in health promotion. Orem's model of self-care has been criticized as it is based on the assumption that individuals are able to exert control over their environments in the pursuit of health. However, many individuals and families do not have control over their physical and social environments, two components that influence health-promotion behaviors. Therefore, it is important to seriously evaluate this assumption when applying the concept to environments in which the ability to change factors may be limited.

The educative-developmental component of nursing practice is now viewed as a reimbursable service by health payors, including managed-care organizations. Major areas of educative-developmental nursing for self-care include enhancing clients' capacities for exercise and physical fitness, nutrition and weight control, stress management, risk reduction, maintenance of family and other social support systems, avoidance of injurious and violent behaviors and substance abuse, and environmental modifications in homes, schools, work sites, and the community to reduce hazards to health and strengthen health-enhancing features. Education, counseling, and environmental interventions directed to these ends are a shared responsibility between the federal government, state and local governments, policy makers, health care providers, community leaders, and individuals.

Broad-based efforts to activate the general public for self-care need to be spearheaded by nurses in collaboration with other health professionals and community members. Activation of consumers to "take charge" of their health is based on the assumptions that consumers need to be:

1. Actively involved in solving health problems.
2. Making rational and informed choices about health and health care.
3. Developing competencies and skills that foster creativity and adaptation amid changing life circumstances.
4. Striving for greater mastery of environmental conditions that influence health and well-being.
5. Promoting public policy to build healthy communities.
6. Advocating for financing plans that pay for self-care education for all people.

Individuals, families, and communities need to be empowered for health promotion. Advances will be achieved when all groups work in concert to make health promotion a coherent social movement that influences the quality and cost of health care delivery. Successful self-care programs for health promotion need to be integrated throughout educational and health care sectors, while tailoring them to fit local needs. In addition, self-care concepts need to be incorporated into the curricula for health professionals.

Self-Care for Health Promotion Throughout the Life Span

Children and Adolescents

Children represent the potential for a healthy society (Earls & Carlson, 2001). This population poses multiple challenges, as almost one-third have a chronic health problem by the time they reach adolescence (Earls & Carlson, 2001). Childhood is a critical period in the adoption of healthy behaviors and a health-promoting lifestyle. Behaviors are developed and learned based on developmental level, social and physical environment, and personal experiences. Thus, health-promotion efforts need to begin before certain behavior patterns solidify.

Childhood is a developmental period during which social and cognitive skills for autonomous decision making and health behaviors are developed. As with adults, health behaviors can be linked to family support and socioeconomic variables and socialization through family, schools, and media. As discussed in Chapter 13, socioeconomic status plays a significant role in health behaviors, as increased socioeconomic status enables the family to provide resources, such as more affluent school systems, nutritional food choices, and access to multiple physical activities (Drukker, Kaplan, Feron, & van Os, 2003). The family environment plays a significant role in self-care for health promotion through positive, stable childhood experiences. A supportive family environment shapes the child's behavior through the use of rewards and punishment in behavior choices. Family support in participating in self-care behaviors has also been shown to facilitate the development of healthy behaviors such as physical activity.

Schools traditionally concentrated on the role of peer pressure in the adoption of self-care behaviors, rather than focusing on health in the curriculum, beginning in the early school years. However, efforts have been expanded based on research showing that targeted education can make a difference in the adoption of healthy behaviors. Most children are exposed to television and electronic media, two health information sources that continue to expand. Children who participated in an Internet-based nutrition program called the 5 A Day Virtual Classroom, which encouraged them to eat more fruits and vegetables, were asked how to get other children across the country to eat "5 a day" (DiSorgra & Glanz, 2000). Suggestions included use of mass media, economic incentives, and social influence. The most frequently mentioned suggestion was to reward children for eating fruits and vegetables. Evaluation of an Internet health site that provides information on drugs, contraception, and other topics of interest to adolescents indicated that the web site was an anonymous, accessible site that provided up-to-date information and help. Over half (55%) of the responders said they had changed their behaviors as a result of answers they had received (Michaud & Colom, 2003). Internet-based programs such as "5 a day" are effective in providing information to promote self-care as well as obtaining valuable information from the consumer's perspective to develop effective health-promotion interventions.

Adolescence is a critical period of physical, cognitive, emotional, and social development in a dynamic and uncertain period between childhood and adulthood (Murray & Zenter, 2000). Developmentally, it is a time characterized by change and transitions. The primary biological transition is puberty. Cognitively, adolescents begin to think more abstractly. However, as children, they lack the ability to apply their cognitive skills to solving problems in stressful situations. This has implications for behavioral choices under stress, such as being pressured by peers to drink alcohol or experiment with illegal drugs. Socially, the family remains an important source of support. Parents can play a positive role in providing emotional support and encouragement and promoting healthy peer interactions, as peers also serve as important role models.

An important area of adolescent health is sexuality. Adolescents have a higher rate of unprotected sex and sexually transmitted infections than adults, and teen pregnancy in the United States is nine times higher than in Europe (Meschke, Bartholomae, & Zentall, 2002). Sexuality is influenced by neighborhood, peers, family, and individual characteristics, making it a complex issue to address. Parents are the primary sex educators for children, and adolescents who feel a positive connection to their family are less likely to participate in risky behaviors. Critical parental factors include communication, values, monitoring and control, and support. The importance of parental factors has resulted in the development of adolescent health-promotion programs with a parent component (Meschke et al., 2002). While these programs vary in the amount of parental involvement, results indicate that programs that strengthen parent-adolescent relationships result in self-care that promotes healthy adolescent sexual behavior.

Health-related factors have been examined that might predict age at first intercourse in African American and white adolescent females (Felton & Bartoces, 2002). African American girls with fewer problem-solving skills than their peers were five times more likely to have early intercourse, three times more likely to practice fewer health-promoting behaviors, and seven times more likely to have fewer years of education. These findings suggest that self-care interventions need to be tailored to high-risk groups of adolescents to promote healthy self-care practices in sexuality.

Approaches to enhance the health-promoting behaviors of children and adolescents should focus on both families and peer groups. This dual approach is critical, since values, attitudes, beliefs, and behaviors of both families and peers influence children's and adolescent's lifestyles. Parents serve as powerful role models of health and health-related behaviors. The rapid developmental changes that occur for children and adolescents and the emerging yet malleable behavioral patterns that will carry into adulthood make the preschool and school-age years an ideal time to enhance skills for preventive and health-promoting behaviors. Many groups and persons influence the lifestyle behaviors of adults, including peers, religious groups, popular singers, athletes, teachers, and other adults in their lives. Peer groups play a critical role in molding lifestyles for school-age children, particularly adolescents. When peers reinforce the active health consumer role, peer pressure becomes a positive force.

An increasing number of school health programs are giving considerable attention to lifestyle education to increase children's health and resilience and teach skills to modify peer group affiliations and resist the pressure of peers who encourage health-damaging behaviors. School-based health-promotion research provides valuable information about effective interventions that promote adoption of healthy self-care behaviors in children and adolescents. The Child and Adolescent Trial for Cardiovascular Health (CATCH), the largest school-based trial ever sponsored by the National Institutes of Health (Perry et al., 1997), was implemented into 56 schools in four states. The interventions consisted of an Eat Smart food service program, a physical education program, classroom curricula, and parental involvement programs. The third- to fifth-grade curricula focused on choosing healthy foods, physical activity, and intentions to smoke tobacco. Two-and-one-half years after implementing the interventions in the schools, significant changes were still evident in the food service program and physical education classes, and the children in the intervention schools had made significant changes in eating and physical activity self-care behaviors. At the 3-year follow-up, significant differences still existed for dietary knowledge, physical activity, and intentions. In addition, differences in fat intake were evident in the fifth- and eighth-grade groups. The findings of sustained physical activity is especially significant in light of accumulating evidence of a decline in physical activity among youth because of television and computer games, which require minimal physical exertion. At 5-year follow-up, although adherence had decreased, the Eat Smart program had been maintained as a result of policy changes in food services (Hoelscher et al., 2004). In addition, elements of the classroom curriculum had been maintained over time, although they were weak. The physical activity materials were also still in wide use. Findings from this large study indicate that self-care behaviors can be initiated and sustained with school-based interventions that include institutional changes, personal changes, and family support for the program and encouragement of their children to actively participate, as well as involvement in the family activities sponsored by the program. Training school personnel appears to be an essential component in promoting institutionalization and implementation of school health education programs. In addition, the programs need to be compatible with the school environment, goals, and mandates. In other words, they need to be flexible so that they can be individualized and compatible with current practices. The primary barriers to institutionalization include a low priority for health-promotion activities, time constraints of schools, lack of mechanisms for training, and lack of funds for materials, equipment, and lower-fat vendor products (Lytle, Ward, Nader, Pederson, & Williston, 2003).

Several nurse researchers are conducting programs of research to promote self-care in adopting health behaviors in children and adolescents. Harrell and colleagues (1998) at the University of North Carolina initially conducted research to promote cardiovascular health in third and fourth graders. The intervention in the Cardiovascular Health in Children (CHIC) study consisted of an 8-week knowledge and attitude program and a physical education program. One year following the intervention significant improvements were noted in both knowledge and cholesterol levels in those who received the intervention. In another study Harrell implemented a school-based intervention in youth ages 11 to 14 years. An intervention that combined exercise and education resulted in the greatest changes on blood pressure and oxygen capacity (McMurray et al., 2002). More recent research by Dr. Harrell and colleagues (2003) indicates that physical activity, measured by MET levels, progressively decreases between the sixth and eighth grades in school. These results point to the need to find ways to encourage adolescents to participate in more vigorous activities and reduce time in sedentary activities. For example, computer and television use time can be limited daily and participation in community and family outdoor physical activities can be planned and fostered. At both the family and community levels, new physical activities need to be developed and fostered that involve participation by peers as well as family members. Walking instead of riding needs to be rewarded in this group.

Felton, a nurse researcher, and her colleagues (2002) also have a sustained program of research that targets child and adolescent health behaviors. Results of their research indicate that families and the community must be included in the intervention with the child. Participation in community sports has been shown to be a self-care activity important for the development of regular physical activity. "Best" friends have also been found to have a significant influence on the adoption of risky behaviors, pointing to the importance of peers in the development of healthy and unhealthy behaviors. Additional research has found that African American girls in middle schools in rural and urban areas were less active physically than white girls, spent more time watching television, and had greater BMIs. Access to sports equipment, perceived safety, and physical activity self-efficacy were higher in white girls. This research points to the need to focus on both the individual as well as the physical and social environments to promote self-care for healthy behaviors. Hendricks (1998), another nurse scientist, found that levels of hope and self-efficacy are critical concepts in developing interventions to empower adolescents to make healthy behavior lifestyle choices. This finding has been validated in a school-based physical activity intervention in adolescent girls, which indicates that self-efficacy can be changed to increase participation in physical activity (Dishman et al., 2004).

Loveland-Cherry (2000) has investigated the role of the family in the use and misuse of alcohol in fourth-grade children. Her results indicate that self-efficacy, parent-child interactions, and family and peer adjustment are correlated with alcohol use/misuse. Results of a family-based intervention to study the effects of changing parental norms and behavior to prevent or delay adolescent alcohol use resulted in later initiation of alcohol use and less subsequent misuse for adolescents who had reported no use of alcohol prior to the intervention. However, there was no change in those who were using alcohol before beginning the program. Dr. Loveland-Cherry's research has shown that family interventions can promote healthy behaviors to prevent substance abuse in adolescents before they begin these unhealthy behaviors (Loveland-Cherry, 2000; Tuttle, Melnyk, & Loveland-Cherry, 2002).

Children and youth who have dropped out of school or are homeless need special attention in developing self-care behaviors for health promotion (Murray & Zenter, 2000; Nies & McEwen, 2001). Education sessions for these children may have to take place in parks, food kitchens, or homeless shelters. Children of one-parent families as well as "latch key youth" of two working parents may also require special attention (Nies & McEwen, 2001). Special sensitivity to the lack of resources for daily living, lack of parental influence and supervision, and low levels of motivation because of life conditions is critical for promoting a healthy lifestyle.

Young and Middle-Age Adults

Young and middle-age adulthood is the time in the life cycle when many persons are intensely involved in careers and child rearing. The momentum of everyday life and demands of dependent others may leave little time for focusing on health in the absence of an illness crisis. Strengthening support within the family for self-care is particularly important at this time. Adults need to accept responsibility for modeling and teaching younger and older children competent self-care; increasing family knowledge and expertise with health-promotion skills; and learning how and when to use health care resources for the family. Adult learners bring many assets to self-care education, including a background of life experiences, self-direction in learning, problem- or interest-centered (as opposed to subject-centered) learning needs, and interest in immediate, rather than delayed, application. Self-care education for adults consists of the following components (Whitehead & Russell, 2004):

1. Provide time to express feelings.
2. Express a supportive attitude.
3. Reinforce client self-esteem.
4. Provide access to health information.
5. Learn self-care skills that can be applied immediately.
6. Present alternative views on health issues.
7. Offer all views related to complementary self-care therapies.

8. Provide timely feedback and reinforcement.

9. Provide flexible learning pathways.

Adults who are tuned in to their own needs for self-care may be more effective in reducing the stress inherent in multiple societal roles, including family and work responsibilities. Systematically planning health-promotion activities into daily routines at work or with family members can both enhance health in a busy lifestyle and model healthy lifestyles to family members. For example, physical activities can be planned prior to dinner rather than watching television. Or, if feasible, the children can be walked to school, rather than driven. Adequate attention to self-care during the young and middle-age years promotes optimal productivity and life satisfaction and lays the groundwork for a healthy and productive retirement and old age.

Activities of everyday life shape and influence the health of family members (Christensen, 2003). Family practices either promote or hinder the development of good health habits and well-being in children. Life transitions, such as having children and beginning paid work, are associated with physical inactivity in women (Brown & Trost, 2003). In addition, inequalities in education between partners is associated with increased health risks, specifically having one partner with low educational attainment (Monden, van Lenthe, De Graaf, & Kraaykamp, 2003). This finding is thought to be due to material (housing quality, living conditions) and psychosocial (social support, stress, coping) factors that in turn affect the spouse's health. Education is strongly associated with lifestyles, such as smoking and dietary behaviors. Nursing interventions need to pay attention to the social context and implement interventions within the family that take into consideration family demands, employment status, and educational levels to promote self-care for healthy behaviors for partners and their children (Artazcoz, Borrell, Benach, Cortes, & Rohlfs, 2003).

Older Adults

Older adults are the fastest growing population group in the United States. Research indicates that chronic health problems associated with old age can be prevented or postponed and controlled with health behaviors such as regular exercise and good nutrition. However, fewer than 10% of persons over age 65 regularly exercise and less than 40% consume the recommended five servings a day of fruits and vegetables (Clark, Nigg, Green, Riebe, & Saunders, 2002).

Self-care for older adults focuses on maximizing independence, vigor, and life satisfaction. Health promotion in this population is vital to prevent complications and decrease risks that reduce life quality (Davidhizer, Eshelman, & Moody, 2002). Ability for self-care is high for many elders and most function well. The ability for self-care must be transformed into self-care activity to maintain and improve health and well-being. Self-care education must take into account the physical, sensory, mobility, sexual, and psychosocial changes that accompany aging as well as feelings of dissatisfaction and helplessness that have been reported in the elderly (Soderhamn, Lindencrona, & Ek, 2000). Physical activity and smoking cessation make a significant difference in morbidity and mortality in older persons (Brawley, Rejeski, & King, 2003). Exercise can enhance the self-esteem of older adults and in some cases decrease depression and anxiety. Sedentary activity, such as television viewing, can be replaced with physical activity. This approach is as useful with the elderly as it has been in children and young adults. In persons age 65 and older, maintaining independence and activity enhances their well-being, pointing to the need for ongoing health promotion to promote self-care to maintain a regular physical activity program. Barriers that the elderly have identified, including psychological and health barriers, need to be addressed in these programs (De Bourdeaudhuij & Sallis, 2002). Psychological barriers such as loneliness and depression are common in this age group. Health barriers may include limited mobility or vision and hearing difficulties.

Personality and coping styles do not appear to change significantly with age. Thus, persons who develop positive coping skills early in life can meet social demands in later years, find meaning in life, and direct ample energy to appropriate self-care activities. Older individuals who have been characterized as information seekers have been found to have greater health-promoting behaviors. Information seeking included reading articles about health, listening to television or radio programs, talking with friends, and performing self-examinations. Other patterns linked with health-promoting behaviors and well-being include positive perceptions of one's health and aging, involvement in groups and organizations, and contact with family members (Benjamini, Idler, Levanthal, & Levanthal, 2000).

Retirement is a significant life event that presents a major challenge for the older population financially, socially, and emotionally. The challenges will be magnified as the length of time an individual will live following retirement continues to increase. Appropriate self-care in the form of anticipatory planning is associated with successful adaptation. Gioiella's (1983) self-care actions that facilitate healthy retirement are still timely:

1. Planning ahead to ensure adequate income.
2. Developing friends not associated with work.
3. Decreasing time at work in the last years before retirement by taking longer vacations, working shorter days, or working part-time.
4. Developing routines, including adequate physical activity, to replace the structure of the workday.
5. Relying on other people and groups in addition to spouse to fill leisure time.
6. Developing leisure time activities before retirement that are realistic in energy and monetary cost.
7. Anticipating that exhilaration will be followed by ambivalence before satisfaction with one's retirement lifestyle develops.
8. Assessing living arrangements and, if relocation is necessary, expending time in developing new social networks.
9. Expecting job role loss will have a short-term effect on self-esteem and one's marital relationship.

Older adults often have more time available for the pursuit of personal wellness than younger adults. They should be challenged to use this time productively and counseled about resources available within the community to facilitate such efforts.

The fastest growing segment of the U.S. population is the group age 85 and over. Less than one-fourth of the persons in this age group live in nursing homes, so these elderly individuals need safe, health-enhancing communities as well as support services to assist them in continuing health-promotion activities that focus on quality versus quantity of life. With adequate support from families and health professionals and access to resources, many older adults choose to remain in their own home throughout their old age. The nation must address the scope of health-promotion services needed by the elderly to support their self-care capabilities. The Study of Exercise and Nutrition In Older Rhode Islanders (SENIOR) project is a community-based intervention to increase physical activity and intake of fruits and vegetables in community-dwelling older adults (Clark et al., 2002). Programs such as this one can facilitate healthy behaviors and provide the support to enable elders to remain independent as long as possible. Cost-effective and efficient methods for developing these services using available technologies, such as web-based communication to augment personal contact, are needed, as the elderly are rapidly becoming computer literate. Major attention is devoted to promoting the health and well-being of older adults, a rapidly growing segment of the U.S. citizenry.

Health and well-being in old age depends on freedom from disease, functional status, and adequate social and environmental supports (Kim, Bengtson, Myers, & Eun, 2000). Promotion of self-care activities to maintain and improve functional status includes strategies for safe mobility and prevention of falls as well as activities to promote social functioning and integration. All evidence to date indicates that the elderly can become physically fit. However, it is much easier to remain physically active if this self-care behavior has been developed earlier in life.

Self-care for health promotion in older women needs attention because of different experiences of aging and old age in women. Women live longer than men and are more likely to live their later years alone with substantially lower incomes, more vulnerability to poverty, and more chronic health conditions than men in the same age group (Department of Health and Human Services, Health Maternal and Child Health Bureau, 2003). Barriers to participation in health-promotion activities in older women include transportation, scheduling, and cost factors (Kim, June, & Song, 2003). However, low-cost interventions can be implemented in communities, such as walking groups. Health-promotion programs for older women should address two issues (Kim et al., 2003). First, it has been established that the physical and mental health of older women is closely related to their place of residence. Institutional environments and living alone are negative influences on the performance of health behaviors. Second, health promotion with older women needs to include strategies for long-term performance of healthy behaviors. Many challenges and opportunities are presented for women as they age in America. Nurses and the health care system must respond to the issues that prevent elderly women from being able to participate in healthy behaviors, such as fear of leaving the security of their home or lack of transportation. Frameworks of women's health may be useful in guiding self-care interventions for women (Kar, Pascual, & Chickering, 1999). These frameworks take into account the social context in which women experience their lives as well as their perceptions of their health and well-being, factors that must be incorporated into all health-promotion activities.

Goals of Health Education for Self–Care

Education of the public for self-care is an integral part of a number of federal documents and policies, including *Healthy People 2010* (U.S. Department of Health and Human Services, 2000), and has begun to be a viable and visible focus for federal health expenditures. Only a small percentage of the federal budget is actually spent on health education activities. Within the federal government, the Office of Disease Prevention and Health Promotion (ODPHP), the Office on Smoking and Health (OSH), the Office of Women's Health, the Center for Minority Health, and the Centers for Disease Control and Prevention are examples of major agencies focused on meeting the health education needs of the public. National goals for health education for self-care are not well articulated in a single document but exist in numerous documents that address various self-care issues, such as those related to cardiovascular health, mental health, child development, nutrition, and elimination of health disparities. Recommended goals in the public and private sectors for self-care education directed toward disease prevention and health promotion include:

1. Continue to increase the consciousness of the American people about major threats to health that are preventable, and provide individual, group, and environmental means to eliminate these threats.

2. Change those who define health as only the absence of disease to expand the definition to high-level wellness among individuals, families, and communities.

3. Create conditions and resources to empower communities for self-care to address social and environmental ills that prevent the achievement of well-being.

4. Create financial and other incentives to foster active health-information seeking and positive health practices.

5. Assist people in developing the requisite knowledge and skills to successfully implement health-promoting and preventive behaviors.

6. Design and implement culturally and socioeconomically appropriate health-enhancing program strategies for health promotion for diverse populations.

7. Implement curricula to provide the educational base in preschool, elementary, and secondary schools to develop behaviors for healthy living throughout the life span.

To achieve these goals, health policy makers and health professionals must be particularly sensitive to the extent to which problems of literacy and poverty present barriers to health education, discussed in Chapter 13. Approaches to self-care education that use community workers and communication media such as radio that do not require reading but are accessible to a vast majority of the population are important in educating low literacy populations about self-care needs and strategies. Competent self-care must also be economically plausible to individuals and families living in poverty. This requires coordination of public, private, and volunteer services to provide coherent self-care education and options to facilitate responsible yet low-cost health-promotion programs and services, such as walking and jogging trails and programs and peer support groups for adolescents and adults who are trying to change unhealthy behaviors.

The Process of Empowering for Self-Care to Promote Health

Empowerment is a process through which individuals gain mastery over their lives (Kar et al., 1999). The aim of empowerment is to enable clients to take proactive actions to promote the positive aspects of their lives. In other words, empowerment is the means to improve quality of life. Empowerment is a multilevel construct (Kar et al., 1999). In the case of self-care, empowerment is an enabling process directed at the individual. However, empowerment can also be directed at the community or the organization. When individuals are empowered, they have the self-efficacy, awareness, knowledge, and competency to take proactive actions to reach their health-promotion goals. Health education empowers individuals, as it provides the tools for self-care.

Responses of individuals and groups to the process of health education for self-care are multidimensional and complex. The client brings to the learning situation a unique personality and learning style, established social interaction patterns, numerous group affiliations, cultural norms and values, proximal and distal environmental influences, and a given level of readiness to adopt self-care behaviors. The nurse also comes with innate personality characteristics, values, attitudes, and social circumstances that affect the nature of the interaction. The self-care education process as a collaborative endeavor between client and nurse is depicted in Figure 12–1. The interaction for self-care education brings the professional expertise of nurses and other health care professionals together with the health care knowledge and goals of the client. Mutual assessment of health care competencies, strengths, and needs by the client and nurse will decide the learning priorities, the pace of learning (long-term and short-term objectives), and the interpersonal and environmental support needed for learning. Barriers to learning and implementing self-care behaviors need to be identified and directly addressed with clients. Failure to identify and

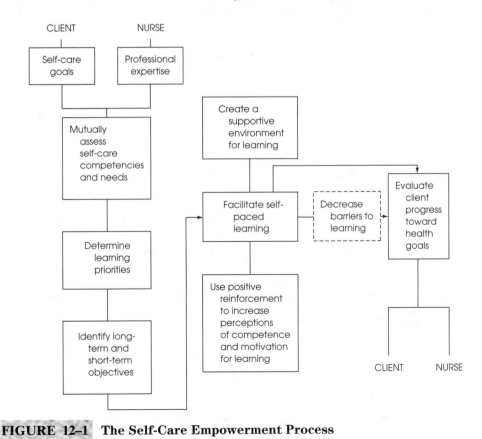

FIGURE 12–1 **The Self-Care Empowerment Process**

decrease barriers can result in frustration and a lack of satisfaction for clients when they evaluate progress toward their self-care goals. Specific components of the self-care empowerment process are described in the following text.

A review of interventions to promote dietary change behaviors indicates that medium-to high-intensity interventions promote larger changes than low-intensity interventions (Pignone et al., 2003). Interventions using self-help materials and interactive communications, including computer-generated telephone or mail messages, along with brief health care provider sessions, reduced fat consumption and increased intake of fruits and vegetables. These types of interventions are feasible to be implemented by nurses in their practice.

Mutually Assessing Self-Care Competencies and Needs

The client often comes to the encounter with health care professionals with certain self-care goals in mind. Competencies related to these goals can be assessed through informal discussion, health-knowledge checklists (as shown in Figure 12–2), or structured tests of

---

In the list below, please check those behaviors that you are comfortable in performing for yourself without assistance from others.

_____ Counting my pulse at the wrist for 1 minute

_____ Counting my pulse at the neck for 1 minute

_____ Selecting comfortable and appropriate shoes for brisk walking or jogging

_____ Selecting appropriate clothing for walking or jogging activities

_____ Planning a progressive schedule of exercise to meet my personal needs

_____ Indicating the ideal weight range for my height

_____ Calculating my maximal heart rate during exercise

_____ Planning time for exercise that is convenient and possible

_____ Selecting warm-up exercises that I could do before brisk walking or running

_____ Selecting procedures for cooling down after vigorous exercise

_____ Exercising at least five times a week for 30 minutes

_____ Integrating physical-fitness activities with my recreational interests

_____ Maintaining a record of my progress in physical activity over a period of several months

_____ Eating appropriately before or after vigorous exercise

_____ Avoiding injuries during exercise

FIGURE 12–2   **Health-Skills Checklist for Exercise and Physical Fitness**

knowledge in specific content areas. The first approach is recommended for low-literacy clients or those uncomfortable with paper-and-pencil tasks. Observation of actual behavior, if this is possible, can also provide useful insights.

The activated client is motivated to seek health information that will assist in self-care. Apathy, lack of interest, and inattention should alert the nurse to a lack of motivation on the part of the client. Reasons for lack of interest should be explored so that the nurse can knowledgeably intervene to increase motivation.

Determining Learning Priorities

Deciding where to begin is often a dilemma for the nurse when the client needs information about many different health topics. Clients have definite ideas about what they wish to know and what is important to them. Sometimes interest may not lie in the area that possesses the greatest threat to personal health. As an example, a client may smoke but be more interested in starting to exercise than in quitting smoking. While the nurse may believe that smoking constitutes a more serious threat to the health of the client than a sedentary lifestyle, it is obviously better to be a physically active smoker than an inactive smoker, since risks are synergistic. If an exercise program is implemented, the client may also develop a heightened awareness of the negative impact of smoking on lung capacity and physical endurance. At a later point, the client may exhibit readiness to discuss approaches to smoking cessation based on concrete experiences with the health- and activity-compromising effects of smoking.

Identifying Long-Term and Short-Term Objectives

Identification of both short- and long-term objectives is important in self-care education. Long-term objectives guide large segments of learning. Short-term objectives identify the specific content or activities that must be progressively mastered to meet the long-term objectives. The objectives should be realistic; neither too easy, resulting in boredom, nor too hard, resulting in discouragement. An example of a goal and objectives identification form is presented in Figure 12–3. The form enables the client to check off each objective as it is

Health Goal: Increased Physical Fitness	
Long-Term Objective: To take a brisk walk for 30 minutes five times a week	
Related Short-Term Learning Objectives	**Objectives Attained**
1. Demonstrate how to check my pulse at the neck by counting beats for 10 seconds and multiplying by six. 2. State heart rate that I should achieve during exercise. 3. Demonstrate two warm-up exercises to use before walking. 4. Demonstrate two cool-down exercises to use after brisk walking. 5. Construct a weekly schedule for brisk walking. 6. Map out three different and interesting routes to take when walking.	

FIGURE 12–3 Goal and Objectives Identification Form

attained and maintain awareness of the desired behavioral and health outcomes. Both the nurse and the client should retain a copy for continuing reference and update.

Facilitating Self-Paced Learning

The pace at which a client learns depends on personal motivation, assertiveness, perseverance, skills, and learning style. The pace of learning may also vary with age, health status, and educational level. Self-pacing is important to allow the client to be self-directed and maintain control over the learning process. The pace at which the client meets each short-term objective will vary, and expectations of both the client and the health professional should be adjusted accordingly. The important factor is not how rapidly knowledge or skill is attained but the extent of mastery.

The nurse must be realistic about teaching and learning and accept both good and bad days in clients of all ages. Sometimes the nurse and client will be elated with the results, sometimes discouraged. When efforts are less rewarding than anticipated, the pace of learning should be reviewed carefully. It is possible that expanding the time frame for learning will result in increased success for the client. This is especially true for young children and adolescents, who have less experience in the learning process than do adults.

Using Positive Reinforcement to Increase Perceptions of Competence and Motivation for Learning

In education for self-care, the client, the nurse, and the family of the client all play important roles in reinforcement. The nurse should be attuned to small steps in client progress and use positive reinforcement such as praise and compliments frequently to enhance the client's feelings of success in developing competence in self-care. Cues should be used to facilitate successful responses and immediate feedback should be provided to correct errors in performance. When cues and error feedback are intermingled with positive reinforcement, they are helpful, nonthreatening, and enhance intrinsic motivation. Immediate and consistent reinforcement facilitates rapid learning and assists the client in deriving satisfaction from learning. Once learning has occurred, intermittent reinforcement of the desired response strengthens the behavior, making it more resistant to extinction.

Family members need to learn to serve as sources of support for one another in developing health behaviors. For example, achievement of a specific goal may be rewarded by a family outing in the park or by the family spending time together in a favorite activity at home. It is important for the family to maintain a balance between support and pressure, which will be negatively perceived. By providing mutual support, a sense of healthy interdependence rather than crippling dependence is created within the family.

Actual performance of new behaviors that lead to success is the most powerful way to strengthen self-efficacy (perceived confidence; De Bourdeaudhuij & Sallis, 2002). Other sources of self-efficacy, such as modeling, observational learning, and verbal persuasion, can be learned from the nurse during the educational sessions.

Clients should be made aware of the importance of self-reward or self-reinforcement in the health education process. It is important that they learn to reward their own efforts and achievements, since much of the time, reinforcement for self-care cannot be supplied by others. A schedule of rewards can be tailored by the client to personal preferences. However, use of foods or negative behaviors for reinforcement should be discouraged. It is important that the client also learn to use internal self-reinforcement such as self-praise and self-compliment. Learning to use internal self-reward in an appropriate manner permits the client to be less dependent on the availability of tangible objects to facilitate the learning process.

Creating a Supportive Environment for Learning

The environment in which health education for self-care is provided is vitally important to the success of educational efforts. If a clinic is used for health education, the classrooms should be warm, comfortable, and informal. A desk should not be placed in the room; instead, tables and chairs or sofa and chairs should be placed in a conversational setting. Walls should be pleasant in color with pictures and textured materials used to create a homelike, supportive, and nonthreatening climate. Visual aids in flip-chart form on an easel at a comfortable height to use while seated in a chair are ideal. If very young children are present during the sessions, an area with toys and books may need to be provided for their use. This will minimize parental distraction. If children are old enough to be included in the sessions, they should be actively involved. Often, use of bright colors and interesting figures or designs on flip charts will amuse children and maintain their interest. Children can play an important role in reinforcing learning or in reminding parents and other family members to engage in the recommended behaviors.

To the extent possible, actual materials available in the home should be used in teaching. If a client is expected to use a booklet on low-cholesterol foods at home in preparing meals, the booklet to be used should be the basis for instruction. If the client is learning relaxation techniques, audiotapes and videos for practice must be usable in the client's home. They should be demonstrated in the classroom or clinic and questions regarding their use should be answered. Well-illustrated materials should be supplied liberally to the client to take home to provide reinforcement of knowledge and skills gained during health education sessions.

The minimal time needed for most health instruction is 15 to 30 minutes, so the nurse needs to decide whether individual or small-group teaching methods are to be used. If health education is provided to groups, the groups should be kept small (four to six individuals) to facilitate interaction and attention to the specific needs of group members. A combination of group and individual instruction may also be helpful. A combined approach allows for efficient use of professional time yet meets the unique educative-developmental needs of clients.

Decreasing Barriers to Learning

Barriers to learning can result from various sources: personal values, beliefs, and attitudes; lack of motivation; poor self-concept; or inadequate cognitive or psychomotor skills. Whatever the source, if the client is not making progress, barriers within the individual, as well as the family and the environment, should be explored. Barriers must be identified and reduced or eliminated before progress can continue.

Strategies to manage obstacles to healthy behavior should be an integral part of the health education plan. In this way, problems are addressed systematically, and progress in decreasing barriers can be periodically assessed. The client may be unaware of what is inhibiting progress or reluctant to share information with the nurse. A climate of trust will facilitate communication between the client and the nurse concerning obstacles to learning and performance.

Evaluating Client Progress Toward Health Goals

Evaluation is a collaborative process by which the nurse and client judge to what degree long- and short-term objectives and health goals have been attained. Evaluation involves direct or indirect observation of behavior. The major source of error in direct measurement is observation of the target behaviors during limited clinic or home visits. A source of error in indirect measurement is that self-report by clients may be inaccurate, or clients may ascribe a "halo effect" to themselves, seeing their performance of health behaviors as more frequent or more intensive than they actually are.

A combination of methods should be used in evaluating progress. These may include checklists of objectives (see Figure 5–3), client progress notes, laboratory measurements, paper-and-pencil tests, verbal questioning, and direct observation. The primary purpose of evaluation is to provide an accurate picture of where clients stand in attaining their health goals. The desired outcome from self-care education is knowledge that will enhance self-care behaviors and lead to a healthy lifestyle.

Other Considerations in Self-Care Empowerment

Each client's desire for competence in self-care must be assessed. Some individuals do not want to be responsible for their own self-care but instead wish to function within society in a highly dependent role. Their desire for competence may have been frustrated by a health care system that makes people feel dependent and helpless. It is critical to assess very early the extent to which clients desire to assume responsibility for their own health when they are given the requisite knowledge and skills to do so.

Clients' conceptualization of health will also decide which content is viewed as meaningful in self-care health-promotion education. When health is defined as maintaining stability or avoiding overt illness, prevention behaviors such as immunization, self-examination for signs of cancer, and periodic multiphasic screening may be most important. When health is defined as self-actualization or well-being, emphasis may be placed on relaxation techniques, enhancing self-awareness, environmental appreciation during outdoor physical activity, or developing aspects of self that represent untapped potential. The role culture plays in self-care for health promotion is discussed in Chapter 13.

The Role of the Internet in Self-Care Education

The growth and improvement in the technology of the Internet has made it an attractive channel for health education and promotion (Winefield, Coventry, & Lambert, 2003). Areas such as telemedicine and telecommunication are expected to continue to increase and create partnerships between clients and health care professionals. Consumers now have access to quality up-to-date information on a variety of topics that were not traditionally available. This information has the potential to enhance personal health and quality of life.

A positive aspect of the Internet for self-care is that extensive information is accessible that may be difficult to obtain elsewhere. This information can be shared at anytime in almost any geographic location. This has important implications for persons living in rural or inaccessible areas, persons who are homebound, and persons who work. The anonymity associated with the Internet is another positive aspect for many. Unresolved issues include quality assurance and confidentiality (King, Stokols, Talen, Brassington, & Killingsworth, 2002). The quality of health information available is highly variable, indicating that clients need to learn to evaluate the information. In addition, the Internet is inaccessible to many who do not have adequate financial resources, or lack computer skills or an appropriate literacy level. The "digital divide," which refers to those who have access and those who do not have access, received attention in the *Healthy People 2010* objectives to emphasize the need for information access for all population segments to eliminate the knowledge gap (U.S. Department of Health and Human Services, 2000). Emerging issues that will have to be addressed by this technology include the possibility of diminished involvement in face-to-face interactions with family members and friends as well as weakening attachments to one's local environment with greater access to remote people and places (King et al., 2002). Another potential is the possibility of information overload and stress.

Self-help and support groups who meet online are called Internet newsgroups, Usenet newsgroups, and Usenet support groups (Michaud & Colom, 2003; Nguyen, Carrieri-Kohlman, Rankin, Slaughter, & Stulbarg, 2003). Self-help groups are usually led by a lay person, while support groups are usually led by a health care professional. These virtual support electronic networks enable persons with similar health interests to converse and pose questions, provide mutual information and support, and minimize feelings of isolation (Michaud & Colom, 2003). Nurses need to share knowledge of effective programs and Internet sites that will strengthen the client's role in their self-care.

Mass education available through advanced technology is changing the way the public relates to health care professionals. Young persons perceive the Internet as a primary source of information, not an adjunct to traditional informational modes. Nurses should work to ensure that the information revolution is used to empower individuals and communities and is accessible to those who do not currently benefit because of poverty or other social, environmental, and cultural conditions. In addition, health care professionals need to monitor the content and quality of the sites they recommend (Nguyen et al., 2003). Finally, although Internet users are searching for information, formal evaluation of participant's health outcomes and satisfaction with the information have lagged far behind. Formal evaluations are needed to evaluate the outcomes of Internet-based programs and information to establish the positive effects of this application to health promotion.

Directions for Research in Self-Care

Although self-care has been practiced for centuries, it has only become the focus of research for health professionals in the last two decades. Theoretical work by Orem has been the primary driving force in nursing for empirical work on the various dimensions of self-care and related nursing care systems. Directions for research in self-care to broaden our understanding of this widely occurring but little understood phenomenon include:

1. Identify developmental changes in self-care agency across the life span.
2. Describe how peers influence self-care practices of preadolescents and adolescents.
3. Critically analyze the long-term health care outcomes of self-care.
4. Explore self-care practices outside the domains of traditional health care.
5. Test culturally appropriate interventions to enhance self-care among diverse individuals and families.

Further work is needed both in developing measures of self-care and in designing intervention studies to test the usefulness of self-care strategies.

Directions for Practice in Self-Care

The changing nurse-client relationship in self-care is reflected in the many changes in the health care system. The nurse's role as facilitator, resource, and teacher has become more important than ever before, as clients are asked to assume more responsibility for their health. In today's cost-containment environment, development of health-promoting behaviors at a young age and maintenance of these behaviors throughout the life span is critical. A multidisciplinary team approach is needed to implement health-promotion programs in schools and at work sites, as well as in community locations, that are easily accessible. These programs should target the individual, the family, and social and environmental factors that may facilitate or inhibit adoption of self-care behaviors. Strategies that strengthen family communication and support need to be implemented to promote adoption of healthy behaviors in children and adolescents. The nurse should encourage school systems to include instruction for healthy nutrition, allow for regular physical education, and create after-school opportunities for sports and other activities. Partnerships with churches and community organizations are needed to guide children and adolescents as well as the elderly in healthy activities. Self-care education is complex. However, use of new technologies and active involvement of individuals and their family members in the educational process can help ensure the adoption of healthy behaviors.

SUMMARY

Empowerment for self-care emphasizes the competencies of clients for self-direction and self-responsibility in planning and managing self-care activities. Environmental constraints that impair self-care need to be addressed and resolved to optimize client success. The client should control the content and pace of learning experiences. Educative-supportive care provided by the nurse will enable clients to achieve their health goals. The nurse, in functioning as a resource person, enhances the success of clients in acquiring knowledge and skills in self-care. Further research on the dimensions of self-care within the context of health promotion will provide important information for facilitating optimum self-care across the age continuum.

LEARNING ACTIVITIES

1. Plan a school-based intervention to promote a decrease in television viewing by adolescents, using peer support.
2. Develop long- and short-term objectives to increase physical activity in elders.
3. Describe how you would evaluate the effectiveness of a physical activity program for the elderly.

SELECTED WEB SITES

Children and Adolescents

Bright Futures

http://www.brightfutures.org

Centers for Disease Control Healthy Youth

http://www.cdc.gov/healthyyouth/index.htm

National Institute of Child Health and Human Development

http://www.nichd.nih.gov

Young and Older Adults

Health and Age

http://www.healthandage.com

Healthfinder R

http://www.healthfinder.gov

HealthWeb

http://www.healthweb.org

MEDLINE plus

http://www.medlineplus.gov

National Institute on Aging

http://www.nih.gov/nia

National Women's Health Education Center

http://www.4women.gov

Senior Net

http://www.seniornet.org

REFERENCES

Artazcoz, L., Borrell, C., Benach, J., Cortes, I., & Rohlfs, I. (2003). Women, family demands and health: The importance of employment status and socio-economic position. *Social Science & Medicine, 59*(2), 263–274.

Benjamini, Y., Idler, E. L., Levanthal, H., & Levanthal, E. A. (2000). Positive affect and function as influences on self-assessments of health: Expanding our view beyond illness and disability. *J Gerontol B Psychol Soc Sci, 55*(2), 107–116.

Boote, J., Telford, R., & Cooper, C. (2002). Consumer involvement in health research: A review and research agenda. *Health Policy, 61*, 213–236.

Brawley, L. R., Rejeski, J., & King, A. C. (2003). Promoting physical activity for older adults. *Am. J Prev Med, 25*, 172–183.

Brown, W. J., & Trost, S. G. (2003). Life transitions and changing physical activity patterns in young women. *American Journal of Preventive Medicine, 25*(2), 140–143.

Christensen, P. (2003). The health-promoting family: A conceptual framework for future research. *Social Science & Medicine, 59*(2), 377–387.

Clark, P. G., Nigg, C. R., Green, G., Riebe, D., & Saunders, S. D. (2002). Members of the SENIOR Project Team. The Study of Exercise and Nutrition in Older Rhode Islanders (SENIOR): Translating theory into research. *Health Education Research, 17*(5), 552–561.

Coulter, A. (2003). An unacknowledged workforce: Patients as partners in healthcare. In C. Davies (Ed.), *The future health workforce* (pp. 33–48). New York: Palgrave McMillan.

Davidhizer, R., Eshelman, J., & Moody, M. (2002). Health promotion for aging adults. *Geriatric Nursing, 23*(1), 30–35.

De Bourdeaudhuij, I., & Sallis, J. (2002). Relative contribution of psychosocial variables to the explanation of physical activity in three population-based adult samples. *Preventive Medicine, 34*, 279–288.

Department of Health and Human Services, Health Maternal and Child Health Bureau. (2003). *Women's health USA 2003.* Washington DC: Health Resources and Services Administration.

Dishman, R. K., Motl, R. W., Saunders, R., Felton, G., Ward, D. S., Dowda, M., & Pate, R. R. (2004). Self-efficacy partially mediates the effect of a school-based physical-activity intervention among adolescent girls. *Prev Med, 38*(5), 628–636.

DiSorgra, L., & Glanz, K. (2000). The 5 a Day virtual classroom: An on-line strategy to promote healthful eating. *J AM Diet Assoc, 100*(3), 349–356.

Drukker, M., Kaplan, C., Feron, F., & van Os, J. (2003). Children's health-related quality of life, neighborhood socio-economic deprivation and social capital. A contextual analysis. *Social Science & Medicine, 57*, 825–841.

Earls, F., & Carlson, M. (2001). The social-ecology of child health and well-being. *Annu Rev Public Health, 22*, 143–166.

Felton, G. M., & Bartoces, M. (2002). Predictors of initiation of early sex in black and white adolescent females. *Public Health Nurs, 19*(1), 59–67.

Felton, G. M., Dowda, M., Ward, D. S., Dishman, R. K., Tros, S. G., Saunders, R., & Pate, R. R. (2002). Differences in physical activity between black and white girls living in rural and urban areas. *J Sch Health, 72*(6), 250–255.

Gioiella, E. C. (1983). Healthy aging through knowledge and self care. *Aging Prev, 3*(1), 39–51.

Harrell, J. S., Gansky, S. A., McMurray, R. G., Bangdiwala, S. I., Frauman, A. C., & Bradley, C. B. (1998). School-based interventions improve heart health in children with multiple cardiovascular disease risk factors. *Pediatrics, 102*(2 Pt 1), 371–380.

Harrell, J. S., Pearce, P. F., Markland, E. T., Wilson, K., Bradley, C. B., & McMurray, R. G. (2003). Assessing physical activity in adolescents; common activities of children in 6th–8th grades. *J Am Acad Nurse Pract, 15*(4), 170–178.

Hendricks, C. S. (1998). The influence of race and gender on health promoting behavior determinants of southern "at-risk" adolescents. *ABNF J, 9*(1), 4–10.

Hoelscher, D. M., Feldman, H. A., Johnson, C. C., Lytle, L. A., Osganian, S. K., Parcel, G. S., Kelder, S. H., Stone, E. J., & Nader, P. R. (2004). School-based health education programs can be maintained over time: Results from the CATCH Institutionalization study. *Preventative Medicine, YPMED-01368*, 4C.

Kar, S. B., Pascual, C. A., & Chickering, K. L. (1999). Empowerment of women for health promotion: a meta-analysis. *Social Science and Medicine, 49*, 1431–1640.

Kim, C. G., June, K. J., & Song, R. (2003). Effects of a health-promotion program on cardiovascular risk factors, health behaviors, and life satisfaction in institutionalized elderly women. *International Journal of Nursing Studies, 40*, 375–381.

Kim, K., Bengtson, V. L., Myers, G. C., & Eun, L. (2000). Aging in east and west at the turn of the century. In V. L. Bengston, K. Kim., & J. C. Meyers (Eds.), *Aging in east and west families, states, and the elderly* (pp. 3–16). New York: Springer.

King, A. C., Stokols, D., Talen, E., Brassington, G. S., & Killingsworth, R. N. (2002). Theoretical approaches to the promotion of physical activity: Forging a transdisciplinary paradigm. *Am J Prev Med, 23*(2s), 15–25.

Lenoci, J. M., Telfair, J., Cecil, H., & Edwards, R. R. (2002). Self-care in adults with sickle cell disease. *Western Journal of Nursing Research, 24*(3), 228–245.

Loveland-Cherry, C. J. (2000). Family interventions to prevent substance abuse: Children and adolescents. *Annu Rev Nurs Res, 18*, 195–218.

Lytle, L. A., Ward, J., Nader, P. R., Pederson, S., & Williston, B. J. (2003). Maintenance of a health promotion program in elementary schools: Results from the CATCH-ON study key informant interviews. *Health Educ. Behav, 30*(4), 503–518.

McMurray, R. G., Harrell, J. S., Bangdiwala, S. I., Bradley, C. B., Deng, S., & Levine, A. (2002). A school-based intervention can reduce body fat and blood pressure in young adolescents. *J Adolesc Health, 31*(2), 125–132.

Meschke, L. L., Bartholomae, S., & Zentall, S. R. (2002). Adolescent sexuality and parent-adolescent process: Promoting healthy teen choices. *Journal of Adolescent Health, 31*, 264–279.

Michaud, P. A., & Colom, P. (2003). Implementation and evaluation of an Internet health site for adolescents in Switzerland. *Journal of Adolescent Health, 33*, 287–290.

Monden, C. W. S., van Lenthe, F., De Graaf, N. D., & Kraaykamp, G. (2003). Partner's and own education: Does who you live with matter for self-assessed health, smoking and excessive alcohol consumption? *Social Science & Medicine, 57*, 1901–1912.

Mulatu, M. S., & Berry, J. W. (2001). Cultivating health through multiculturalism. In M. MacLachlan (Ed.), *Cultivating health: Cultural perspectives on promoting health* (pp. 1–12). New York: John Wiley & Sons.

Murray, R. B., & Zenter, J. P. (2000). *Health promotion strategies through the life span* (7th ed.). Upper Saddle River, NJ: Prentice Hall.

Nies, M. A., & McEwen, M. (2001). *Community health nursing* (3rd ed.). Philadelphia: WB Sanders Company.

Nguyen, H. Q., Carrieri-Kohlman, V., Rankin, S. H., Slaughter, R., & Stulbarg, M. S. (2003). Internet-based patient education and support interventions: A review of evaluation studies and directions for future research. *Computers in Biology and Medicine, 34,* 95–112.

Orem, D. E. (1995). *Nursing: Concepts of practice* (5th ed.). New York: McGraw Hill, Inc.

Perry, C. L., Sellers, D. E., Johnson, C., Pedersen, S., Bachman, K. J., Parcel, G. S., Stone, E. J., Luepker, R. V., Wu, M., Nader, P. R., & Cook, K. (1997). The child and adolescent trial for cardiovascular health (CATCH): Intervention, implementation, and feasibility for elementary schools in the United States. *Health Education & Behavior, 24*(6), 716–735.

Pignone, M. P., Ammerman, A., Fernandez, L., Orleans, C. T., Pender, N., Woolf, S., Lohr, K. N., & Sutton, S. (2003). Counseling to promote a healthy diet in adults: A summary of the evidence for the U.S. Preventive Service Task Force. *American Journal of Preventive Medicine, 24*(1), 75–92.

Soderhamn, O., Lindencrona, C., & Ek, A. C. (2000). Ability for self-care among home dwelling elderly people in a health district in Sweden. *International Journal of Nursing Studies, 37,* 361–368.

Tuttle, J., Melnyk, B. M., & Loveland-Cherry, C. (2002). Adolescent drug and alcohol use. Strategies for assessment, intervention, and prevention. *Nurs Clin North Am, 37*(3), 443–460.

U.S. Department of Health and Human Services. (2000, January). *Healthy People 2010* (conference edition in two volumes). Washington, DC: U.S. Government Printing Office.

Whitehead, D., & Russell, G. (2004). How effective are health education programmes—resistance, reactance, rationality and risks: Recommendations for effective practice. *Internal J of Nurs Studies, 41,* 163–172.

Winefield, H. R., Coventry, B. J., & Lambert, V. (2004). Setting up a health education website: Practical advice for health professionals. *Patient Education and Counseling, 53*(2), 175–182.

13

Health Promotion in Vulnerable Populations

OBJECTIVES

1. Discuss the major factors that play a role in health disparities.
2. Describe the concepts in the Vulnerable Populations Model to eliminate health disparities.
3. Describe the continuum of interpersonal skills for cultural competence.
4. Define the major categories or factors that affect health-promotion programs in vulnerable populations.
5. Describe strategies to ensure culturally competent programs.

OUTLINE

- Health Status and Health Behaviors of Vulnerable Groups
- Eliminating Health Disparities
- Planning Culturally Competent Health-Promotion Interventions
- Essential Characteristics to Consider in Designing Programs
- Strategies for Implementing Culturally Appropriate Interventions
- Directions for Research in Vulnerable Populations
- Directions for Practice in Vulnerable Populations
- Summary
- Learning Activities
- Selected Web Sites
- References

As the 21st century unfolds, all health care professionals will be increasingly expected to provide health care to individuals who are poor, socially marginal, or culturally different from the traditional mainstream of society. The values, attitudes, culture, and life circumstances of these individuals and the communities in which they reside must be taken into consideration when planning health-promotion and prevention activities. Taking into account the factors that reflect the diversity of these populations is a key to promoting successful behavior change.

In spite of the improvements in health in the United States during the last century, disparities in health between the majority (white) population and minority populations continue to exist. Health disparities refer to the incidence, prevalence, mortality and burden of diseases, and other adverse health conditions that exist among certain groups of populations in the United States (National Center for Minority Health and Health Disparities, 2001). A report by the National Center for Health Statistics (2001) has documented these disparities for certain racial and ethnic groups. There is growing consensus that health disparities are a result of psychosocial and cultural factors as opposed to genetic differences at the population level (Hogue, 2002). Major reasons for the disparities include socioeconomic factors, language, discrimination, lack of access to care, environmental hazards, and cultural barriers. Eliminating health disparities will require health-promotion and prevention programs that are culturally tailored to enhance our ability to promote effective self-care behaviors. Elimination of health disparities is one of the two major themes of the *Healthy People 2010* objectives (U.S. Department of Health and Human Service, 2000). Although many of the causes of these disparities need the input of society and government, development of health-promotion programs tailored for diverse communities is a realistic goal for nursing.

Health Status and Health Behaviors of Vulnerable Groups

Vulnerable populations are diverse groups of individuals who are at the greatest risk of poor physical, psychological, and/or social health outcomes (Aday, 1999). Vulnerable populations are more likely to develop health problems, usually experience worse health outcomes, and have fewer resources to improve their conditions. Various terms have been used to describe vulnerable populations including *underserved populations*, *special populations*, *medically disadvantaged*, *poverty-stricken populations*, and *American underclasses* (Aday, 1999). Vulnerable groups include persons who experience discrimination, stigma, intolerance, and subordination, and those who are politically marginalized, disenfranchised, and often denied their human rights. Vulnerable populations may include people of color, the poor, non-English-speaking persons, recent immigrants and refugees, homeless persons, mentally ill and disabled persons, gay men and lesbians, and substance abusers.

Societal and environmental factors play major roles in characterizing vulnerable populations (Flaskerud & Winslow, 1998; U.S. Department of Health and Human Services, 2000). Specifically, low socioeconomic status has been documented to be the most consistent predictor of disease and premature deaths in this country. Class-related inequities in mortality rates for three-fourths of all deaths are observed across the life span in almost every country in the world (Sebastian, 1999). Those at greatest risks for increased morbidity and mortality are ethnic and racial minorities, two highly vulnerable groups (Sebastian, 1999). Although there is great diversity among minority populations, overall, minorities have substantially lower incomes than whites. Income is a powerful variable that explains health status. Higher incomes facilitate access to care, better housing in safer neighborhoods, and increased opportunities for healthy food purchases as well as health-promotion programs. The poverty rate continues to be almost three times greater for African Americans and Hispanics than whites (DeNavis-Wait, 2003). Educational attainment is also lower in minority groups. High-risk behaviors have been inversely correlated with lower educational levels (National Center for Health Statistics, 2001). Higher educational levels also enable persons to obtain health-related information at understandable levels.

Socioeconomic status (SES) accounts for much of the observed disparities in health, as a socioeconomic gradient exists for almost every health indicator for every racial and ethnic group (National Center for Health Statistics, 2001). The socioeconomic differences are apparent in risk factors such as smoking, obesity, elevated blood pressure, and sedentary lifestyle as well as insurance coverage, physician visits, and avoidable hospitalizations. However, racial differences persist at equivalent levels of SES (Ward, 2003). Socioeconomic status in minority populations may involve a time component (Anderson, 2003; Nickens, 1997; Spector, 2004). Nichons suggests that populations who have been poor over several generations, suffering ongoing discrimination and frustration without substantial upward movement, may feel powerless and perceive their conditions differently from recently arrived immigrants who are poor but hopeful about their future. Evidence for this hypothesis comes from studies related to birth outcomes and infant mortality. Black-white differences in infant low birth weight and infant mortality have existed for decades and in African Americans is twice that of whites (National Center for Health Statistics, 2001). The differences persist even when the effects of social class, prenatal care, and living conditions are controlled, or when only middle-class populations with access to care are studied. The most significant predictor of black-white differences in infant mortality has been found to be an index of housing segregation, independent of black-white differences in median family income or the prevalence of poverty (Roach, 2000). Thus, racism can affect health status directly as well as indirectly in the stress of experiences of discrimination and the societal stigma of inferiority (Ren, Amick, & Williams, 1999; Ward, 2003).

The health status of Hispanics declines among immigrants as their stay in the United States increases and with succeeding generations (Guendelman, 2000). Rates of infant mortality, adolescent pregnancy, and cigarette, alcohol, and illicit drug use all increase with acculturation. For example, Hispanic women in southern California have been reported to have poorer birth outcomes as they become more acculturated (Guendelman, 2000). Acculturation may increase risk factors for birth outcomes. In addition, acculturation involves abandonment of one's cultural beliefs and assimilation of the dominant society's values.

Access to care can be measured by the proportion of a population that has health insurance. Racial and ethnic minorities are much more likely to be underinsured or lack health insurance (Aday, 1999). When they do have insurance it is likely to be public insurance, primarily Medicaid. Health insurance contributes to the amount and type of health services obtained. Lack of health insurance has important implications for health-promotion and prevention efforts, such as screening and access to wellness programs. Insurance status has been correlated with reported health status. Those who rated their health as fair or poor were more likely to be uninsured than those who rated their health as good or excellent

(Aday, 1999). Racial and ethnic minorities also experience greater barriers in accessing their usual source of care, have more difficulty getting an appointment, and wait longer during appointments. These factors are compounded by the fact that most minority communities mistrust the government and government-controlled programs. Thus, financial and nonfinancial barriers to access of care exist for vulnerable populations. These barriers need to be eliminated to ensure access to quality health care.

Eliminating Health Disparities

The Vulnerable Population Model focuses on the major personal and environmental resources needed to achieve and maintain health, thereby eliminating health disparities, and is shown in Figure 13–1. The model, adapted from Flaskerud and Winslow (1998) and *Healthy People 2010* (U.S. Department of Health and Human Services, 2000), incorporates social capital, socioeconomic status, sociocultural context, access to and quality of care, risk factors for disease, and health outcomes. Social capital, socioeconomic status, sociocultural context, and access/quality of care are factors that may affect individuals, either positively or negatively, and indicate the availability or lack of resources thereby predicting vulnerability. *Social capital* refers to features of social relationships, including levels of interpersonal trust and norms of reciprocity and mutual aid. Social capital reflects the quantity and quality of interactions with family, friends, coworkers, and others in the community. When these ties are weak or absent, vulnerability may result. *Socioeconomic status*, including income, employment, and education, is considered a human factor that influences vulnerability. A higher education level correlates with greater decision making, a better economic situation, and a higher awareness about the benefits and risks to health. However, education cannot achieve its potential if young people do not attend school because of poverty and other social conditions. In addition, children cannot learn effectively

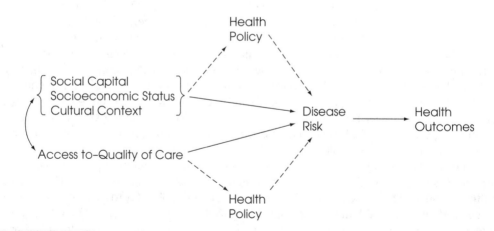

FIGURE 13–1 **Vulnerable Populations Model**

(Adapted from J. Flaskerud and B. Winslow, 1998, "Conceptualizing Vulnerable Populations Health-related Research," *Nursing Research*, 47(2), 69–78.)

if they are hungry or suffer from undue stress. The *cultural context* refers to cultural beliefs, values, and customs, including cultural explanations of illness, language, religious or spiritual beliefs, and personal life experiences that play a role in health outcomes. *Access to care* depends on health insurance, transportation, and understanding of the health care system. *Quality of care* is also related to health outcomes, and those who receive a lower quality of care, including poor access, have poorer health outcomes. *Risk for disease* refers to factors that increase one's susceptibility for disease. Risk factors may be personal or present in the physical environment. Vulnerable groups have higher risk behaviors related to dietary intake, weight, activity level, cigarette smoking, and alcohol and illicit drug intake (Resnicow, Braithwaite, Dilorio, & Glanz, 2002). The relationship between availability of resources (social capital, socioeconomic status, cultural context) and disease risks proposes that fewer resources increase one's risks. This relationship has consistently been documented in adolescents and adults (National Center for Health Statistics, 2001). Second, risks are related to health outcomes. Birth and death rates, life expectancy, morbidity from specific diseases, life expectancy, accessibility of health care, and many other factors can be used to measure *health outcomes.* The relationship between risks for disease and morbidity and mortality has been observed in all populations. Risk factors are higher in those who live in poverty and lack resources. As risk factors increase, morbidity also increases. The relationship between resources, risk factors, and mortality has also been documented. Health policy is proposed to mediate the relationships between social capital, socioeconomic status, and risks and between access to and quality of care and disease risks. *Health policy* can promote individual and community health through health-promotion campaigns, mandates, and accessible services. The role of policy in influencing both risks and health outcomes points to the need for a community and societal perspective. Aday (1999) also proposes that a community perspective offers the most promise to reshape policy to eliminate the health disparities in vulnerable populations.

The Office of Minority Health, the National Center for Minority Health and Health Disparities (NCMHD), and the U.S. Department of Health and Human Services (USD-HHS) were established to focus on closing the gap in health disparities (Fiscella, Franks, Gold, & Clancy, 2000). The NCMHD supports research to uncover knowledge to eliminate the disproportionate burden of ill health among minority Americans. African Americans, Asian and Pacific Islanders, Hispanics and Latinos, and Native Americans and American Indians are recognized groups who suffer from health disparities. No simple solutions are easily available to eliminate health disparities in this country, or the world, for that matter. However, nurses, as frontline providers with a person-environment perspective, can implement culturally competent individual, family, and community-based programs to begin to tackle this major problem.

Planning Culturally Competent Health-Promotion Interventions

Expertise in cultural competence and sensitivity to differences among cultures is a needed skill, considering the diversity of vulnerable populations and the number of interacting factors operating to create health disparities (Huff & Kline, 1999). Cultural competence is defined as appropriate and effective communication that requires one to be willing to listen and learn from members of diverse populations, and the provision of information and services in appropriate languages, at appropriate comprehension and literacy levels, and in the context of the individual's health beliefs and practices (Chin, 2000). In culturally competent health-promotion programs, the beliefs, interpersonal style, attitudes, and behaviors of individuals and families are respected and incorporated into program planning, implementation, and evaluation activities. Nurses and other health care professionals need to be aware of their own cultural values and beliefs and recognize how these influence their attitudes and behaviors toward another group.

Bushy (1999) describes cultural-linguistic competence as a continuum of interpersonal skills ranging from *ethnocentrism* on one end of the continuum to *enculturation* at the other end of the spectrum. *Ethnocentrism*, one anchoring point on the continuum, refers to assumptions or beliefs that one's own way of behaving or believing is the most preferable and correct one, and therefore the standard by which all cultural groups will be judged. Thus, the beliefs of other cultural groups are devalued or treated with suspicion or hostility. *Cultural awareness*, the next stage on the continuum, refers to an appreciation of and sensitivity to another person's values, beliefs, and practices. Next, *cultural knowledge* refers to gaining understanding and insight of different cultures. The continuum progresses to *cultural change* and then *cultural competence*, the level at which the health care provider is aware, sensitive, and knowledgeable about the other culture, and has the skills to employ appropriate health-promotion activities. *Enculturation*, the opposite anchoring point on the continuum, refers to fully internalizing the values of the other culture. Enculturation is evident when the health care provider develops culturally sensitive health-promotion programs in collaboration with individuals in the cultural group and incorporates members of the cultural group to deliver and evaluate the intervention.

Developing cultural competence is not a linear process. Progress depends on life's experiences, exposures to other cultures, and receptivity to learning about new cultures. Acquisition of cultural competence skills is an ongoing process to ensure the delivery of health-promotion interventions that are appropriate, acceptable, and meaningful for persons of diverse backgrounds. Diversity is embedded in cultural competence, but it is just one component. Accepting and understanding differences in customs and patterns of thinking are ways in which diversity is valued.

Essential Characteristics to Consider in Designing Programs

Characteristics of vulnerable populations that may affect successful health promotion efforts need to be identified in order to achieve goals established by the nurse and client. Huff and Kline (1999) categorize these factors as demographic, cultural, and health care system variables. These characteristics or factors are listed in Table 13–1. Culturally relevant interventions related to some of the characteristics are described in Table 13–2.

Demographic factors are self-explanatory. Language is probably the most salient demographic difference among diverse groups, so knowledge of language spoken is a key feature in the delivery of wellness programs. The inability to communicate creates barriers in

TABLE 13–1 **Characteristics to Assess in Vulnerable Populations***

Demographic Factors	Cultural Factors	Health Care System Factors
Age	Age	Access to Care
Gender	Gender, Class	Insurances, Financial resources
Ethnicity	Worldview	Response to illness
Primary language spoken	Primary language spoken	Orientation to prevention services
Religion	Religious beliefs, practices	Perception of need for services
Education, literacy level	Communication patterns	Distrust of Western medicine
Occupation, income	Social customs, values	Experience with system
Area of residence	Traditional health beliefs and practices	Western vs. folk health beliefs and practices
Transportation	Dietary preferences and practices	Communication concerns
Duration in United States	Generation in United States	

*Adapted from K.M. Huff and M.V. Kline, 1999, *Promoting Health in Multicultural Populations*, Thousand Oaks: Sage Publications.

accessing wellness or screening programs as well as health care, or it may result in errors and/or inappropriate care. Even in English-speaking minority clients, communication may be problematic, as clients may not fully understand the information and avoid further verbal communication to get their questions answered. In 2001, the Office of Minority Health published standards for cultural and linguistic services in health care. Three standards specifically address the need to provide language assistance services, including bilingual staff and interpreter services, verbal and written notices of their rights in their preferred language, and assurances of competent language assistance to those with limited English proficiency (Anderson, Scrimshaw, Fullilove, & Frelding, 2003).

Geographic location is another major barrier, as the physical environment plays a major role in promoting healthy behaviors (Cohen, Farley, & Mason, 2003). Poor neighborhoods are likely to be associated with areas that are unattractive and dangerous. Research on "walkability" indicates that attractive, aesthetically pleasing settings are more conducive to physical activity (Brownson et al., 2000). Fear may be a major factor in limiting outside activities due to such things as drug sales or violence. Poor neighborhoods have fewer services available, such as clinics or community centers and public transportation. In addition, limited services, such as grocery stores, often result in higher prices paid for fresh fruits and vegetables that may be scarce and of lesser quality.

Cultural factors that may affect the success of health education also need to be identified. For example, some cultures may believe that life is predetermined, and nothing can be done to change things. Social customs and norms need to be known, as such things as touching, shaking hands, eye contact, or smiling may have different connotations. Religious practices may also serve as potential barriers, and certain practices may need to be taken into consideration when planning for health promotion. For example, prayer and chanting, dancing rituals, and purification ceremonies are important in the Native American culture to reestablish harmony in one's physical, mental, and spiritual life. The nurse must work within the cultural religious framework in the health-promotion encounter.

TABLE 13–2 Culturally Relevant Intervention Strategies for Vulnerable Populations

Characteristic	Strategy
Communication	- Assess primary language spoken, knowledge of English, literacy level - Use same language as target culture - Understand cultural meanings of health terms - Explore cultural explanations of health - Use culturally specific medias to deliver messages - Involve community in developmental activities
Family relationships	- Understand role of family and extended family in health - Involve family in health-promotion activities - Assess religion and its role in family - Acknowledge role of church and incorporate church network
Time orientation	- Explore time orientation of target culture - Understand meaning of "clock" time - Tailor message to dominant time orientation (i.e., present, past, future)
Access/acceptance of health-promotion programs	- Assess barriers to accessibility of health-promotion programs - Assess environmental resources of community - Use existing community sites to deliver programs, such as churches and schools - Incorporate health-promotion activities into ongoing community activities - Explore cultural values about participating in health-promotion activities such as exercise

Adapted from C. Keller and K. Stevens, 1997, "Cultural Considerations in Promoting Wellness," *Journal of Cardiovascular Nursing, 11*(3), 15–25.

Verbal and nonverbal communication, body language, and word meanings vary across cultures. In low-literacy groups, abstract concepts may not be understood, so traditional written communication will not be appropriate. Health-promotion programs are more successful when they are delivered in the same language as that of the participants. Therefore, persons who represent the target culture and speak the same language should be involved in the development and implementation of interventions. In addition, culturally specific newspapers, as well as radio and televisions stations, can be targeted to deliver health messages in the meaningful language. Many people will hide their illiteracy due to the stigma attached, so it should never be assumed that someone can read or follow written or complex verbal instructions. Functional literacy is the ability to read at a fifth-grade level. In the United States, almost half of the population is either functionally illiterate or possesses marginal literacy skills. This has many implications for the choice of communication channels used to deliver wellness interventions.

Family relationships and the concept of family differ in many cultures. In some cultural groups, for example, it is common for the family to include more than the immediate relatives. The needs of the family may be considered subordinate to the needs of the individual in some cultures, such as Asians and Hispanics. In these groups, support from family members is more important than external support. Family members need to be intimately involved to support the individual in lifestyle change or wellness interventions. Family-oriented approaches using family and extended family networks, rather than individual ones, are more likely to be successful in behavior change in African American and Hispanic cultures (National Literacy and Health Program, 1999). In cultures where the woman's role is subordinate, it may be important to emphasize the value of the woman's behavior change for the entire family. Family networks may also include church relationships in certain cultures, because of the social support and communication networks offered (Coe & Keller 1996). In these cultures, the church may be an effective place to implement health-promotion programs. In addition, knowledge of and respect for religious customs is important to promote desired outcomes. Educational strategies should capitalize on the powerful effects of family and church networks to promote behavior change.

Time orientation refers to how the perception of time varies among cultures. Kluckhohn and Strodtbeck (1961), two anthropologists, identified three major time orientations that exist in every society: past, present, and future. A past orientation is based on the importance of tradition and is noted in Asian groups and American Indians. In these cultures deceased relatives are part of the extended family, so the perspective of a deceased family member may be incorporated into their health practices. In the present orientation, the focus is on the here and now. A present orientation is common in vulnerable populations, as the focus is on surviving today and short-term consequences, so the future may have no meaning. Persons with a present orientation have more difficulty changing behaviors, as the current activity is the priority. The future orientation emphasizes planning for time extending from the present. Middle-class Americans are considered to be more future oriented, as they work and plan for retirement and often delay present gratification. Health-promotion programs may appeal to future-oriented persons who want to be healthy in their retirement. However, these people may be so busy working for the future, health and wellness may not be a priority. Knowledge of one's dominant time orientation as well as adherence to "clock" time will eliminate the misunderstanding of response to appointments. Nurses also need to understand how the individual prioritizes time to plan for successful attendance at programs and screening services. Interventions need to take into consideration one's time orientation. For example, present-oriented persons need help in connecting their present lifestyle behaviors with future consequences. Asking for examples of persons in their family or community who may be suffering from the consequences of an unhealthy lifestyle may help make the connection.

Health care system factors are also important to assess prior to health-promotion efforts. Access to programs is an issue because of existing cultural barriers in accessing systems of care (Chin, 2000). Vulnerable populations have more problems accessing care and accepting therapeutic interventions because of costs, distance, transportation, language, and perceived lack of acceptance by health care providers (Murdaugh, Russel, & Sowell, 2002). Missed appointments or program sessions may not mean the individual is not interested in health promotion. Transportation or child care may not be available, or bilingual support may not be adequate. Acceptance of interventions depends on multiple factors, including distrust, interactions with health care providers, and incorporation of the cultural values and lifestyle of the community. Culturally sensitive approaches based on individual and family values enhance access and acceptance of health interventions. Conducting focus groups with individuals in the target community to learn culturally relevant information on which to base interventions has become a successful strategy (National Literacy and Health Program, 1999). Community priorities, problems, and resources need to be identified and resources allocated to promote successful health-promotion efforts. Churches or other sites within the community should be used whenever possible to facilitate easy access as well as a comfortable environment. Mobile clinics that go door to door to screen and provide information are another option.

The Office of Minority Health's (2000) standards for culturally and linguistically appropriate health care services are also relevant for the delivery of health-promotion programs and are summarized in Table 13–3. Health care providers have accepted the need for culturally competent programs. Now standards need to be developed to monitor and evaluate outcomes of culturally competent programs. Programs that improve the quality of life of individuals in the community will lead to the development of competent communities, in which members can identify and begin to solve their own issues.

Giger, Davidhizar, and Poole (1997) propose that health-promotion needs vary across groups based on six cultural phenomena. These phenomena, which are used to assess clients prior to any health-promotion activities, include communication, space, social organization, time, environmental control, and biological variations. Communication and time are described similar to the previous discussion of communication and time characteristics. Space refers to personal space or the area surrounding a person's body that determines the personal boundaries. Individuals in various cultures differ in their need for personal space. Social organization refers to patterns of social behavior that provide explanations for behavior related to life events such as birth, illness, and death. Environmental control refers to the ability to direct activities that influence the natural

---

TABLE 13–3 Recommended Standards for Culturally Appropriate Health-Promotion Programs

1. Acquire the attitudes, behaviors, knowledge, and skills needed to work respectfully and effectively with individuals in a culturally diverse environment.

2. Use formal mechanisms to involve communities in the design and implementation of health-promotion programs.

3. Develop strategies to recruit and retain culturally competent staff who are qualified to address the health-promotion needs of the racial and ethnic communities.

4. Provide ongoing education and training in culturally and linguistically competent program delivery.

5. Provide all participants with limited English proficiency programs conducted in their primary language.

6. Translate and make available signage and commonly used written educational material.

7. Ensure that the participants' birthplace, religion, cultural dietary patterns, and self-identified race/ethnicity are documented.

8. Undertake assessments of cultural competence, integrating measures of satisfaction, quality, and outcomes of health-promotion programs.

Adapted from D. Chin, 2000, "Culturally Competent Health Care," *Public Health Reports, 115*, 25–33.

environment. Finally, biological variations refer to physiologic differences that exist within a racial group. Assessment of the six cultural phenomena enables nurses and other health care providers to respond to the needs of vulnerable populations with appropriate interventions. Research is needed on the significance of these phenomena in promoting behavior change in diverse populations.

Strategies for Implementing Culturally Appropriate Interventions

Strategies to make health-promotion programs and materials more culturally appropriate have been described. These strategies are based on the experiences of health care professionals working with diverse populations. Krueter and colleagues (2002) have divided the strategies into six categories, including *peripheral, evidential, linguistic, constituent involving, socio-cultural,* and *cultural tailoring.*

Peripheral strategies involve packaging programs or materials to give the appearance of cultural appropriateness (Kreuter et al., 2002). Colors, images, pictures, or titles are used to reflect the social and cultural world of the targeted group. Thus, the materials are seen as familiar and comfortable (Bechtel & Davidhizer, 2000). Materials that are matched to one's culture also help establish credibility and create interest, increasing acceptance and receptivity of the information. Herman, a nurse scientist, and Mock, Blackwell, and Hulsey (2004) used ethnocentric colors and pictures of African American women in a brochure to recruit young women for a study to promote healthy behaviors in pregnant African American women.

Evidential strategies are those used to present information to increase the perceived relevance of the topic for the specific cultural group. For example, provision of information on the prevalence of diabetes in some Native American groups compared to other racial/ethnic groups has been used to raise awareness of the issue and promote lifestyle change. The message becomes more meaningful when it is perceived to be applicable to those who are receiving the message.

When materials and programs are provided in the dominant language of the cultural group, *linguistic* strategies are being applied. As mentioned earlier, appropriate language is essential to effective communication. Strategies, such as translating materials or delivering the program in the target culture native language, are essential. Guidelines are available for translating information from one language to another.

Constituentinvolving strategies are implemented to capitalize on the experiences of those within the target population. For example, training and using peers or lay helpers as well as professional members of the target population provides the nurse with additional knowledge about cultural beliefs and values. In addition, members of the population of interest participate in the planning and development of the health education program for members of the community.

Sociocultural strategies involve building upon the group's values and beliefs. In other words, the program is developed to be culturally sensitive for the target population. Implementing sociocultural strategies facilitates the cultural meaningfulness of the material or programs. For example, nurse scientists who are testing interventions to change dietary behaviors in African Americans with Type II diabetes have been more successful when the church site has been used. Anderson-Loftin, Sullivan, Barnett, and Burn (2000) have developed a dietary change intervention that incorporates traditional foods and the social functions of eating for African Americans to promote weight loss. Programs that are culturally meaningful have been shown to be more effective to change behavior in vulnerable populations (Jenkins et al., 2004).

Cultural tailoring strategies are described as any combination of change strategies intended to reach one individual based on characteristics unique to that person. Change strategies are based on an assessment of the individual. Kreuter et al. (2003) differentiate targeted strategies from tailored strategies, in that the group is the focus when targeted strategies are used. Targeted and tailoring strategies should be used in combination, as one takes the individual's (group) culture into account as well as individual differences within the culture. When individual differences are small, the group can be targeted. However, when differences within the culture need attention, cultural tailoring strategies that focus on the individual are also needed.

Directions for Research in Vulnerable Populations

Although evidence indicates that health disparities exist for vulnerable populations, little research has been conducted to define the most effective strategies to eliminate these disparities. In addition, the relative absence of basic information about health behaviors in vulnerable populations limits the development of culturally appropriate health-promotion and disease-prevention interventions. The effects of changing social capital, socioeconomic status, and access and quality of care on health outcomes need continued, rigorous investigation. Interventions that target subpopulations such as adolescents, women, and the elderly also need to be designed and tested, as these subgroups have received even less attention. Research is especially needed to identify and test the most effective ways to recruit vulnerable populations to participate in research and how to keep them involved until the end of the study. Although successful recruitment and retention strategies have been identified, additional strategies need to be identified and implemented.

All types of interdisciplinary research are needed. Qualitative research must be conducted to better understand the influence of cultural beliefs and practices on health behaviors. In addition to studies that focus on individuals and families, community intervention models are needed to effectively evaluate the contribution of communities in improving and promoting health. Research is needed to translate and adapt measurements that have been standardized in the dominant white population for the target culture to ensure sensitive measures of the variables under study. Health service research is another area of opportunity as the effects of organizational change in providing culturally competent health promotion and prevention programs also need to be evaluated. The research questions are endless, and the issues are complex. Vulnerable groups have traditionally been underrepresented in research for many reasons, including ineffective recruitment and retention strategies, lack of attention to culturally sensitive measures and literacy levels, and lack of trust. However, the significance of the questions that need to be asked and the complex issues that must be addressed offer many opportunities for research collaboration among nurse scientists, other health care researchers, and vulnerable populations.

Directions for Practice in Vulnerable Populations

Nurses have multiple opportunities and challenges with vulnerable populations because of the diversity, poverty, and increased risk factors for disease. Prior to working with diverse populations, nurses must become culturally competent by first examining their own attitudes and values and how these may either facilitate or impede culturally appropriate health-promotion efforts. Next, they should make a commitment to become culturally competent as they work with the minority group or subgroup. This may mean becoming immersed in the culture before attempting any health-promotion efforts. Prior to planning health-promotion activities, characteristics mentioned in this chapter need to be assessed in order to develop successful strategies for lifestyle change. Lifestyle change in vulnerable populations is complex due to such factors as potential language difficulties, educational level, poverty, potentially unsafe housing or neighborhoods, and different cultural beliefs. This means that the cultural relevance of health-behavior models that may guide one's practice needs to be examined. New dimensions, such as health care system factors and ecological factors, need to be added to ensure that the models are comprehensive to guide practice interventions in vulnerable populations. In addition, understanding of potential intervening barriers is needed to plan programs that encourage and facilitate healthy lifestyles.

SUMMARY

In the last century, tremendous progress was made in the health of the American people, due to such basic improvements as safe drinking water, advances in sanitation, more nutritious food, and advances in medical care. However, the health status of the poor and minority populations have lagged behind the health of white Americans. Disparities are noted in infant mortality, cardiovascular disease, cerebrovascular disease, diabetes, kidney disease, AIDS, prostate cancer, and other health problems. Vulnerable populations have diverse threats to health that require attention from clinicians, researchers, and policy makers. Although the contributing factors are multiple and complex, many behaviors are due to personal habits as well as social and environmental factors and are amenable to nursing interventions. Nurses, as holistic care providers, are well positioned to take a critical leadership role in designing and implementing culturally competent health-promotion programs for behavior change in diverse populations.

LEARNING ACTIVITIES

1. Perform an assessment of a specific cultural group of your choice using concepts in the Vulnerable Populations Model.
2. Develop a plan describing how you would become culturally competent in a culture different from your own.
3. Develop a program to promote physical activity in Mexican American women using the six strategies discussed in the chapter.

SELECTED WEB SITES

Center for Research on Minority Health

http://www.ncmhd.nih.gov

EthnoMed

http://www.ethnomed.org

Healthy People 2010

http://www.health.gov/healthypeople

Office of Minority Health

http://www.omhrc.gov

Opening Doors

http://www.openingdoors.org

Resources for Cross Cultural Health Care

http://www.diversityrx.org

The Cross Cultural Health Program

http://www.Xculture.org

National Literacy and Health Program

http://www.brhp.cpha.cd

REFERENCES

Aday, L. A. (1999). Vulnerable populations: A community-oriented perspective. In J. G. Sebastian & A. Bushy (Eds.), *Special populations in the community: Advances in reducing health disparities* (pp. 313–330). Maryland: Aspen Publications, Inc.

Anderson, L. M., Scrimshaw, S. C., Fullilove, M. T., & Fielding, J. E. (2003). Task force on community preventive services. The community guide's model for linking the social environment to health. *Am J Prev Med, 24*(3S0), 12–20.

Anderson, R. T. (2003). Quality of care among disadvantaged women: Adding income level to health datasets. *Women's Health Issues, 13*, 177–179.

Anderson-Loftin, W., Sullivan, P., Barnett, S., & Burn, P. S. (2000). Culturally competent dietary education for southern, rural African Americans with Type 2 diabetes. *Diabetes Educator, 28*(2), 821–832.

Bechtel, G., & Davidhizer, R. (2000). Integrating cultural diversity in patient education. *Semin Nurse Manag, 7*, 193–197.

Brownson, R. C., Eyler, A. A., King, A. C., Brown, D. R., Shyu, Y. L., & Sallis, J. F. (2000). Patterns and correlates of physical activity among U.S. women 40 years and older. *American Journal of Public Health, 90,* 264–270.

Bushy, A. (1999). Resiliency and social support. In J. G. Sebastian & A. Bushy (Eds.), *Special populations in the community: Advances in reducing health disparities* (pp. 189–195). Maryland: Aspen Publications, Inc.

Chin, J. L. (2000). Culturally competent health care. *Public Health Reports, 115,* 25–33.

Coe, K., & Keller, C. (1996). Health protective behaviors of young African-American women: Should we be using a kinship model to teach health behaviors? *Journal of Human Ecology, 5,* 61–70.

Cohen, D. A., Farley, T. A., & Mason, K. (2003). Why is poverty unhealthy? Social and physical mediators. *Social Science & Medicine, 57,* 1631–1641.

DeNavis-Wait, C. (2003). U.S. Census Bureau, current population reports, series, 60–226. *Income, poverty, and health insurance in the United States: 2003.* Washington DC: U.S. Government Printing Office.

Fiscella, K., Franks, P., Gold, M. R., & Clancy, C. M. (2000). Inequality in quality: Addressing socioeconomic, racial, and ethnic disparities in health care. *JAMA, 283*(19), 2579–2584.

Flaskerud, J. H., & Winslow, B. J. (1998). Conceptualizing vulnerable populations health-related research. *Nursing Research, 47*(2), 69–78.

Giger, J., Davidhizar, R., & Poole, V. L. (1997). Health promotion among ethnic minorities: The importance of cultural phenomena. *Rehabilitation Nursing, 22*(6), 303–307.

Guendelman, S. (2000). Immigrants may hold clues to protecting health during pregnancy. In M. S. Jamner & D. Stokols (Eds.), *Promoting human wellness* (pp. 222–257). Berkeley: University of California Press.

Herman, J., Mock, K., Blackwell, D., & Hulsey, T. (2004). Use of a social support web site by low-income pregnant African American women. (Unpublished manuscript).

Hogue, C. J. (2002). Toward a systematic approach to understanding and eliminating African American women's health disparities. *Women's Health Issues, 12*(3), 222–237.

Huff, R. M., & Kline, M. V. (1999). *Promoting health in multicultural populations.* Thousand Oaks, CA: Sage Publications.

Jenkins, C., McNary, S., Zheng, D., et al. (2004). Reducing health disparities for African Americans with diabetes. Progress made by the REACH 2010 Charleston and Georgetown Diabetes Coalition. *Public Health Reports;* 119(3), 322–330.

Kluckhohn, F. R., & Strodtbeck, F. L. (1961). *Variation in value orientations.* Westport, CO: Glenwood Press.

Kreuter, M. W., Lukwago, S. N., Bucholtz, D. C., Clark, E. M., & Thompson, V. S. (2003). Achieving cultural appropriateness in health promotion programs: Targeted and tailored approaches. *Health Education and Behavior, 30*(2), 133–146.

Murdaugh, C. L., Russel, R. B., & Sowell, R. (2002). Using focus groups to develop a culturally sensitive videotape interaction for HIV positive women. *Journal of Advanced Nursing, 32*(6) 1507–1513.

National Center for Health Statistics (2003). *Health, United States, 2003 with chartbook on trends in the health of Americans.* (PHS) 2003–1232.

National Center on Minority Health and Health Disparities (2001). Annual Report on health disparities. Available online at: *http://ncmhd.gov/our_programs/strategies/AnnRptHealthDisparities.asp*

National Literacy and Health Program. (1999). *Directory of plain language health information.* Canadian Public Health Association: Ottawa, Canada.

Nickens, H. W. (1997). The role of race/ethnicity and social class in minority health status. In C. Harrington & C. Estes (Eds.), *Health policy and nursing* (2nd ed., pp. 31–40). Boston: Jones and Bartlett.

Office of Minority Health Resources Center. (2000). Assessing culture competence in health case: Recommendations for national standards and an outcome-focused research agenda [accessed December 22, 2000]. Available online at: *http://www.omhrc.gov/clas/index.htm*

Ren, X. S., Amick, B. C., & Williams, D. R. (1999). Racial/ethnic disparities in health: The interplay between discrimination and socioeconomic status. *Ethn Dis, 9*(2), 151–165.

Resnicow, K., Braithwaite, R. L., Dilorio, C., & Glanz, K. (2002). Applying theory to culturally diverse populations. In K. Glanz, B. K. Rimer, & F. M. Lewis (Eds.), *Health behavior and health education* (3rd ed., pp. 485–509). San Francisco: Jossey-Bass.

Roach, M. (2000). Race and health. In M. S. Jamner & D. Stokols (Eds.), *Promoting human wellness* (pp. 258–293). Berkeley: University of California Press.

Sebastian, J. G. (1999). Definition and theory underlying vulnerability. In J. G. Sebastian & A. Bushy, *Special populations in the community: Advances in reducing health disparities* (pp. 3–9). Maryland: Aspen Publications, Inc.

Spector, R. E. (2004). *Cultural diversity in health and illness* (6th ed.). New Jersey: Pearson Prentice Hall.

U.S. Department of Health and Human Services. (2000, January). *Health People 2010* (conference edition). Washington DC: U.S. Department of Health and Human Services.

Ward, L. S. (2003). Race as a variable in cross-culture research. *Nursing Outlook, 51*, 120–125.

Part 6

Approaches for Promoting a Healthier Society

14

Health Promotion in Community Settings

OBJECTIVES

1. Discuss the role of the family unit in promoting the health of individuals in the family.
2. Describe four components of a successful school health-promotion program.
3. Discuss four advantages of the workplace as a setting for health-promotion programs.
4. Explain the rationale for nursing centers to increase their emphasis on health promotion.
5. List the factors that facilitate successful community health-promotion programs.
6. Discuss the domains of expertise needed to develop community partnerships.

OUTLINE

- Health Promotion in Families
- Health Promotion in Schools
- Health Promotion at the Work Site
- Health Promotion in Nurse-Managed Community Health Centers
- The Community at Large as a Setting for Health Promotion
- Creating Health Partnerships
- The Role of Partnerships in Education, Research, and Practice
- Directions for Research in Multilevel Health-Promotion Settings

The value of health-promotion services for improving the health of populations is recognized worldwide but insurance companies continue to be reluctant to include health-promotion benefits in their reimbursement plans. Integrated services among providers in a variety of settings are needed if people of all ages are to benefit from quality, gender, and culture-sensitive health-promotive care. These services should be delivered at sites where people are and where they spend many of their waking hours. This chapter provides an overview of health-promotion settings from families and schools to the community at large. Partnerships to foster health-promotion services in the community, as well as multi-agency collaboration, are also explored as keys to fostering healthy lifestyles within diverse populations.

Health Promotion in Families

Health values, attitudes, and health-related behaviors are learned in the family context. Factors that influence values, attitudes, and behaviors include the family structure, employment patterns, gender and age differences, stage of parenting, family dynamics, communication patterns, power relations, and decision-making processes (Christensen, 2004). Just as individuals must assume responsibility for their own health status, so must families assume similar responsibilities for the health of the family as a unit. The essential role of the family is to build human capital by investing in the health, education, values, and skills of its members to enable them to have productive roles in society (Bubolz, 2001). The family is the major social unit responsible for the socialization of children, so it is an ideal target for health-promotion and prevention efforts.

Traditional approaches to families have either focused on family structure or family functioning. The structural approach defines how family members are by their relationship to each other, such as a parent. The focus on family functioning offers a way to describe what families do together in order to meet their needs within a context of mutual responsibility. Another theoretical approach for understanding families is the ecocultural approach, which places a strong emphasis on how families maintain their everyday routines (Christensen, 2004). Three factors are important to assess in the ecocultural approach: (a) the relationship of the family to earning a living, neighborhood safety, transportation, and so forth, and how the family balances these issues with efforts to sustain daily routines; (b) the meaningfulness or moral and cultural significance of everyday routines; and (c) the congruence or balance between the family's needs and goals. This approach enables the nurse to obtain a detailed view of the health practices of families, as it enables one to assess if the daily family routines hinder or promote the development of good health.

Specific questions that should be explored in relation to family values, beliefs, and lifestyle include the following: (a) How does the family define health? (b) What health-promoting behaviors does the family engage in regularly? (c) What health-promoting behaviors are particularly enjoyable to family members? (d) Do all family members engage in these behaviors or are patterns of participation highly variable throughout the family system? (e) Is there consistency between stated family health values and their health actions? (f) What are the explicit or implicit health goals of the family? (g) What factors are operating to prevent health-promoting behaviors? (h) What resources are available to facilitate health-promoting behaviors?

Variant family forms are common in today's society. Family units may be traditional two-parent families, one-parent families (most often mother only), blended families (parts of two preexisting families), extended families (nuclear plus a relative, often older), augmented families (additional members, not blood relations), married adults, and unmarried adults (blood and non-blood relations). Families are as diverse as individuals. The nurse working with families in health promotion must be sensitive to both the commonalities and differences across varying family forms. Understanding the milieu for the promotion of health in nontraditional families is essential to successful family health promotion counseling and behavioral interventions.

The family is a pivotal group to decrease risky behaviors and increase healthy behaviors among its members. Families exert three types of influences: cultural/attitudinal, such as church attendance or current school success; social/interpersonal, including social support and family caring; and intrapersonal, such as self-esteem, coping, depression, self-efficacy, and loneliness (Grunbaum, Tortolero, Weller, & Gingiss, 2000). Because of the importance of family, interventions have focused on improving parenting skills and family relationships. There are less disruptive behaviors of children in families that improve parenting skills and solve marital problems (Loveland-Cherry, 2000). Home-based family interventions that focus on parenting, as well as the adolescent at risk, to decrease alcohol use and misuse among adolescents have also been successful. Loveland-Cherry, a nurse scientist, has shown that family interventions can reduce adolescent alcohol use and misuse that can be sustained for up to 4 years (Loveland-Cherry, Ross, & Kaufman, 1999). The GREAT Families Program was designed to address parenting practices and family relationships to prevent and reduce violent and aggressive behavior in students at risk for these behaviors (Phillips-Smith et al., 2004). All of these programs support the importance of connectedness of children and adolescents with caring families.

Families demonstrate a spectrum of abilities, insights, and strengths. The challenge for the nurse is to assist the family unit to identify relevant health goals, plan for positive lifestyle changes, and capitalize on their strengths to achieve desired health outcomes. Nursing care directed at improving health behaviors in the family unit should include assessing current family lifestyle; planning collaboratively with the family for positive and enjoyable behavior change; promoting knowledge and skills, and increasing the collective efficacy of family members to implement change; and evaluating family health behavior and health outcomes. Prenatal and postnatal visits with families offer windows of opportunity to initiate discussions of family health promotion. Motivation to create healthy family environments is optimal during parenting in early infancy and childhood. Health-promotion counseling and strategic support enables family members to exert control over family health behaviors and health status.

Health Promotion in Schools

Since the majority of the nation's children are enrolled in elementary and secondary schools, school-based health-promotion programs can be implemented to increase the health-promoting behaviors among children and adolescents before certain behavior patterns solidify. Schools should be health-enhancing environments that build resilience and assist children to develop healthy behaviors such as positive nutrition and regular exercise. Teachers and school health personnel set the normative expectations for healthy behaviors and serve as role models for health-enhancing lifestyles. Positive peer influences need to be nurtured to foster health-promoting rather than health-damaging behaviors. Parents who are interested and involved in creating healthy school environments and model healthy lifestyles in the home environment are also crucial to the success of school-based health-promotion programs.

The "Five C's," competence, confidence, character, connection, and caring/compassion, are key attributes of positive youth development (Lerner & Thompson, 2002). Programs that focus on developing these attributes help children and adolescents develop into healthy, productive adults. Key features of effective programs have been identified that take into account both individuality and social context. Programs that are known to be effective have the following components (Lerner & Thompson, 2002). The programs:

1. are predicated on a vision of positive development.
2. focus on participation in all facets of the program, including design, conduct, and evaluation.
3. pay attention to group diversity.
4. are conducted in accessible, safe settings.
5. recognize the interrelated challenges facing children and adolescents.
6. provide integrated support services.
7. provide training to adult leaders.
8. emphasize life-skills development.
9. incorporate program evaluation.

These features offer a gold standard by which to measure the adequacy and sensitivity of programs to promote healthy behaviors for diverse populations. The first programs to target health promotion in schools focused on the individual and provided information about potential health threats and risks of certain behaviors (Maes & Lierens, 2003). In the second phase of program development, the influence of parents, peers, and other environmental influences began to be addressed. Both of these phases were based on the assumption that individuals determine their lifestyle. Most school-based interventions focused on specific topics such as physical activity, smoking cessation, or dietary behaviors and were based on individual-level theories, such as social cognitive theory, to promote change. These programs usually provided health education within the confines of the school curriculum. More recently, influences of the social and physical environment have been fully recognized and are beginning to be incorporated into school-based programs. More diverse theories are also being applied that take into consideration the social context. The Gatehouse Project is a program that targeted three aspects of the school social context: security, communication, and participation (Patton, Bond, Butler, & Glover, 2003). School-wide strategies, such as mentoring programs, promotion of positive classroom climates, and introduction of a curriculum to promote social and emotional skills, were the main components. Substantial positive changes were noted in behaviors of children in the intervention schools, including a reduction in health-risk behaviors. The findings document the value of including the individual as well as the social context of the school, where young people spend over a third of their waking hours.

The Child and Adolescent Trial for Cardiovascular Health (CATCH) is one of the largest school-based health education studies conducted in the United States (Hoelscher et al., 2004). The study was designed to decrease risk factors for heart disease in children and included a curriculum component augmented by a family component, a physical activity component, a school food service component, and a program to promote smoke-free school policies. Evaluation 5 years following the intervention indicates that changes in the environment to support healthy behaviors can be maintained. However, compliance was less than desired. The researchers concluded that staff training is a significant factor in achieving institutionalization of these programs.

Physical activity, a major public health concern, has been the focus of many larger-scale school-based interventions. These interventions are based on the rationale that physical activity during childhood may enhance health, both short term and throughout later life. The "Move It Groove It" school-based intervention for children 7 to 10 years old was shown to improve fundamental movement skills as well as increase vigorous exercise in both boys and girls (van Beurden et al., 2003). A 2-year follow-up of 24 middle schools that participated in an intervention to increase physical activity and decrease high-fat food consumption showed that the intervention was effective in increasing physical activity in boys, but not girls (Sallis et al., 2003). A better understanding is needed of gender differences in health promotion as well as barriers to implementation and participation.

Health-promoting behaviors are acquired more readily in childhood, when routines and habits are being formed. Habits or behaviors developed in childhood and adolescence are more likely to persist as an integral part of one's lifestyle than changes made in health behaviors later in the adult years. Development of healthy behaviors in very young children is critical to increasing the prevalence of healthy lifestyles in the total population.

Health Promotion at the Work Site

The escalating costs of health insurance benefits have motivated employers to implement work-site prevention and health-promotion initiatives to control costs and maintain a healthy and productive workforce. Work sites offer access to large numbers of adults and serve as a vehicle for delivering interventions at multiple levels, including individual, interpersonal, environmental, and organizational (Sorensen, Linnan, & Hunt, 2004). These programs can create and maintain social norms for healthy behaviors. These programs may increase productivity, decrease absenteeism, decrease use of expensive medical care, and lower disability claims, resulting ultimately in a more productive and globally competitive workforce. Comprehensive programs are more likely to have successful long-term results if they address risk-reduction counseling, modify workplace policies, and make changes in the physical work environment.

Work-site wellness programs range from annual events, such as health fairs, to ongoing comprehensive programs (Shephard, 2000). Some programs are only available to employees of a certain rank, or the work site may subsidize membership at an independently operated facility. Programs typically include on-site exercise capabilities, and opportunities to improve diet, quit smoking, control substance abuse, relieve stress, and control obesity (Shephard, 2000). A multifaceted on-site program is likely to attract and retain a broader spectrum of workers and is more cost effective. Offering a variety of health-promotion programs at the work site, using differing approaches, increases the appeal of the program to employees of varying cultural backgrounds and of differing ages. Although work-site programs are increasing in major corporations, they remain rare in companies that employ less than 50 people (Shephard, 2000).

Work-site programs create a cultural milieu that supports health-promoting behaviors. For example, smoke-free workplaces have made major contributions to recent declines in cigarette smoking in both the United States and Australia. Policy changes also result in a decrease in exposure of nonsmokers to environmental tobacco smoke at the work site.

Workplace programs have many strengths including access to employees during the workday over an extended period of time. Opportunities are increased to change policies and promote environmental support to enhance employees' healthy behaviors. The potential is increased to modify social norms and increase interpersonal support for coworkers who are motivated to change. Finally, employers have opportunities to offer incentives to reward healthy behaviors. Change in workplace cultures is important to achieve broad-based support for health-promotion programs. Examples of changes at the work site following management training for health promotion included availability of health materials, healthier foods in cafeterias and vending machines, healthier snacks at meetings, discounted rates at fitness centers for employees and families, periodic health screening, and on-site health fairs.

Work-site programs offer a range of approaches that may be used to promote wellness at the work site. Work-site behavioral skill interventions have been shown to increase physical activity and enjoyment of exercise if employees are encouraged to exercise and taught behavioral skills to maintain exercise such as goal setting, time management, self-talk, social support building, relapse prevention, and environmental modification (Nichols et al., 2000). In addition, work-site-based initiatives to increase fruit and vegetable consumption have been effective (Beresford et al., 2001; Sorensen et al., 2004). Effectiveness increases if programs are based on a social ecological approach, address multiple risk factors for change, and integrate families and neighborhoods. Nurses need to identify barriers and facilitators to change within work sites as well as key policy and program components that are most effective in promoting change.

Including families in work-site health-promotion programs is of interest because many employers also pay health care costs for family members. Smokers are more likely to have spouses who smoke, and individuals with physically active spouses are more likely to be active themselves. Their children are also likely to be more active. Some companies have also invited teachers from local schools to participate in work-site programs to ensure consistency and integration of health-promotion concepts across schools and work sites. This effort, if expanded, may give rise to "seamless" health-promotion programming in communities that would accelerate behavior change efforts across the life span.

The major weakness of work-site programs is that they attract only a limited number of employees (Shephard, 2000). Barriers that are usually mentioned include the time commitment and availability of on-site facilities and programs. Nurses who are employed in these settings are challenged to integrate the programs so that as many employees as possible can benefit.

Work-site health-promotion programs are projected to expand in the future, as healthy lifestyles help contain health care costs. Programs that include attention to physical and mental health, as well as social health, increase the overall effectiveness of the company as well as the health and life quality of the employee. Exciting possibilities exist for integrating these programs into a coordinated community effort.

Health Promotion in Nurse-Managed Community Health Centers

Nurse-managed community health centers represent an ideal setting for offering a spectrum of services including health-promotion and prevention counseling, behavioral interventions to promote healthy lifestyles, and screening to detect health risks. The hallmark of nurse-managed community health centers is primary care delivered by nurses. A focus on the "individual and family" rather than "the presenting illness" has enhanced the appeal of nurse-managed centers to deliver care to a growing segment of the population. Many families prefer to obtain health care from nurse practitioners in a setting that is user friendly and respectful of their unique assets and needs. Nurse-managed centers provide family-oriented, culturally sensitive care to diverse populations. Many families need assistance with healthy parenting or meeting the health-promotion needs of family members. Nurse-managed centers may include direct care services as well as education classes, small group support sessions, and family and individual counseling. Family-focused activities of nurse-managed centers address a growing community need. Computerized systems to track client outcomes must be accessible to collect information needed to evaluate the quality and cost effectiveness of health-promotion services and programs delivered in nurse-managed centers as well as provide evidence for future reimbursement of nursing practice.

The University of South Carolina founded the Children and Family Healthcare Center in 1998 to provide primary health care to children who were placed in protective custody because of abuse or potential abuse. The Center has been expanded to offer comprehensive services to children and families in the surrounding community. Pediatric and family nurse practitioner faculty members provide immunizations, well-baby checkups, and health-promotion and preventive services for children and adults, as well as 24-hour primary care services. The Center also serves a large population of adolescents who are in foster care. This nurse-managed center is located in a former shopping center in a low-income area of town. Local artists have painted colorful murals on the walls. Children who attend the Center for the first time may visit the "secret closet" to select a stuffed animal or toy donated by community groups. Girl Scout troops and church groups keep the closet stocked. Reimbursement from Medicaid and other third-party reimbursement, private pay and various state and federal programs, and grants and contracts support the Center to maintain fiscal stability.

Nurse-managed centers are located in diverse environments in order to be accessible to populations served. Some centers are located at or near schools to help meet the health needs of children and adolescents in a confidential and developmentally appropriate manner. Nurse-managed centers are also located in malls, storefronts, or housing developments to provide access to people where they congregate or spend time when not at school or work. Nurse-managed centers offer care that enhances the health and well-being of all family members. The centers also offer interdisciplinary care that provides a range of health and social services and integrated care that covers the life span of families and individuals.

The continued national emphasis on cost containment in health care has made nurse-managed centers appealing as an integral component of the health care system. Evaluation of nurse-managed centers indicates that participants are highly satisfied with services, health outcomes can be improved, the quality of care is good, and cost savings can be realized (Badger & McArthur, 2003; Hildebrandt, Baisch, Lundeen, Bell-Calvin, & Kelber, 2003). Opportunities to link university nursing programs and nurse-managed centers are particularly attractive, as the latest scientific developments may be implemented to improve services through evidence-based practice. In addition, the primary practice settings are ideal clinical practice sites for students, as they offer preceptors, nursing models of care are role modeled, and students are exposed to diverse populations and community-based care.

Nurses need to address legislative impediments that constrain the establishment of nurse-managed centers and the provision of reimbursed health-promotion and prevention services to individuals and families. Nurse-managed centers are uniquely positioned in the health care system to negotiate with managed care organizations to be primary care providers to a growing segment of the population. Both professional and lay organizations should continue concerted efforts to bring nurse-managed community health centers into the mainstream of health-promotion and prevention services.

The Community at Large as a Setting for Health Promotion

Changing the health behavior of communities rather than individuals is based on the premise that community organizing and community building are central to community health education and promotion (Minkler, 2002). Community-based health-promotion and prevention programs encompass a range of activities such as health education, risk-reduction intervention programs, environmental awareness and improvement programs, and initiatives to change laws or regulatory policies to be supportive of health.

Four basic values influence the success of health care professionals who work in communities (Minkler, 2002). Communities are different from health care systems, so skills and values needed in the community are not the same as those that have been effective in the medical system. The values are as follows.

1. Health care professionals respect the wisdom of the community.
2. Health care professionals share health information in an understandable form.
3. Health care professionals use their capacities, skills, contacts, and resources to strengthen the power of the community.
4. Health care professionals focus on capacities, not needs and deficiencies.

Community activation, a health-promotion strategy, includes organized efforts to increase community awareness and consensus about health problems, coordinate health-promotion partnerships to plan environmental change, allocate resources across organizations within the community, and promote citizen involvement in these processes. Community activation matches programs to "real" community needs identified by those who reside in the community. The community is a "living" organism with interactive webs among organizations, neighborhoods, families, and friends. The challenge of community activation is to involve community members in all aspects of planning to achieve goals they have defined.

An implementation model for community programs needs to be responsive to issues and problems raised during program planning and implementation. Four principles facilitate community capacity building and ownership of the project (Potvin, Cargo, McComber, Delormier, & Macaulay, 2003).

1. Community members are integrated as equal partners.
2. Intervention and evaluation components need to be integrated.
3. Organizational and program flexibility is necessary to be responsive to demands in the community environment.
4. The program should be a learning project for all involved.

These principles were confirmed in a community project in which a malaria vaccine was tested (Reeder & Taime, 2003). Words of wisdom from the malaria vaccine research trial included having ongoing knowledge of the community and viewing the community as partners in the work. A community partnership takes a lot of time, people, and resources, and must be based on honesty and respect. Community programs are dynamic processes defined through an ongoing negotiation process among all members.

Community-based health-promotion programs offer an excellent approach to reach impoverished communities with limited resources. Health-promotion services must be provided in the settings where people live, work, and play. Offering nutrition services in churches and mammography screening in malls brings valuable services to people in real-life settings. The synergy of bringing community strengths and resources together and the empowerment that subsequently results from early successes warrant continued attention in designing innovative and culturally sensitive health-promotion programs for large aggregates.

Creating Health Partnerships

Health partnerships across settings are a major strategy to optimize the health of communities. Many economic, social, and health incentives for organizational partnerships exist in the current health care system. Partnerships promote continuity of care in health promotion and prevention and synergistic use of resources to achieve optimal effectiveness and efficiency. Partnerships may consist of any combination of work sites, schools, nursing centers, and other health agencies and universities working together to improve the health of an entire community.

A community partnership is defined as a relationship between collaborating parties (people and organizations) committed to work together to achieve a common purpose

(Roussos & Fawcett, 2000). Community partnerships recognize the value of community members and health care providers working together to create new health care systems that are user friendly, accessible, and culture sensitive. Partnerships optimize the combined resources of all partners so that mutually valued goals are achieved. Health partnerships use community organizations to achieve health empowerment, to improve health in communities of color, and to eliminate health disparities. Thus, community health partnerships incorporate an ecological approach. Partnerships have been organized around a variety of community concerns including adolescent pregnancy, violence, and substance abuse.

In establishing successful health partnerships, a relationship is established that clearly communicates respect for the community's right to identify problems and potential solutions to those problems. Initially the community's norms for participation must be assessed with the following questions.

Is current community problem solving an individual or collective effort?

How in touch are citizens with each other?

What are the units of interaction (e.g., neighborhoods, townships, housing complexes)?

Does crime or other factors deter citizens from interacting?

Some communities have established structures for community planning to address health concerns. Current patterns of citizen involvement, existing relationships among community organizations, and organizations known for activating community involvement (e.g., churches, recreation centers, service clubs) are analyzed to learn how partnerships for health promotion might be shaped in any given community. For some communities, flexible coalitions are the appropriate organizing framework to address community health needs, whereas for others, a leadership board or council is needed to combine the power of key community activists.

An important goal of community partnerships focused on health promotion is empowerment. Community empowerment is defined as social-action processes in which individuals and groups act to gain mastery over their lives through changing their social and political environment (Minkler, 2002). Members of a partnership create conditions that empower their joint efforts. Community partnerships for health promotion have the potential to bring about institutional and policy changes that affect many people. The commitment of partnerships to the broader goals of positive social, structural, and individual change is essential to improving the overall health of communities.

Building partnerships requires substantial time and effort. It is important to acknowledge the diverse interests of partners in the early stages of the partnership and implement strategies to address any cultural gaps that exist. Practice principles that need to be addressed include (Baker, Homan, Schonhoff, & Kreuter, 1999):

1. Find the right mix of ownership and control among partners.
2. Recognize the assets of all partners.
3. Develop relationships based on mutual trust and respect.
4. Acknowledge and honor different partner agendas.
5. Acknowledge the difference between community input and active community involvement.
6. Resolve ethnic, cultural, and ideological differences between and among partners.

A shared vision among partners creates a common identity and a shared purpose. A vision is an image of what partners see as outcomes of their collaboration. A shared vision facilitates a shared mission that identifies the primary reasons for the existence of the partnership. An example of a mission statement is as follows.

To assist individuals and families in the community to adopt healthy lifestyles, and to assist the community to develop culturally sensitive, cost-effective health-promotion and prevention services.

The potential for fostering healthier lives for citizens of all ages lies in the power of partnerships that are multisectoral and reach beyond the bounds of traditional medicine. Partnerships enable members to appropriately plan, implement, and evaluate community-based health-promotion interventions.

A community organization approach to health-promotion partnering is based on concepts of self-determination, shared decision making, bottom-up planning, community problem solving, and cultural relevance. The philosophy underlying this approach is that health promotion is likely to be more successful when the community at risk identifies its own health concerns, develops its own intervention programs, forms a board to make policy decisions, and identifies resources for program implementation. Communities that are empowered through organization and active participation in partnerships develop the skills and abilities to solve problems that compromise their health and well-being. Individual behavior-change efforts are limited without efforts to bring about systematic change through health partnerships.

Community health partnerships bring greater "rationality" to health care expenditures by advocating funding of prevention and health-promotion services by national, state, and private insurers. Politically active partnerships can redirect public and private health care dollars so that they are allocated as depicted in Figure 14–1 with major emphasis on population-based health care services and clinical preventive services. Community participation and positive health policies are key elements for successful community health partnerships.

The Role of Partnerships in Education, Research, and Practice

Multidisciplinary education and collaborative practice experiences with community residents help prepare health professional students for the diversity of health care roles that they will assume over their careers. As care moves from traditional institutions, except for the critically ill, to the community, knowledge and skills to function in diverse community settings are essential to meet the health needs of individuals and families. Gaining access to community educational experiences for students and faculty is a win–win situation for both schools of nursing and communities. For example, students in the early stages of baccalaureate nursing education can experience various aspects of the role of community health worker by distributing health education materials in a community, participating in screening programs, helping organize health fairs, collecting health data from communities, and surveying the use of vending machines and fast-food stores to assess availability

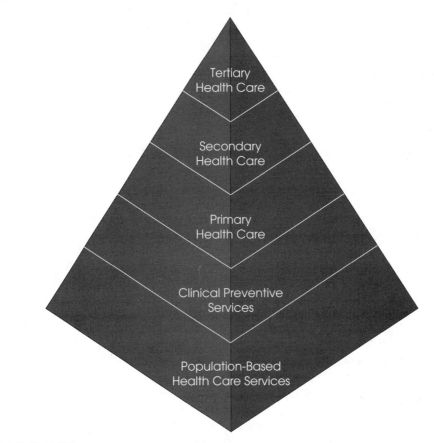

FIGURE 14–1 Health Services Pyramid

(From U.S. Public Health Service, December 1994/January 1995, *A Time for Partnership: Report of State Consultations on the Role of Public Health, Prevention Report,* Washington, DC: U.S. Public Health Service.)

and cost of health-promoting options. Advanced baccalaureate students with a greater understanding of the role of culture and socioeconomic class on health behaviors can provide education classes at schools and work sites, assist community residents in identifying environmental health risks, and provide self-care education to groups of individuals who have similar health-risk profiles.

Graduate students, faculty, and community member representatives provide a strong team for training community health workers in underserved communities. In order to build a successful cohort of community health workers, schools of nursing must (a) establish rapport with the community; (b) collaborate with the community to assess health needs; (c) hire workers from the community to gain the trust and participation of community residents; (d) share program ownership and decision making with community health care workers, empowering them to develop program goals and design strategies for greater effectiveness; (e) facilitate program flexibility so workers are able to adapt to changing needs; and (f) closely link workers with community health and social service agencies so that professional backup is available as necessary (Baker et al., 1999; Roussos & Fawcett, 2000).

The need has never been greater for nursing programs to take an active role in developing enduring health-promotion partnerships. The holistic view of nursing provides the orientation necessary to work collaboratively with communities to accomplish health goals. The escalating need for reform in health care and the economic pressures for cost-effective, multidisciplinary, quality care places nurses in a unique position to make changes in community health care systems.

Community–academic health partnerships are also valuable allies in research. Partnering with universities throughout all stages of assessing, planning, and conducting health-promotion interventions creates a sense of community ownership of the study and takes advantage of the expertise of university faculty. Research community–academic partnerships foster enthusiastic participation, attentiveness to recruitment, thoughtful interpretation of findings, and commitment to dissemination of results to the community.

Community partnerships play a strategic role in creating community capacity to respond to health needs. In addition, partnerships set expectations that the health care system will function as a co-partner with other systems in the community to shape public policy that will foster conditions for healthy living.

Directions for Research in Multilevel Health-Promotion Settings

There is no single method to evaluate the success of interventions that go beyond the individual level. Nurse scientists need to apply diverse evaluation strategies that are effective for families, schools, and communities as units of analysis. Attention to process as well as outcome evaluation is also needed to identify implementation strategies that are most effective in promoting healthy behaviors. Suggested directions for research include:

1. Describing health-promotion and disease-prevention beliefs and practices in diverse families and communities as a basis for designing culturally sensitive interventions.
2. Testing the synergistic effects of school, family, and community health-promotion efforts for adolescents on individual- and community-level health outcomes.
3. Identifying facilitators and barriers to participating in work-site programs.
4. Testing community partnership strategies that optimize community and environmental change.
5. Designing valid and reliable community-level health outcome indicators.
6. Developing uniform methods and measures to assess health outcomes and cost outcomes across a range of programs and communities.

Anecdotal evidence suggests that community partnerships make a difference in health practices and the health of the community. However, few systematic studies have been conducted to test the effectiveness and sustainability of community partnerships, particularly in communities with underserved populations. Partnership intervention studies are critically needed. Interventions need to be carefully documented to identify the effective components. Multiple measures should be used to assess the behavioral, social, and environmental outcomes of partnership activities.

Directions for Practice to Promote Health in Diverse Settings

Multiple settings offer opportunities to provide health-promotion services. Nurses with an understanding of community health issues and problems are ideally suited to provide leadership in the development, implementation, and evaluation of health-promotion programs in schools, work sites, nursing centers, and other community settings. Financial support for such programs should be sought from a variety of public and private sources. The health problems of today are best addressed by many sectors coming together in partnerships to improve social and environmental conditions that compromise health. Partnerships offer a way to communicate, collaborate, and empower to achieve solutions not attainable by single groups or organizations. Particularly exciting is the opportunity for schools of nursing to join with other health professions' schools, health care provider groups, and communities in building health partnerships. These partnerships, designed in a community-sensitive manner, will improve prevention and health-promotion services provided to diverse populations.

SUMMARY

Health-promotion services should be offered in multiple settings to reach diverse populations. Development and maintenance of healthy lifestyles and healthy environments must be a central goal. Programs that involve the community and are tailored to its needs enhance cultural appropriateness and the likelihood of success. Formation of community partnerships creates a network of community residents and health care providers to offer quality health-promotion and prevention services.

LEARNING ACTIVITIES

1. Identify a community-based health-promotion program in your community and assess its effectiveness by interviewing two citizens who live in the community (e.g., the Red Dress Campaign to recognize heart disease as the major killer of women in the United States).

2. Investigate the level of interagency collaboration in a program to promote health or prevent disease in your community. What agencies are present? What agencies need to be involved?

3. Describe the steps you would take to work with an impoverished community to improve access to immunizations for children.

4. Identify a work-site program in your community. Assess its strengths and limitations from the perspective of both the employer and the employee.

SELECTED WEB SITES

Centers for Disease Control and Prevention, National Center for Chronic Disease Prevention and Health Promotion

http://www.cdc.gov/nccdphp/index.htm

Centers for Disease Control and Prevention: The Planned Approach to Community Health (PATCH)

http://www.cdc.gov/nccdphp/patch

Centers for Disease Control Prevention Guidelines

http://www.phppo.cdc.gov/cdcrecommends

Guide to Community Preventive Services

http://www.thecommunityguide.org

REFEWRENCES

Baker, E. A., Homan, S., Schonhoff, R., & Kreuter, M. (1999). Principles of practice for academic/practice/community research partnerships. *American Journal of Preventive Medicine, 16*(3S), 86–93.

Badger, T. A., & McArthur, D. B. (2003). Research briefs: Academic nursing clinic: Impact on health and cost outcomes for vulnerable populations. *Applied Nursing Research, 16*(1), 60–64.

Beresford, S. A. A., Thompson, B., Feng, Z., Christianson, A., McLerran, D., & Patrick, D. L. (2001). Seattle 5 a Day worksite program to increase fruit and vegetable consumption. *Preventive Medicine, 32*, 230–238.

Bubolz, M. M. (2001). Family as source, user, and builder of social capital. *The Journal of Socio Economics, 30*, 129–131.

Christensen, P. (2004). The health-promoting family: A conceptual framework for future research. *Social Science & Medicine.* In press.

Grunbaum, J. A., Tortolero, S., Weller, N., & Gingiss, P. (2000). Brief report: Cultural, social, and intrapersonal factors associated with substance use among alternative high school students. *Addictive Behaviors, 25*(1), 145–151.

Hildebrandt, E., Baisch, M. J., Lundeen, S. P., Bell-Calvin, J., & Kelber, S. (2003). Eleven years of primary health care delivery in an academic nursing center. *Journal of Professional Nursing, 16*(1), 279–288.

Hoelscher, D. M., Feldman, H. A., Johnson, C. C., Lytle, L. A., Osganian, S. K., Parcel, G. S., Kelder, S. H., Stone, E. J., & Nader, P. R. (2004). School-based health education programs can be maintained over time: Results from the CATCH institutionalization study. *Preventive Medicine.* In press.

Lerner, R. M., & Thompson, L. S. (2002). Promoting healthy adolescent behavior and development: Issues in the design and evaluation of effective youth programs. *Journal of Pediatric Nursing, 17*(5), 338–344.

Loveland-Cherry, C. J. (2000). Family interventions to prevent substance abuse: Children and adolescents. *Annu Rev Nurs Res, 18*, 195–218.

Loveland-Cherry, C. J., Ross, L. T., & Kaufman, S. R. (1999). Effects of a home-based family intervention on adolescent alcohol use and misuse. *Stud Alcohol Suppl, 13*, 94–102.

Maes, L., & Lievens, J. (2003). Can the school make a difference? A multilevel analysis of adolescent risk and health behavior. *Social Science & Medicine, 56*, 517–529.

Minkler, M. (2002). *Community organizing and community building for health.* New Brunswick: Rutgers University Press.

Nichols, J. F., Wellman, E., Caparosa, S., Sallis, J. F., Calfas, K. J., & Rowe, R. (2000). Impact of a worksite behavioral skills intervention. *Am J Health Prom, 14*(4), 218–221.

Patton, G., Bond, L., Butler, H., & Glover, S. (2003). Changing schools, changing health? Design and implementation of the gatehouse project. *Journal of Adolescent Health, 33*, 231–239.

Phillips-Smith, E., Gorman-Smith, D., Quinn, W. H., Rabiner, D. L., Tolan, P. H., Winn, D. M., and the Multisite Violence Prevention Project. (2004). Community-based multiple family groups to prevent and reduce violent and aggressive behavior: The GREAT Families Program. *American Journal of Preventive Medicine, 6*(IS), 39–47.

Potvin, L., Cargo, M., McComber, A. M., Delormier, T., & Macaulay, A. C. (2003). Implementing participatory intervention and research in communities: Lessons from the Kahnawake Schools Diabetes Prevention Project in Canada. *Social Science & Medicine, 56*, 1295–1305.

Reeder, J. C., & Taime, J. (2003). Engaging the community in research: Lessons learned from the malaria vaccine trial. *Trends in Parasitology, 19*(6), 281–282.

Roussos, S. T., & Fawcett, S. B. (2000). A review of collaborative partnerships as a strategy for improving community health. *Annu. Rev. Public Health, 21*, 369–402.

Sallis, J. F., McKenzie, T. L., Conway, T. L., Elder, J. P., Prochaska, J. J., Brown, M., Zive, M. M., Marshall, S. J., & Alcaraz, J. E. (2003). Environmental interventions for eating and physical activity: A randomized controlled trial in middle schools. *American Journal of Preventive Medicine, 24*(3), 209–217.

Shephard, R. J. (2000). Worksite health promotion and the older worker. *International Journal of Industrial Ergonomics, 25*, 465–475.

Sorensen, G., Linnan, L., & Hunt, M. K. (2004). Worksite-based research and initiatives to increase fruit and vegetable consumption. *Preventive Medicine.* In press.

van Beurden, E., Barnett, L. M., Zask, A., Dietrich, U. C., Brooks, L. O., & Beard, J. (2003). Can we skill and activate children through primary school physical education lessons? "Move It Groove It"— a collaborative health promotion intervention. *Preventive Medicine, 36*, 493–494.

15

Promoting Health Through Social and Environmental Change

OBJECTIVES

1. Justify the rationale for describing health as a social goal.
2. Describe the common health-damaging factors in the environment and their etiology.
3. Discuss the two opposing approaches to behavior change and the pros and cons of each approach.
4. Describe the role of financial incentives in behavior change.

OUTLINE

- Health as a Social Goal
- Health in a Changing Social Environment
- Promoting Health Through Public Policy
- Promoting Health Through Environmental Change
  A. Eliminating Health-Damaging Features of the Environment
  B. Augmenting Health-Promoting Features of the Environment
- Voluntary Change Versus Legislative Policy
- Economic Incentives for Disease Prevention and Health Promotion
- Directions for Research in Social and Environmental Change
- Directions for Practice to Promote Social and Environmental Change
- Summary
- Learning Activities
- Selected Web Sites
- References

Recognition that health behavior is influenced by the social and physical environments in which people live has resulted in new ways to achieve behavior change (Anderson, Scrimshaw, Fullilove, & Fielding, 2003). As mentioned in earlier chapters, large-scale change is best accomplished by focusing on altering social and environmental structures that influence health as well as individual and group behaviors. Effective health-promotion efforts must take into consideration the dynamic relationships between individuals and families as well as changing social and environmental contexts. Health and social policies that fail to directly address harmful living conditions such as poverty, abuse, violence, hunger, and unemployment; environmental threats such as pollution in work sites and communities; and disparities in access and care will not result in changes that will promote the health of individuals and communities. Individual and family efforts to adopt healthy behaviors are also likely to be ineffective as a result of environmental constraints and policies that do not promote healthy living. Any strategy for health promotion that focuses only on individual behavior change will fail without simultaneous efforts to alter the physical and social environment as well as the collective behavior of the community. In the Health Promotion Model described in Chapter 2, interpersonal influences and situational factors are proposed to affect decisions to engage in health-promoting behaviors. Creative initiatives to foster social and environmental conditions that actively promote health are addressed in this chapter.

Health as a Social Goal

Health needs to be identified as a social goal as well as an individual goal, as the health of societies, communities, families, and individuals are integrated and inseparable. Health is influenced by social, cultural, economic, and political factors as well as biological and psychological factors (Hancock, 1999). Health-promotion efforts involve working with communities to ameliorate conditions that contribute to poor health such as inadequate housing, an unsafe water supply, poor nutrition or interruptions in the food supply, chemical toxins, poor recreational facilities, inadequate access to care, and lack of economic opportunity, as these issues directly impinge on health. Therefore, behavior-change strategies need to be redirected beyond the individual to include community- and policy-level factors (Roussos & Fawcett, 2000).

Health as a social goal requires the integration of theories that address social change (Chapter 3) with theories that address individual behavior change (Chapter 2) and family change (e.g., family stress theory, family development theory, family systems theory). The three theoretical perspectives are complementary. When nurses think only in terms of one-to-one relationships, the range and success of intervention possibilities are severely limited. Individual-level approaches have been reported to be successful in persons with chronic diseases (Whitehead & Russell, 2004). However, health behavior change is more likely to be successful when the social context in which the individual acts is targeted as well. For example, smoking cessation programs must not only target the individual addictive properties of smoking. The social conditions in which smoking occurs must also be addressed, including the advertising and sale of cigarettes, the influence of the tobacco industry on certain sectors of the population, and the role of public policy in changing smoking behaviors. Tobacco public policy interventions have been successful in changing smoking behaviors through laws that reduce exposure to secondhand smoke in public facilities, excise taxes that increase the costs of cigarettes, limiting youth access to cigarettes, and regulating advertising and promotion of tobacco products (Mileo, 2003; U.S. Department of Health and Human Services, 2000). Similar strategies that target the obesity problem in the United States are needed. Environmental changes for obesity, such as modifying how food is marketed and priced, establishing standards for foods served in cafeterias and vending machines on city or county property, levying taxes on high-sugar foods to fund subsidies for fruits and vegetables, increasing mass-media promotion of healthy food and activity, creating pedestrian zones in cities, and adding drinking water fountains, will help counter obesity. Individuals, communities, and government need to form alliances and have a sustained commitment to stop the increasing trend in obesity in children and adults (French, Story, & Jeffry, 2001). Enduring, large-scale behavior change is best achieved by changing the standards of acceptable behavior in a community rather than by attempting to change the behavior of individuals against overwhelming social odds.

The pursuit of health as a social goal requires that people of a shared community engage together in the process of change to accommodate various social, political, and economic developments. Central concepts in community-building models include participation, empowerment, critical consciousness, community competence, and issue selection (Minkler & Wallerstein, 2002). Empowerment is a social action process through which individuals and communities gain control over their lives and their environment to improve their health and quality of life. Community competence, a closely related concept of empowerment, focuses on problem-solving ability as a central goal of the community. Competent communities can identify the problems and needs of the community, achieve a working consensus on goals and priorities, agree on ways to implement goals, and collaborate effectively in actions that need to be taken (Minkler & Wallerstein, 2002). Health care providers can assist in the development of community competence by identifying natural leaders in a community who will undertake their own community assessments and actions necessary to strengthen the community. Leadership development is also a critical component in developing community competence. Leaders are needed who can stimulate people in the community to identify problems and solutions and act as facilitators to build group effectiveness. As a community gains competence in negotiating for resources to address a particular problem, the community becomes empowered, which enhances its problem-solving ability and capacity to cope with other problems that may arise. In addition, the community members gain a sense of ownership in that they have a sense of responsibility for and control over the programs promoting change, as they have been involved in initiating and promoting them (Lichtenstein, Thompson, Nettekoven, & Corbett, 1996).

Ecological models focus on changing the environmental context, including regulatory changes to support healthy behaviors (Sallis & Owen, 2002). The *Healthy People 2010* objectives incorporate an ecological model of health promotion to address the social and physical context in which negative behaviors occur (U.S. Department of Health and Human Services, 2000). Social ecological models focus on the social context to produce large-scale social change. Social change refers to altering the social structures of a community (Anderson et al., 2003). Social change is generally followed by changes in the normative structures, or the shared rules and expectations (rules of conduct) that govern everyday life. When rules that govern behavior are modified, normative change takes place. Social change may occur through a functionalist view or conflict view (Anderson et al., 2003). The functionalist view sees change as a gradual adaptive process oriented toward community reform and is based on cooperation and consensus. As the community changes, social norms change and new rules of conduct arise for the changed community. Social change focuses on the community's strengths and how these strengths can be used to the best advantage in fostering continuing development of community competence. In the conflict view, the system changes by coercive means or social control, in which those who control important parts of the community attempt to change social norms. A functionalist perspective is consistent with an expansive view of health. These two perspectives are contrasted in Figure 15–1. Social ecological models hold promise for successful health promotion. More research is needed on environmental influences on behavior and evaluation of health-promotion programs that target the social context.

In summary, when health is considered a social goal as well as an individual goal, the focus for health promotion includes the community as well as the individual (Anderson et al., 2003). Individuals can govern their own behavior and should do so. Government can formulate broad policies and allocate funding. However, priority decisions and strategies

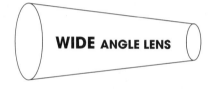

Models for Intervention

Social change	*Social control*
Social analysis	Epidemiologic and demographic analysis
Focus on strengths	Focus on weaknesses
Goal is health outcome and increased community competence	Goal is health outcome
Organized around human categories	Organized around disease categories
Asks what people's motives are	Asks how can we motivate people

FIGURE 15–1 **Comparison of Social Change with Social Control Models**

(From E. Eng, M.E. Salmon, and F. Mullen, 1992, "Community Empowerment: The Critical Base for Primary Care, *Fam Community Health, 15*[1], 1–2. Used with permission.)

for social change for more complex lifestyle issues can best be made collectively by members of the community. This strategy ensures that programs are relevant and appropriate for the people involved, and encourages greater involvement in the planning and implementation process.

Health in a Changing Social Environment

Despite the absence of comprehensive enabling legislation, health care reform in the United States continues to proceed at a rapid rate, propelled by social, environmental, and economic forces. The rise of managed care and market competition in the 1990s produced major changes in health care financing and delivery and resulted in a shift in power from providers to purchasers (Oliver, 2000). However, the financial downturn of managed care organizations has resulted in an uncertain future for this approach as a way to manage health care costs. New models of care are based on various cost-containment strategies, as national health care expenditures continue to be a major concern. The currently evolving model, labeled "defined contributions," means that rising health care costs are shifted from employers onto their employees (Bodenheimer & Grumbach, 2002). In this model, employees bear the risks of increased health costs, as employers pay a fixed sum for each employee. The defined contribution approach is favored by the current government administration for persons on Medicare. This type of program raises serious concerns, as employer and government incentives to control overall health care costs have been removed, passing the costs on to the employee. The single most important factor explaining the continued upward trend in the number of uninsured is decreasing private insurance coverage (Leaffer & Gonda, 2000). The defined contributions approach will certainly increase the inequities in health care coverage and access.

Absence of guaranteed access to care has also been a major factor in the push for health care reform. Access to health care increases (a) physical capacity, (b) personal resources to realize aspirations, and (c) ways to cope with the environment to improve one's health and quality of life (Gulzar, 1999). Every community should be able to provide services to monitor the health status of its members; inform, educate, and empower community members; and assist its members in accessing personal health services (Speers & Lancaster, 1998). Successful reforms in health care systems are needed to create new opportunities for communities, health care providers, and health systems to develop linkages to improve health. However, this remains a major challenge.

In addition to health care reform, the communication revolution resulting from rapid digital and mobile technological advances has changed our society to an information- and knowledge-based one. Information is available at the click of a mouse, and the news media can now deliver health education and counseling to individuals as well as the public. Based on comprehensive, computerized health assessments, information systems can tailor health-promotion programs to the knowledge, beliefs, motivations, and prior health-behavior histories of diverse individuals and families. Health-promotion activities are taking advantage of computer-based technologies such as CD-ROM and the Internet to target audiences, tailor health-promotion messages, and promote interactive ongoing exchanges about health (U.S. Department of Health and Human Services, 2000). Personal computers in the home offer informational resources, answer questions, and provide electronic access to support and discussion groups. One major issue will continue to be the scientific credibility of the information accessed on the Web in relation to the existing state of knowledge (Mechanic, 1999). Information must be carefully screened and delivered with quality programs if it is to contribute to improving health-promotion efforts.

Information systems are now enabling large segments of any community to be in touch with each other about the social problems that they face and their potential solutions. Furthermore, a composite plan for addressing health-related social and environmental conditions can be jointly developed by citizens without leaving their homes. Information technology offers the possibility of direct contact with policy makers in relation to health issues, formation of national networks to enhance local coalitions, and development of multiple communication links between health facilities and grassroots community groups.

The information era has also begun to bring about changes to empower families. Parents now often work at home as well as receive health information and health care at home by taking advantage of interactive computer technology (Nguyen, Carrieri-Kolman, Rankin, Slaughter, & Stulbarg, 2004). Research results indicate that the Internet revolution is reshaping education, as individuals conduct health-information searches and share information with their families and talk about it with their health care providers (Leaffer & Gonda, 2000). Computer-assisted health education is also being successfully implemented by means of the Internet (Winzelberg et al., 2000).

The information revolution is challenging health professionals to think creatively about the future of health care and new ways to educate health professionals in a multicultural society, as well as the potential consequences of this technology on society (Stokols & Montero, 2003). Futurist perspectives need to be critically analyzed so that the nursing profession stays at the forefront in helping clients to enhance health amid conditions of rapid social and environmental change.

Promoting Health Through Public Policy

The importance of shaping healthy policies in the public and private sectors as the primary vehicle for achieving major improvements in health status for populations has been widely advocated. Policies set goals and limits and define choices; therefore, policy plays a vital role in achieving the goals of health promotion (Cohen, Farley, & Mason, 2003). Personal, social, and political factors all influence the development and implementation of health policy. For example, at the personal level, changes in public sentiment have influenced the development of health policy related to smoking in public places in this country. At the political level, food lobbyists have been successful in maintaining the economic interests of the food and drug industries to prevent accurate labeling of foods and lower drug costs. On a more positive note, public policy has resulted in the removal of cigarette commercials from television.

The idea of developing policies for healthier communities is not new. Historically, local governments provided environmental safeguards against infectious diseases. However, the parameters of a healthy community have been expanded to include social and economic factors as well as environmental ones (Cohen et al., 2003). An underlying assumption of developing healthy communities is that local government plays a significant role through the development and implementation of policies to improve health, while community members actively participate in the decision-making process. Thus, policy formulation to promote health begins at the local level, through identification of problems and development of local ordinances to implement change.

The role of government in regulating health behavior remains nebulous. State and federal policies regulate a range of health behaviors, including alcohol, tobacco, seat belt use, food safety, and drug use. In addition, state and federal governments play a major role in the payment of health services. However, in many cases, a uniform health policy is missing, as in the case of immunization for measles or helmet use in motorcycle riding. One question that continues to be debated is how far policy should go in terms of individual behavior. The *Healthy People 2000* objectives emphasized individual responsibility, thus avoiding large-scale health policy mandates. However, an underlying premise of the *Healthy People 2010* objectives is that individual health is inseparable from the health of the larger community, which in turn determines the health status of the nation. The *Healthy People 2010* objectives and the national goal to eliminate health disparities challenge local, state, and federal governments, as well as policy makers, to be active participants in the development of policies to improve the health of communities. For example, local governments can limit youth access to tobacco in local markets and vending machines. Local and state policies can also be developed to target economic development in communities with high unemployment or promote safe housing in poor neighborhoods (Mileo, 2003). Health policies have direct and indirect effects on health (Mileo, 2003). Long-term changes occur as a result of modifying the conditions under which people live.

Although policy making is usually thought to occur at the national and international level, local and regional policy making can be just as fruitful in health-promotion efforts. Local and regional policy making can occur through social service agencies, local transportation authorities, public safety commissions, economic development zones, and professional organizations. An advantage of beginning at the local level for policy making is that the policy will have an influence in the community almost immediately, as trickle-down time is eliminated. Community and political leaders, along with the local and state health departments, can advise and advocate large-scale changes to promote health.

Policy making is driven by the interplay of stakeholder interests and uses both science-based and nonscience-based information (Mileo, 1998). Policy making is value driven, dynamic, and often chaotic and is about social influence, as it involves persuasion, attitude change, decision making, and compromise. Facts, or science-based information, are usually used in the early phases of policy development to identify problems and solutions, including the economic costs. However, nonscience-based or less verifiable information presented by stakeholders who offer their informed judgments and personal experiences is also used to promote the legitimacy of a proposed policy. Both types of knowledge are needed to gain support for successful policy making. Although scientific knowledge is critical, stakeholders also need other information such as the political costs as well as the resources needed to implement the policies. This additional information assists in the development of consensus to achieve policy development.

Health policies are needed that encourage individuals and communities to place a higher value on health and provide them with resources necessary to make healthy changes. This means that the necessary capacity and infrastructure relevant to health promotion must be developed and sustained in communities. Collaborative partnership models to develop health policy need to be implemented and tested to reduce disparities in access to information and resources. The value of individuals, communities, and local and state government, as well as national government, as active partners in this effort is critical.

Promoting Health Through Environmental Change

The quality of the physical environment in which people live is critical to the health of populations. Traditionally, environmental health practices have focused on controlling factors that are beyond the power of most people. However, individuals and communities have control over many external factors. The goal is to help people change these factors in order to promote healthy environments. Not only should health-damaging features of the environment be eliminated, but health-enhancing features should be augmented and actively used to promote improved health and well-being.

Eliminating Health-Damaging Features of the Environment

The harmful effects of toxic substances in the environment are vividly illustrated by the fact that 1 in 20 children have blood lead levels that exceed acceptable levels, and the risks are greatest for low-income racial and ethnic groups living in older housing (Feinberg, Glymour, & Scheines, 2003; Salazar, 2000). Although there has been a dramatic reduction in the number of children with elevated lead levels due to screening and public education campaigns, much more remains to be done. Lead can be found in urban areas not only in paint but also in dust and soil. Exposure to high levels of lead can be fatal, but even low exposures can be toxic to the central nervous system, resulting in delayed learning, impaired hearing, and growth deficits. Such disorders severely limit the potential of children to successfully compete in school and make affected children prone to early dropout and compromised adult lives.

Leading indoor air hazards to which many thousands of people are exposed each year are tobacco smoke and radon. Environmental tobacco smoke is a cause of disease including lung cancer in nonsmokers. Children of parents who smoke are more likely to develop lower respiratory tract infections and middle ear infections than are children of parents who do not smoke. Asthma and other respiratory diseases are triggered or worsened by tobacco smoke and other substances in the air. Since the mid-1980s, asthma rates in the United States have risen to the level of an epidemic (U.S. Department of Health and Human Services, 2000). Other indoor hazards include tight building syndrome, which is attributed to recycled air in buildings that may breed fungi and bacteria (Marcott, 2002).

The second leading cause of lung cancer, after smoking, is exposure to radon, a natural by-product of the breakdown of uranium that is found in many homes, offices, and schools (U.S. Environmental Protection Agency Web site). Radon from soil gas is the main cause of radon problems. The Environmental Protection Agency reports that although inexpensive kits are available for radon testing, only 5% of homes have actually been tested. As many as 8 million homes may have radon at a level requiring correction.

Outdoor air quality continues to be a widespread environmental problem nationally as well as internationally. The effects are noted in premature deaths, cancer, and respiratory and cardiovascular diseases. Motor vehicles account for one-fourth of emissions that produce ground-level ozone, the largest problem in air pollution. The estimated annual costs of human exposure to outdoor air pollutants range from $40 billion to $50 billion, and an estimated 50,000 premature deaths (U.S. Department of Health and Human Services, 2000). Changes are beginning to occur by encouraging and rewarding individuals not to drive their cars, but to walk or use public transportation, such as the Rail Trail in western Sydney, Australia, which promotes walking and cycling (Merom, Bauman, Via, & Close, 2003). Local and regional governments can devise public transportation systems that are amenable to communities and design streets that facilitate bicyclists and pedestrians. The increasing popularity of hybrid automobiles that use alternative fuels is a positive development. Nationally, support needs to be increased for the development and use of alternative fuels such as ethanol by commercial and private vehicles.

Water quality remains a major issue because of protozoa and chemical contaminants. Industry and agricultural runoff may contaminate water. For example, the development of intensive animal feeding operations has resulted in the discharge of improperly treated animal wastes into recreational and drinking water. The development of new molecular technologies to detect and monitor water contamination has eliminated the inability to detect parasitic contamination. These new technologies will greatly improve water monitoring and surveillance techniques.

Hazardous substances in the environment also pose significant health risks. For example, the Agency for Toxic Substances and Disease Registry (ATSDR) continues to publish a list of the most hazardous waste sites that need extensive cleanup (U.S. Department of Health and Human Services, 2000). Low-level radiation wastes deposited in landfills or carried from their source by air, groundwater, or surface runoff accumulate and have the capacity to affect surrounding populations. New jobs need to be created at hazardous waste sites to facilitate closure and cleanup of these sites. The widespread use of pesticides also continues to pose a threat, and children are at increased risk for pesticide poisoning.

Work-related injuries and illnesses result in billions of dollars in lost wages, lost productivity, and health care costs. The *Healthy People 2010* objectives target preventive practices to reduce latex allergy, effective tuberculosis control programs, and rollover protective structures for agriculture tractors. In addition to occupational hazards in the work environment, as the economy continues to evolve from an industrial to a service-oriented one, the workforce is changing. Younger children (16 to 17 years), as well as women, minorities, and the elderly, who are now in the workforce present new challenges for work safety and health.

Environmental variables have three functions important to health promotion. First, environmental variables are part of a complex group of factors that lead to healthy and unhealthy behaviors as previously described. Second, environmental variables moderate the effects of health-promotion efforts. If the environment is not taken into account, the health-promotion program may be ineffective. For example, local neighborhoods affect health, as the neighborhood resources, or lack thereof, may either increase or reduce stress, mobilize or isolate individuals, and provide access to resources, such as fire protection and safe water, or limited access to such needed resources (Altschuler, Somkin, & Adler, 2004). Finally, environmental variables can be changed to achieve health-promotion goals. Changing environmental variables requires targeting policy makers in private industry as well as in government. Accomplishment of the *Healthy People 2010* objectives warrants attention to these factors.

Nursing as a health care profession must take responsibility for protecting and maintaining an environment that is health strengthening rather than health damaging. For example, noise is a feature of the environment that can be potentially stressful and health damaging. Hearing loss is a priority research area identified by NIOSH, as it ranks among the top 10 occupational hazards. Developing interventions to foster the use of hearing protection at work sites has been the target of ongoing research efforts by Lusk and her colleagues (1997; Lusk et al., 2003; Lusk, Eakin, Kazanis, McCullagh, 2004) at the University of Michigan. Based on her findings, Lusk, an occupational health nurse and clinical researcher, recommended that workers play a role in the selection of hearing protection devices instead of basing their choice exclusively on noise reduction in order to increase use. In addition, training programs need to be tailored to the level of education and trade group, as the percentage of workers who do not wear protective devices continues to be alarmingly high.

Risk assessment is the means by which currently available information about environmental public health problems can be organized and understood. Four major steps are involved in the risk assessment process:

1. Hazard identification
2. Dose–response assessment
3. Exposure assessment (estimation of human exposure over time)
4. Risk characterization (determination of risk for human populations under various exposure scenarios)

In hazard identification, the range of toxic effects for a substance is identified from the literature. The second step, dose–response assessment, is used to describe as accurately as possible the relationship between magnitude, duration, frequency, and timing of chemical exposure and the frequency of manifestation of the chemical's adverse effects. Human exposure assessment identifies the range of exposures experienced by the target population of concern. In the fourth step, risk characterization, the particular risks that are likely to be experienced by the population of interest under actual expected exposure conditions, are described. This four-step assessment framework can be applied to many types of health threats that arise within the environment, including potential threats arising from the introduction of new technologies. Comprehensive risk assessment directs attention to those sources of risk that, if reduced, will yield the greatest public health benefits.

Health professionals should note that the tolerance for risks on the part of individuals and families is based on the characteristics of the risk itself. For example:

1. Voluntarily assumed risks are tolerated better than those imposed by others.
2. Risks over which scientists debate and are uncertain are more feared than those in which scientific consensus endorses a risk.
3. Risks of natural origin are often considered to be less threatening than those created by humans.

Responses differ according to the characteristics of the risk being considered, alternating from undue alarm to apathy. Individuals should be encouraged to consider objective information about the nature and extent of various environmental risks, rather than relying on feelings and emotions. Further, some societies base risk-reduction priorities on the relative ease with which risk reduction can be achieved. Ease of resolution sometimes has a poor correspondence to the public health importance of the risks being attacked. Environmental risk-reduction objectives should be based on the best available scientific knowledge about the relative risks of various pollutants to health rather than on what is emotionally appealing or politically attractive at a particular point in time.

Many major environmental risks require intensive, multifaceted, and often long-term interventions to influence related attitudes and to reallocate resources for their control. By focusing on environmental change in the local community and its work sites, such as methods to reduce environmental pollutants; safe waste disposal; monitoring and surveillance to ensure quality water; worker protection from toxic substances, diseases, and injuries, such as prevention of noise-induced hearing loss; nurses can play a proactive role in promoting health through environmental management.

Augmenting Health-Promoting Features of the Environment

The environment can nurture, comfort, relax, strengthen, and add to a sense of well-being (Herzog, Maguire, & Nebel, 2003). Important elements of a health-promoting environment include color, lighting, furnishings, temperature, texture, nature, art, music, scents, and privacy. Appropriate colors can improve mood and relax or energize. Natural lighting increases serotonin production and has a positive effect on mood, decreasing the potential for depression. Adequate lighting is necessary for the health and safety of elderly individuals as well as communities. Adequate privacy is important, as crowding, especially with inadequate environmental resources in neighborhoods and cities, is associated with increased crime and violence. Viewing natural elements or nature scenes has been shown to promote a shift to a more positive emotional state and an increased attention span. Understanding the uses of nature and its health-enhancing properties may result in the development of innovative health-promotion modalities for use by care providers in optimizing health and well-being.

Characteristics of the environment also promote restoration, or a renewing of diminished functional resources and capabilities. Four features of restorative environments have been identified (Herzog et al., 2003). The first feature is being away. This refers to settings that call on different mental content; in other words, getting away from it all. The second feature of a restorative setting is extent. Extent refers to sufficient content and structure of a setting to occupy the mind to allow rest to occur. Third, fascination refers to effortless attention. Fascination is restoration when it is characterized by effortless attention and aesthetic beauty in the setting. The last feature is compatibility. A setting is compatible if there is a good fit between the individual's purpose and activities supported or demanded by the setting. Environments need to be assessed to realize the beneficial effects of restorative components. Interventions can then be implemented to improve the restorative elements to improve health and well-being.

Discovery of strategies to foster health and well-being through use of health-enhancing environments in inner cities, at work sites, and in school settings is important for prevention and health promotion. For example, community gardens have been shown to improve psychological well-being and social relations and to facilitate healing as well as increase the supply of vegetables. A survey of community gardens in New York found that the gardens improved social networks and facilitated community organizing to promote change (Armstrong, 2000). Several important questions arise, including: What are the significant health-promoting aspects of the environment? How can features of the environment be enhanced to improve mental and physical health? Areas of the environment, including housing, water quality, food quality, waste disposal, and air quality, all need attention to promote the health of its citizens. In addition, the components previously mentioned need further exploration and application to learn how changing aspects of one's living and working environments can promote health.

Voluntary Change Versus Legislative Policy

In a democratic society, it is widely assumed that matters of risk critical to survival and security are predominantly subject to regulatory decisions, whereas risks that are not clearly vital to general health and welfare are issues for personal decision and action. In a democracy, even vital risks may be left to individual decision, providing that they do not infringe on the rights of others. The role of government continues to be questioned in relation to legislating environmental and behavioral changes that promote good health and increase longevity. If the government uses the means at its disposal to regulate changes in behavior, it may be faced with problems of an ethical nature. However, voluntary, individual approaches may fall short of achieving widespread change in self-damaging behaviors.

Government involvement in lifestyle reform is to some extent supported by the long-standing role of the federal government as a health care provider. In the face of high costs of health care, it may be cost-effective for the government to consider legislation that requires individuals to assume more self-care responsibility. Although such federal regulations might be cost effective if health-promotion interventions are shown to substantially reduce health care costs, many individuals may resist legislation of preventive and health-promotion measures as unethical or undue intrusion upon their individual freedom. Ethical issues, including individual autonomy, must be thoughtfully considered in matters of health.

Two philosophical views of the role of government are often labeled "individualism" and "paternalism" (Ribisl & Humphries, 1998). Individualism is the American ideal, in which individuals are given maximum freedom in the area of health promotion. Health habits are considered personal, so outside interventions by governmental policy are not warranted. Poor health is attributed to individuals; thus, society's responsibility is minimized. Paternalism, the counterpoint, holds that experts (professionals and policy makers) have a moral responsibility to solve health problems because individuals lack the ability to do so. Therefore, interventions, such as laws and public policies, are justified for the health of society. The role of individuals in this model is to adhere to policies. Individuals are not blamed for their problems as they are viewed as victims of circumstance. Both views have strengths that deserve mentioning. In the individualism model, control of health promotion is shared, as control is in the hands of the individuals, promoting a sense of efficacy and empowerment. Second, diversity of opinions is respected in the individualistic view. The strength of the paternalistic view is that it is intended to reduce health disparities. Health policies are socially responsible as they apply to all segments of the population. In addition, problems greater than the individual, such as environmental issues, are recognized and addressed.

Both approaches have limitations as well. The overriding emphasis on individualism or personal responsibility for health results in victim blaming, which becomes problematic for poor people, because poverty is now widely accepted as a significant risk factor for illness and premature death (Minkler, 2000). However, overemphasis on paternalism or social responsibility ignores individual and group differences in human responses as well as the contributions of individuals to lifestyle change. The strengths of both approaches need to be combined to promote health in individuals and communities. Collaborative models of health promotion will promote community control, allow diversity, incorporate environmental issues, and reduce health disparities in different segments of the community.

Over two decades ago, Pellegrino (1981) suggested guidelines in considering trade-offs between individualism and social responsibility (paternalism) in relation to health. These guidelines remain timely.

1. Certain lifestyles result in disease, disability, and death, with economic consequences for the whole society. Thus, there is a social mandate to encourage healthier lifestyles in all citizens.

2. In a civilized and democratic society, individual freedom must be protected and is to be limited only when it violates the freedom of others. In an interdependent society, free acts are subject to justifiable restriction.

3. Coercive measures should be considered only when their effectiveness is unequivocal for large numbers of people and when control extends over a limited sector of life.

4. Even if a societal control measure meets all of the previous criteria, it must accommodate as closely as possible the democratic principle of self-determination. Voluntary measures must be clearly inadequate at the outset or must have failed before coercive measures are contemplated.

While government regulation is sometimes deemed necessary for the public good, self-direction is valued by Americans. Most individuals believe that they are the best judge of what is good for them, and the process of choosing is considered a good in itself, even when the outcomes may be health damaging. Some persons may voluntarily opt for a brief life span full of unhealthy practices. It can be argued that if the practices are not detrimental to others and are carried out in full awareness of the consequences, these people should be allowed to pursue the course they want. For these individuals, the role of the nurse is to make sure that they have as much information as possible on which to base informed decisions concerning lifestyle and health-related behavior.

Deciding whether social changes to enhance health should be voluntary or mandatory presents society with a complex dilemma. Is coercion ever appropriate? If so, how and to what extent? Is it coercive to increase cigarette taxes in order to help defray the cost of smoking-induced disease? Should highly refined sugar products and high-cholesterol foods also be taxed more heavily to pay for the cost of health problems induced by obesity and atherosclerosis? Should taxes on large, high-speed automobiles be proportionately higher than taxes on smaller cars with limited speed and greater fuel economy? Which lifestyle, organizational, and social changes should be voluntary and which should be mandated through legislation? A balance of voluntary and mandatory action is needed, while continuing to pay close attention to the ethical dimensions of such health-related decisions.

Economic Incentives for Disease Prevention and Health Promotion

The dependence of the American people on diagnosis and treatment of disease to improve health and increase longevity is economically and socially rooted in our culture. Until recently, Americans were willing to spend escalating proportions of both personal and public dollars on an increasing array of medical services, hoping for "magic bullets" to cure all ills. However, the availability of health care technology and medical interventions exceeds society's ability to afford them. In addition, medical care is considered to account for only 10% to 15% of the declines in premature death in the 20th century, while factors that help to prevent illness have been responsible for the remaining decline. Health care systems are now undergoing restructuring and new health care policies are being implemented to attempt to achieve a balance among prevention, health promotion, and disease treatment services.

Health-promotion programs continue to be at a competitive disadvantage for time and money, in spite of mounting evidence that health-promotion and prevention efforts reduce morbidity and mortality (Stave, Muchmore, & Gardner, 2003). Those allocating resources require evidence of cost savings, indicating that health-promotion programs will receive increased scrutiny in the era of declining resources. The public must be convinced of the value of staying well, the effectiveness of environmental and behavioral change in promoting health and preventing disease, and the economic and human advantage of shifting a portion of health care dollars from treatment of illness to keeping people healthy. Nurses should be particularly sensitive to the need to evaluate costs as well as health outcomes of their health-promotion programs.

Cost-effective analysis (CEA), *cost–benefit analysis* (CBA), and other economic evaluations discussed in Chapter 13 have assumed an important role in research and health care policy decisions (Muenning, 2002). These methods, particularly CEA, are useful for evaluating and comparing different health-promotion strategies and providing health care professionals with important information related to patient preferences and priorities for prevention and health promotion. However, the results of these analyses may also be controversial if the social implications are not taken into account. This issue was raised in the state of Oregon when health interventions were prioritized based on cost-effectiveness analysis. Interventions that were considered unaffordable were not paid, creating both statewide and national attention for social reform.

Positive effects from any health-promotion program require a chain of events: a structured program, participation continuing over time, and health enhancement or reduction of risk, measured by specified outcome criteria. For many disease-prevention and health-promotion programs, costs are incurred as the program is implemented while benefits may be obtained in the future. An extended time period between costs and benefits can be reconciled with cost-analysis procedures. However, consumers may not be willing to spend to protect themselves from a health problem with a 20-year latency when they feel well. Emphasizing short-term as well as long-term benefits may enhance consumer acceptance of disease-prevention and health-promotion interventions that require marked environmental and individual behavioral change (Brown & Garber, 2000).

High demands for medical services result in high rates of use of resource-intensive services and less emphasis on self-care, preventive, and health-promotion services. Traditional insurance coverage has offered little in the way of incentives to increase motivation for engaging in prevention and health-promotion activities. Individuals and families who have insurance rarely have coverage for disease-prevention and health-promotion services, because such services cannot be related to a specific diagnosis or medical complaint. Even more distressing is the higher incidence of preventive screening in low-risk groups than in high-risk groups, when the latter group could benefit more from such services but does not have insurance to access them. This is referred to as reverse targeting. As mentioned earlier, the number of Americans who are uninsured or underinsured for health care costs continues to rise. Those who are mainly affected include children and young adults, poor and middle-income families, African Americans, and Hispanics. States in the South and Southwest continue to have the highest rates of uninsurance. Lack of insurance has been associated with difficulties with access to the health care system, unmet medical needs, and less likelihood of obtaining preventive services such as mammograms. It is obvious that the *Healthy People 2010* objectives will not be achieved unless the financial barriers to receiving preventive and health-promotion services are removed.

Rather than discouraging prevention and health promotion, as our present reimbursement system does, economic advantages for using such services are needed. Financial incentives, such as the following, need to be offered, particularly under the new approaches to health care costs, such as the defined contribution payment plan, as these financial incentives will help to decrease costs as well as promote health.

1. Expand insurance coverage to include primary health care services for prevention and health promotion.
2. Offer partial insurance premium refunds or reduced premiums for maintaining good health or improving health status.
3. Develop a sliding scale for insurance premiums based on documented attendance at education programs to promote healthy lifestyles and use of early detection screening services.

Nurses are in a key position to work with consumer groups to shape health and social policies to offer more incentives for prevention and health promotion. Further, because of nursing's person–environment orientation, nurses can work in collaboration with other professionals and with diverse populations and communities to promote local, national, and global changes supportive of health and healthy lifestyles.

Directions for Research in Social and Environmental Change

Social and environmental change approaches to promote health offer new vistas for nursing research. The significance of social change approaches that realize human health potential are beginning to be realized. New models that test public and organizational policy in managing risk and fostering health need rigorous evaluation. Suggested directions for nursing and interdisciplinary research efforts are as follows:

1. Test the effects of both family and community health-promotion interventions on positively altering health-related social norms among children and adolescents.
2. Develop and test models that proactively manage the environment to reduce health threats.
3. Analyze the cost effectiveness of financial incentives in health care plans that focus on health-promotion and disease-prevention services.
4. Test the effectiveness of eliminating environmental barriers to healthy food choices and active lifestyles to treat and prevent obesity.

The study of interactive effects of human and environmental factors in health and disease is complex and requires interdisciplinary research collaboration to address the many gaps in knowledge that now exist.

Directions for Practice to Promote Social and Environmental Change

Health promotion and prevention interventions can no longer focus exclusively on the individual if large-scale behavior change is to be achieved. The social and physical environments, as well as individual behaviors, must be targeted. The comprehensive view of health promotion emphasizes the need for collaboration between health care professionals, health care organizations, and policy makers at the local, state, and national levels. Nurses will need to help build healthy communities by implementing interventions that focus on community development. Skills are needed to be able to work with communities to identify resources, problems, and opportunities. The nurse also needs to know how to implement strategies to involve community members and provide them with training to develop the leadership necessary to play an active role in the change process.

Because of the multiple factors involved in behavior change that go beyond the individual, nurses also need to become active in the promotion of health policy to decrease social and environmental risk factors present in many communities. This can be accomplished by working with local health departments and state legislatures to make changes as well as lobbying efforts to increase funds and services. Health promotion in the 21st century brings many challenges due to the rapid, ongoing changes in the population, workforce, technology, and health care environment. However, these challenges bring new opportunities for nurses, who, with other members of the interdisciplinary health care task force, will create innovative plans to improve health.

SUMMARY

The focus of this chapter has been on society as a collective and the impact of public policy and social and physical environments on the health status of individuals, families, and communities. Attempts to change health behaviors without changes in the environments in which people live will result in frustration and failure of health-promotion efforts. A balanced approach to disease prevention and health promotion requires attention to the (a) quality of the social and physical environments, (b) disparities in health-promoting options available within the environment, and (c) changes in health policy to create healthier communities. Because health is no longer viewed as an aim in itself, but as a resource for personal and social development as well as a product of social conditions, changes in public policies should become part of any effort to promote health.

LEARNING ACTIVITIES

1. Conduct a home assessment to identify a health-damaging environmental factor. Describe the history of the problem, its effects on the health of the family, barriers to solving the problem, resources needed to solve the problem, and resources available to solve the problem.
2. Develop at least three community strategies to solve the problem identified above and an evaluation plan of your possible solutions.
3. Write a letter to your state legislators voicing your concerns about the above environmental problem and how they might help solve the problem.

SELECTED WEB SITES

Clearinghouse for Occupational Safety and Health Information

http://www.cdc.gov/niosh/homepage.html

Drug Policy Information Clearinghouse

http://www.whitehousedrugpolicy.gov

Food and Drug Administration

http://www.fda.gov

Health Resources and Services Administration

http://www.hrsa.gov

Indoor Air Quality Information Clearing House

http://www.epa.gov/iaq

National Lead Information Center

http://www.epa.gov/lead/nlic.htm

Office on Smoking and Health

http://www.cdc.gov/tobacco

Additional Web Sites

Kaisernetwork Health Policy as it Happens

http://www.kaisernetwork.org

National Academy for State Health Policy

http://www.nashp.org

REFERENCES

Altschuler, A., Somkin, C. P., & Adler, N. E. (2004). Local services and amenities, neighborhood social capita, and health. *Social Science & Medicine.* In press.

Anderson, L. M., Scrimshaw, S. C., Fullilove, M. T., & Fielding, J. E. (2003). The task force on community preventive services. The community guide's model for lining the social environment to health. *Am J Prev Med, 24*(3S), 12–20.

Armstrong, D. (2000). A survey of community gardens in upstate New York: Implications for health promotion and community development. *Health & Place, 6*, 319–327.

Bodenheimer, T. S., & Grumbach, K. (2001). *Understanding health policy: A clinical approach* (3rd ed.). New York: McGraw-Hill.

Brown, A. D., & Garber, A. M. (2000). A concise review of the cost-effectiveness of coronary heart disease prevention. *Medical Clinics of North America, 84*(1), 279–282.

Cohen, D. A., Farley, T. A., & Mason, K. (2003). Why is poverty unhealthy: Social and physical mediators. *Social Science & Medicine, 57*, 1631–1641.

Feinberg, S. E., Glymour, C., & Scheines, R. (2003). Expert statistical testimony and epidemiological evidence: The toxic effects of lead exposure on children. *Journal of Econometrics, 113*, 33–48.

French, S. A., Story, M., & Jeffry, R. W. (2001). Environmental influences on eating and physical activity. *Annu Rev Public Health, 22*, 309–335.

Gulzar, L. (1999). Access to health care. *J Nurs Schol, 31*(1), 13–19.

Hancock, T. (1999). Future directions in population health. *Can J Public Health, 90*(Suppl 1), S68–S70.

Herzog, T. R., Maguire, C. P., & Nebel, M. B. (2003). Assessing the restorative components of environments. *Journal of Environmental Psychology, 23*, 159–170.

Leaffer, T., & Gonda, B. (2000). The Internet: An underutilized tool in patient education. *Comput Nurs, 18*(1), 47–52.

Lichtenstein, E., Thompson, B., Nettekoven, L., & Corbett, K. (1996). Durability of tobacco control activities in eleven North American communities: Life after the community intervention trial for smoking cessation (COMMIT). *Health Educ Res, 11*, 527–534.

Lusk, S. L. (1997). Effects of hearing and protection of noise induced hearing loss. *AAOHN Journal, 45*(8), 397–405.

Lusk, S. L., Ronis, D. L., Kazanis, A. S., Eakin, B.L., Hong, O., & Raymond, D. M. (2003). Effectiveness of a tailored intervention to increase factory workers' use of hearing protection. *Nursing Research, 52*(5), 289–295.

Lusk, S. L., Eakin, B. L., Kazanis, A. S., & McCullagh, M. C. (2004). Effects of booster intervention on factory workers' use of hearing protection. *Nursing Research, 53*(1), 53–58.

Marcott, R. T. (2002). Environmental factors related to health promotion. In J. A. Maville & C. G. Huerta (Eds.), *Health promotion in nursing* (pp. 115–143). New York: Delmar Thomson Learning.

Mechanic, D. (1999). Issues in promoting health. *Social Science and Medicine, 48*, 711–718.

Merom, D., Bauman, A., Via, P., & Close, G. (2003). An environmental intervention to promote walking and cycling—the impact of a newly constructed Rail Trail in Western Sydney. *Preventive Medicine, 36*, 235–242.

Mileo, N. (1998). Priorities and strategies for promoting community-based preventive policies. *Journal of Health Care Management Practice, 4*(3), 14–28.

Mileo, N. (2003). *Public health in the market.* Ann Arbor: The University of Michigan Press.

Minkler, M. (2000). Health promotion at the dawn of the 21st century: Challenge and dilemmas. In M. S. Jamner & D. Stokols (Eds.), *Promoting human wellness* (pp. 349–377). Berkeley: University of California Press.

Minkler, M., & Wallerstein, N. (2002). Improving health through community organization and community building. In K. Glanz, F. M. Lewis, & B. K. Rimer (Eds.), *Health behavior and health education* (3rd ed., pp. 279–311). San Francisco: Jossey-Bass.

Muenning, P. (2002). *Designing and conducting cost-effectiveness analysis in medicine and health care.* San Francisco: Jossey Bass.

Nguyen, H. Q., Carrieri-Kolman, V., Rankin, S. H., Slaughter, R., & Stulbarg, M. S. (2004). Internet-based patient education and support interventions: A review of evaluation studies and directions for future research. *Computers in Biology and Medicine, 34*, 95–112.

Oliver, T. R. (2000). Dynamics without change: The new generation. *Journal of Health Politics, Policy and Law, 25*(1), 225–232.

Pellegrino, E. D. (1981). Health promotion as public policy: The need for moral grounding. *Prev Med, 10*, 371–378.

Ribisl, K. M., & Humphries, K. (1998). Collaboration between professionals and mediating structures in the community: Towards a "Third Way" in health promotion. In S. A. Shumaker, E. B. Schron, J. K. Ockene, & W. L. McBee (Eds.), *The handbook of health behavior change* (2nd ed., pp. 535–554). New York: Springer.

Roussos, S. T., & Fawcett, S. B. (2000). A review of collaborative partnerships as a strategy for improving community health. *Annu Rev Public Health, 21*, 369–402.

Salazar, M. K. (2000). Environmental health: Responding to the call. *Public Health Nurs, 17*(2), 73–74.

Sallis, J. F., & Owen, N. (2002). Ecological models of health behavior. In K. Glanz, F. M. Lewis, & B. K. Rimer (Eds.), *Health behavior and health education* (3rd ed., pp. 462–484). San Francisco: Jossey-Bass.

Speers, M. A., & Lancaster, B. (1998). Disease prevention and health promotion in urban areas: CDC's perspective. *Health Education and Behavior, 25*(2), 226–233.

Stave, G. M., Muchmore, L., & Gardner, H. (2003). Quantifiable impact of the contract for health and wellness: Health behaviors, health care costs, disability, and workers' compensation. *J Occup Environ Med, 45*(3), 109–117.

Stokols, D., & Montero, M. (2002). Toward an environmental psychology of the Internet. In R. B. Bechtel & A. Churchman (Eds.), *Handbook of environmental psychology* (pp. 661–675). New York: John Wiley & Sons.

U.S. Department of Health and Human Services. (2000, January). *Healthy People 2010* (conference edition in two volumes). Washington DC: U.S. Government Printing Service.

U.S. Environmental Protection Agency Web site: *http://www.epa.gov/radon*

Whitehead, D., & Russell, G. (2004). How effective are health education programmes—resistance, reactance, rationality and risk? Recommendations for effective practice. *International Journal of Nursing Studies, 41*, 163–172.

Winzelberg, A. J., Eppstein, D., Eldredge, K. L., Wilfley, D., Dasmahapatra, R., Dev, P., & Taylor, C. B. (2000). Effectiveness of an Internet-based program for reducing risk factors for eating disorders. *J Consult Clin Psychol, 68*(2), 346–350.

Index

U

Undernutrition, role of, 179
Unitary man, theory of, 22
Upper fat limits, 178
Upstream, 267
U.S. Department of Health and Human
　　Services (USD-HHS), 307

V

Vicarious learning, 41
Voluntary change *versus* legislative policy,
　　348–350
Vulnerable Population Model, 306
Vulnerable populations, health promotion in
　access to care, 307
　constituent-involving strategies, 313
　cultural awareness, and, 308
　cultural change, and, 308
　cultural context, role of, 307
　cultural factors in designing programs, 309
　cultural knowledge, and, 308
　cultural tailoring strategies, 314
　culturally competent interventions, planning,
　　307–308
　culturally relevant intervention strategies,
　　310–311
　demographic factors in designing programs,
　　309
　designing programs, characteristics for,
　　308–313
　eliminating health disparities, 306–307
　enculturation, and, 308
　environmental factors of, 304–305
　ethnocentrism, and, 308

　evidential strategies, 313
　factors of, 304
　health care system factors in designing
　　programs, 309
　health outcomes, measuring, 307
　health policy in, 307
　health status and health behaviors, 304–306
　implementing culturally relevant
　　interventions, 313–314
　linguistic strategies, 313
　peripheral strategies, 313
　practice suggestions, 315
　quality of care, 307
　research suggestions, 314–315
　risk for disease, 307
　social capital, role of, 306
　societal factors of, 304–305
　socio-cultural strategies, 313–314
　socioeconomic status (SES), role of,
　　304–305, 306
　standards for culturally appropriate health-
　　promotion programs, 312

W

Waianae Diet Program, 191
Ways of Coping Questionnaire, 108
Weight-reduction program, initiating a,
　193–194
WHO definition of health, 17–18
Work site, health promotion at the, 325–327
Work Site Intervention Study, 190–191

Y

Yoga, relaxation through, 217